# The Heart of Power

*Health and Politics in the Oval Office*

David Blumenthal and
James A. Morone

With a New Preface

UNIVERSITY OF CALIFORNIA PRESS
*Berkeley · Los Angeles · London*

University of California Press, one of the most
distinguished university presses in the United States,
enriches lives around the world by advancing
scholarship in the humanities, social sciences, and
natural sciences. Its activities are supported by the UC
Press Foundation and by philanthropic contributions
from individuals and institutions. For more
information, visit www.ucpress.edu.

University of California Press
Berkeley and Los Angeles, California

University of California Press, Ltd.
London, England

ISBN 978-0-520-26809-8

The Library of Congress has cataloged an earlier
edition as follows:

Blumenthal, David, 1948–
   The heart of power : health and politics in the
Oval Office / David Blumenthal and James A. Morone.
      p.  ;  cm.
   Includes bibliographical references and index.
   ISBN 978-0-520-26030-6 (cloth: alk. paper)
   1. Medical policy—United States—History.
   2. Presidents—United States—Health. I. Morone,
James A., 1951– II. Title.
   [DNLM: 1. Health Policy—history—
United States.   2. Federal Government—
history—United States.   3. History, 20th
Century—United States.   4. History, 21st Century—
United States.   5. Leadership--United States.
6. Policy Making—United States.   7. Politics—United
States.   8. Public Health Practice—history—United
States. WA 540 AA1 B648h 2009]

RA395.A3B68   2009
362.10973—dc22                         2008054361

Manufactured in the United States of America

18   17   16   15   14   13   12   11   10
10   9   8   7   6   5   4   3   2   1

The paper used in this publication meets the minimum
requirements of ANSI/NISO Z 39.48-1992 (R 1997)
(*Permanence of Paper*).

# Contents

*Preface to the 2010 Edition* / v

*2009 Preface and Acknowledgments* / xiii

INTRODUCTION / 1

1. FRANKLIN DELANO ROOSEVELT
   *The Enigmatic Angler* / 21

2. HARRY S. TRUMAN
   *We'll Take the Starch Out of Them—Eventually* / 57

3. DWIGHT D. EISENHOWER
   *Compassionate Conservative* / 99

4. JOHN F. KENNEDY
   *The Charismatic with a Stricken Father* / 131

5. LYNDON B. JOHNSON
   *The Secret History of Medicare* / 163

6. RICHARD NIXON
   *A Flower That Bloomed Only in the Dark* / 206

7. JIMMY CARTER
   *The Righteous Engineer* / 248

8. RONALD REAGAN
   *Socialized Medicine and the Working Stiff* / 283

9. GEORGE HERBERT WALKER BUSH
   *Stick to the Running Game* / 319

10. BILL CLINTON
    *Kicking the Can down the Road* / 346

11. GEORGE W. BUSH
    *Bring It On—Reforming Medicare* / 385

CONCLUSION
    *Eight Rules for the Heart of Power* / 409

*Notes* / 421

*Index* / 471

*Illustrations follow page 162*

# Preface, 2010

President Obama hushed the audience at a Democratic fundraiser in February 2010 with a story he did not tell lightly. An uninsured Obama volunteer from St. Louis was dying from breast cancer. (Unspoken: just like my mother died from ovarian cancer while struggling with an insurance company.) "She insisted she is going to be buried in an Obama T-shirt," the president continued. "How can I say to her, 'You know what, we're giving up'? How can I say to her family, 'This is too hard'? How can Democrats on the Hill say, 'This is politically too risky'? How can Republicans on the Hill say, 'We're better off just blocking anything from happening'?"[1]

The faithful sprang to their feet and the familiar incantation filled the hall: "Yes we can! Yes we can!"

A month earlier it had looked like they could and they would. The House had squeezed out its version of national health reform (220–215) on November 7, 2009, the Senate managed its own bill on December 24 (without a single vote to spare), and Congressional leaders began negotiating the differences between the two bills. Suddenly, in mid-January, one of the strangest twists in health reform's long, tortured history sent the president's program sprawling just inches from the finish line. A little-known Republican who had pledged to stop Obama's health plan won a special election in an upset and took the seat long held by Senator Ted Kennedy, the lion of health care reform. Newly elected Senator Scott Brown looked like he could deliver on his campaign promise. He

gave the united Republicans the 41st vote that could sustain the filibuster that would greet the final plan when it came up for a last vote in the
Senate.

Democrats panicked. If Republicans could win in Massachusetts,
they could win anywhere. Health reformers could feel the plan's
momentum evaporating into the frigid Washington winter. The Democrats, it seemed, were about to fail again. No matter how close they
got, no matter how clever their legislative maneuvering, no matter how
shrewdly they negotiated with the interest groups (and this time most
past opponents signed up for reform), health care—the signature Democratic issue for more than sixty years—always eluded the reformers. It
was always a bridge too far.

President Obama faced a choice. He had spent his administration's
first year fighting for health care. But public opinion had gone south
on the reform. Opponents were in full cry, moderates were wary, and
polls showed that the public had no idea what was actually in the bill.
Many Democrats urged Obama to make the expedient choice and pivot
from health care to the issue that seemed to preoccupy most Americans:
jobs. Perhaps he could propose a modest health care compromise—
cover children, for example, or regulate insurance companies to curb
practices like denying coverage to patients with preexisting illnesses.

Or he could go for broke. He could put his presidency—and perhaps
his legacy—on the line for a complicated, heavily compromised, and
increasingly unpopular reform. What would he do? Which way would
the cool, cerebral, calculating man—no drama Obama—decide to go?

Future historians will search for the motivations that led Barack
Obama to take his big gamble and push ahead with an intricate but
ultimately successful maneuver around the Senate filibuster. Few presidents have put as much on the line for a single reform, for a single vote.
Did the gamble pay off? Did the legislation improve American health
care? Did it tip the balance of power between the parties?

Time will answer these questions, of course. But one thing, we
believe, is already clear. President Obama accomplished what almost
every Democratic president—Harry Truman, John Kennedy, Jimmy
Carter, and Bill Clinton—aspired to and failed. His accomplishment
invites us to revisit some of the central lessons of health reform. In many
ways, he followed those history lessons. In at least one big way he fell
short. But his most impressive moment came—like Harry Truman's—
after his reform was imperiled.

Begin with what this president did right.

First, he cared about health care—far more than his cool demeanor suggests. From campaign stories about his mother's illness, through countless setbacks and crises over the long Congressional deliberations of 2009, to that evocative tale of a dying uninsured loyalist, health care clearly stuck in Obama's gut. He would not, did not, give up. In East Room remarks before finally signing the hard-won legislation on March 23, 2010, he listed the reasons he had persisted. The first was closest to home: "I did this for my mother."

Second, he acted fast. After a brief postinaugural detour to pass an economic stimulus bill (which contained several important health reform provisions), the administration pressed to get health reform in Obama's first year in office. Here was a president who had learned the lessons of LBJ's success with Medicare—move during the honeymoon, don't let dead cats stink up the porch (see chapter 5). The Obama team also understood the Clinton administration's catastrophic delay. Contrast the Clinton and Obama reform clocks: Obama's legislation made it through the Senate—after nine months of turbulent politics—in late December, year 1, at precisely the same point (late December, year 1) that the Clinton team finally submitted its proposal to Congress.

Third, Obama had a plan on arrival—not a 2,000-page bill, but an approach, a set of principles, that he announced in May 2007 and from which he did not depart. The legislation would dramatically extend coverage by correcting defects in the private insurance market and by providing uninsured Americans the means to purchase private coverage. Employers had to step up, in some form, to guarantee coverage to employees. Health delivery reform through prevention, chronic disease management, and health information technology had to be part of the program. Costs had to be addressed. Ironically, the plan was well to the right of Nixon's 1974 proposal. In fact, its closest predecessor was the Dole-Chafee plan constructed as a Republican alternative to Clinton in 1994. It fell short of what the party faithful had hoped for, but it was a foundation to build on.

Fourth, Obama managed his economists and the economics. Though future scholars will shed light on the memos and the meetings, the administration's decision to expend hundreds of billions on health care—on top of the nearly $900 billion stimulus plan—must have caused sweaty palms and palpitations among dismal scientists in the White House. When the president carved out space for health reform in his proposed economic program for 2009, the die was cast. Later, in September, he calmed jittery nerves among moderate congressional

Democrats by promising a bill that would cost less than $1 trillion and not add "a dime" to the deficit.

Fifth, he went public. He had campaigned on health care, talked about it in Spring 2009, and repeatedly set public deadlines for Congressional action. Even so, the Democrats lost control of the public debate during a long, hot summer of Tea Party activism. Even a powerful September speech before a joint session of Congress—where Congressman Joe Wilson's (R-SC) audible "you lie!" reflected the heat of the controversy—did not turn national sentiment toward health reform. But in the chaotic weeks after the Democrats lost their 60th Senate vote, the president found his voice. He rallied his party in a way reminiscent of Harry Truman giving 'em hell in 1948 or John Kennedy stumping for Medicare after his father's stroke in 1962.

Sixth, the president managed the Congress. He has been criticized for standing back and letting Congress do the drafting. This view, we believe, is naïve about both congressional process and history. Lyndon Johnson and George W. Bush each got results with firm principles and deference on the details. ("I am not trying to go into details," LBJ repeatedly told Ways and Means chair Wilbur Mills in 1964.[2] Johnson always called Medicare "the Mills Bill.") In contrast, the Clinton administration tried to write a detailed bill that congressional committee chairs promptly rewrote or replaced. Presidents Johnson, Bush, and Obama got much further by asking Congress to work from the administration's broad campaign blueprint. The legislative process was not pretty, but it did the job.

Seventh, unlike Jimmy Carter and Bill Clinton, Obama seemed to stay out of the health policy weeds. During convoluted technical debates—about Cadillac health plan taxes, public options, the design of health insurance exchanges, or the power of Medicare cost-containment commissions—the White House batted away pleas to jump into the mud wrestling. Occasionally the president would lob a pronouncement down Pennsylvania Avenue: he supported a public plan, he was flexible on an individual mandate. But for the most part, when he rolled up his sleeves, it was to do what only presidents can do: manage the politics, stiffen the backs of skittish Blue Dog Democrats, or bring disappointed liberals back to the table. Future historians will puzzle out whether President Obama got it exactly right—perhaps he might have intervened more or sooner. But he avoided the temptation to "dive into the PSROs" (see chapter 7)—the nitty-gritty, wonky details that had beguiled some of his failed predecessors.

Finally, the president confronted the toughest lesson that history offers Oval Office health reformers: know how to lose. In the January 2010 State of the Union Address, his party in chaos after the loss of its filibuster-proof Senate majority, Obama stepped back into the fray: "Don't walk away from reform," he told the Congress and the American people. "Not now. Not when we are so close. Let us find a way to come together and finish the job for the American people. Let's get it done." In 1994, Clinton fled the field, ceding the ground to his enemies and leaving health care in the policy wilderness for over a decade. In 2010, Obama did the reverse. His voice grew louder, clearer, more confident as the Democrats fell into disarray. He pushed to get Republicans, as well as Democrats, to own this issue and to take responsibility for fixing a broken system. If he had failed, perhaps his loss—like Truman's or Kennedy's—would have set the stage for another round of health care debate, rather than marking the issue as radioactive. In the end, Obama uncovered a great irony: by knowing how to lose, he won.

We see failings as well as successes in Obama's management of health reform. Lyndon Johnson, the master of the Senate, might very well have found a way to short-circuit the prolonged unsuccessful negotiations between Senators Charles Grassley (R-IA) and Max Baucus (D-MT) that stalled health reform in the Senate, breaching Obama's deadlines and allowing the debate to slip into the near disastrous summer of opposition. Perhaps Obama—and Democrats like Senator Baucus—permitted the chimera of bipartisanship to cloud his political judgment. Perhaps Obama simply didn't have the magic touch, the deeply honed personal instincts and relationships, that gave LBJ the sense of when and how far to push his former Senate colleagues.

While the White House and Democrats focused too long on the inside game of congressional negotiation, they lost control of the public debate. The right-wing populists, self-styled Tea Party activists, roared into the health policy discussion with the 2009 version of "socialized medicine"—the government-run "death panels." The charges—new variations on the trusty old blasts against big government—were simple, pungent, and effective. The administration never found a way to recapture public attention or offer a simple counter to the charges. Like Truman or Clinton before them, the Democrats tried denial (this is not socialized medicine, there are no death panels), backtracking (striking the counseling provisions in the House bill that had set off the storm), and delving into the details (here is what is really in the bill). Once again—yet again—the opposition won the battle of popular perception.

Moreover, the inevitable wheeling and dealing in the House and Senate—there is no other way to pass legislation—was easily ridiculed by
the bill's opponents. President Obama never found a way to explain—to
connect—how and why his health reform principles were being translated into action by the congressional maneuvers. The White House
never managed to sell a persuasive narrative to counter the Tea Party
percussion. That failure, in turn, set the scene for the Massachusetts
election that almost derailed health reform at the very last moment.

Perhaps health reform also got caught up in larger problems that
President Obama struggled to manage. We still live in the philosophical
climate set during Ronald Reagan's first inaugural address: celebrate
individualism, cheer free markets, and bash the government. This is not
fertile ground for national health reform. President Obama campaigned
with an alternative. As he told Joe the Plumber, things are better when
we spread the wealth around. He invoked the old social gospel vision of
community and sharing. Once in office, perhaps wary of the backlash
against "welfare" and "handouts," he lost his rhetorical counter to Reagan-
era individualism. Franklin Roosevelt and John Kennedy had offered a
new ideal of politics and society. They lent a framing, a logic, to the eras
that followed. Future reformers from both parties might do well to learn
that lesson: explain the philosophy that frames your programs.

What next? One story that runs through *The Heart of Power* focuses
on the changes in the political process itself. The most recent edition of
health care reform features something brand new: the ferocious politics
continues even after the legislation is won. Congressional opponents
pledge to fight on—through the courts and into the implementation
process.

That fight will further complicate the huge implementation effort.
For example, the new legislation includes one provision that bars insurers from "unreasonable premium increase[s]" and another that requires
them to spend a minimum amount on "activities that improve health
care quality." These vague mandates have to be defined (what is "unreasonable"? how do we set that "minimum"? what counts as improving
"quality"?). Then officials have to write the rules that put them into
effect.[3] Implementing any ambitious law is difficult. The political and
legal fights that still swirl around the Obama health reform signal an
especially rocky road to implementation.

How will we look back on this health care reform? Back in 1965,
the two parties cooperated once Medicare was won. Even so, implementation was difficult and involved a massive mobilization of national

resources, the desegregation of the hospitals, a threatened physician strike, and reimbursement deals that built a new level of inflation into the medical system. The final result, of course, was an extremely popular and important program burdened by rising costs. On the other hand, the Reagan administration's Medicare catastrophic care coverage was not even fully implemented before Congress unceremoniously buried the entire thing. Now, the Obama administration will try its hand at implementation. What lies ahead is a mix of politics, negotiation, technical decisions, and court rulings that will determine the political legacy of the Obama administration's signature reform.

Still, we end this preface as we did our first, impressed by the person in the Oval Office. Here is a president who learned the lessons of history. Most important, he internalized the great lesson of Harry Truman: learn to face and manage failure, keep fighting despite defeats. Facing a lost election—and leading a dispirited party—President Obama articulated, clearly and insistently, just what was at stake, why he believed in it, and how to negotiate the path ahead. It may well be the first great lesson of his administration. Again, time will tell.

For now, we watch the Obama health reform experience with renewed humility and respect for the political leaders in the eye of the storm. Health care reform continues to grow more important. It remains politically treacherous. And it still trains an unflinching spotlight on the presidency, on the individual standing at the heart of power.

David Blumenthal and James Morone
Brookline, Massachusetts, and Lempster, New Hampshire
March 2009

1. Robert Pear and David M. Herszenhorn, "Democrats Ask, Can This Health Care Bill Be Saved?" *New York Times,* February 6, 2010.

2. Wilbur Mills, telephone audiotape, 9:55 A.M., June 9, 1964, "Recordings and Transcripts of Conversations," Citation 3642, LBJ Library.

3. Robert Pear, "Health Insurers Lobbying to Shape Overhaul Rules," *New York Times,* May 16, 2010.

# 2009 Preface and Acknowledgments

This book began during a walk across the Harvard campus forty-two years ago. Professor Richard Neustadt—short and slim, a pipe between his teeth, a beret atop his head, an easy smile across his face—had just finished a lecture in his popular course on the American presidency. David Blumenthal—tall, serious, slightly diffident, definitely shaggy—had gotten swept up by his teacher's infectious good humor and expansive warmth. The conversation went on as they walked, leaning into the raw New England wind, the actual topic now lost to memory.

Richard Neustadt would pen (back in that era, he wrote in longhand) books that redefined our understanding of presidential power. But Blumenthal, like so many students, was also drawn to this professor by the glow of Camelot—long before we'd heard about its dark side. Richard Neustadt had been there in John Kennedy's White House, and he conjured up the youth, glamour, and call to service that were still inspiring young Americans.

Time passed. Neustadt continued to counsel presidents and inspire students, Blumenthal immersed himself in medicine and health policy research. Their families grew close, sharing marvelous weekends in the soft sunlight at the Neustadt summer home beside a tranquil Cape Cod pond. And then, after years of warm friendship and happy memory, Blumenthal was hit by a bolt from the blue.

Why not a book about how presidents deal with health care issues? There were many fine books on the history of health policy. But none told the story from the presidents' viewpoint. None captured the drama of national campaigns, the sparring in the Oval Office, or that most elusive quality—presidential leadership. None reflected on how these powerful men balanced their hurts with their health policies. And certainly no one had scanned the modern presidencies for the dos and don'ts of winning health care reform.

David mulled over the project. It was missing something. He needed a partner who could bring the perspectives of political science and history. He called Jim Morone—David knew Jim as a scholar who had written ambitious political histories. Morone responded with a tour of presidential scholars who might help the project. David calmly listened to the rendition and, when it was over, said simply: "How about you?" By the time their conversation had ended, *The Heart of Power* was under way.

It proved a magic collaboration. As we haunted the archives, did our interviews, and pored over our notes in the country calm of the Hanover Inn, the presidents turned into flesh-and-blood characters—robust and sickly, wise and foolish, triumphant and defeated. The gentlemanly (if mildly cranky) Dwight Eisenhower became one of David's unexpected favorites. Lyndon Johnson dazzled us both as he pushed, cajoled, and hustled the political establishment toward his Great Society. And Franklin Roosevelt remained awe-inspiring and elusive as we tracked him across his three terms. Each president leaped out of the archives, for better and (in a few cases) for worse, each becoming our companion as we wrestled over the great arc of health and politics in the Oval Office.

However, something else gave our studies a special savor. We studied the presidency during the most exciting presidential campaign of our lives. Like many Americans we felt the inspirational rush that had once been known as Camelot. David had been tapped as a health advisor to the Obama campaign. Meanwhile, Republican John McCain's camp also proposed deep changes in health policy, promising to repeal some rules that—as you'll see in chapter 3—had stood since the Eisenhower administration. As we reflected on Nixon's tormented genius, Reagan's success with Congress, and Truman's earthy wisdom, we knew we were pondering lessons that might prove useful sooner rather than later. The campaign gave our conversations a special electricity. We were thrilled by a mix of discovery and hope.

We are indebted to many, many people. The Robert Wood Johnson Foundation and its Investigator Awards Program made all of this possible. We are most grateful to the program's director, Dr. David Mechanic, and his deputies, Lynn Rogut and Cynthia Church. The Investigator Award Program is far more than a grant program. It creates a family of investigators and invites them to pursue bold new ideas that break the usual mold. David, Lynn, and Cynthia are a constant source of inspiration to their company of scholars.

We visited the archives of all the presidents since Franklin Roosevelt except for Bill Clinton's (which is still getting organized) and George W. Bush's (which doesn't yet exist). Wonderful archivists helped us everywhere we went. In almost every case, they pointed to hidden gold mines. Each archive has its own ambiance. The unpretentious Truman library looks out on an eternal flame (burning by Harry's grave) that seems to symbolize his dreams of a fair society; the Kennedy library juts out into the bay—open to the sea and the sky that JFK loved; the Reagan library, set on a majestic ridge north of Los Angeles, is a great shrine to the president's vision of Americana, with video images of the Gipper looping constantly in many corners of the adjacent museum. But, for all the differences, there is a great constant across the presidential archives: the attentiveness, helpfulness, and diligence of the professionals who staff them. We owe them all an enormous debt. The greatest thanks we can give them is to urge you to visit these wonderful American places.

We also owe special thanks to our agents, Shannon O'Neil and Rafe Sagalyn of the Sagalyn Agency. Rafe has an extraordinary ability that Shannon shares—getting to the real heart of the story, sometimes even before his authors. Lynne Withey and Hannah Love gave our book a warm publishing home; Lynne and her team at the University of California Press brushed away every publishing problem almost as quickly as we could articulate it. Ashley Hubert guided us gracefully through production. And special thanks go to Lara Heimert, executive editor at Basic Books, who generously extended Jim's deadline for the book he was meant to be finishing.

A series of wonderful assistants at Harvard and Brown also helped make the book possible. Our cheers and thanks to Kelli Auerbach, Jason Barnosky, Nick Cetrulo, Tony Dell'Aera, Dan Ehlke, Sarah Johnson, Jeremy Johnson, Ellie MacDonald, Robert Rogers, and Amy Schoenfeld. They have moved on with their lives, or will shortly, but a part of them remains between these pages. We expect to be recommending their books before long.

Many participants provided valuable insights into the events we describe, or commented on individual chapters. We are indebted to Ted Sorensen, Joe Califano, Paul O'Neill, Frank Carlucci, Stuart Altman,

Jim Cavanaugh, Stan Jones, Karen Davis, Jim Mongan, Tom Scully, Gail Wilensky, Judy Feder, Atul Gawande, David Nexon, Mark McClellan, Mark Peterson, Nancy Johnson, and many others who prefer to remain anonymous. All were generous with their time and reflections on the events that we attempted to reconstruct and interpret. We are also indebted to Dr. Jerome Groopman, who read some of the early chapters and gave us invaluable advice on how to make them more cinematic and appealing.

David owes incalculable thanks to Anne Fulton, his long-suffering assistant, who kept him on track with this project, as she has on so many others, with grace and efficiency.

Ellen Blumenthal and Deborah Stone lived with the presidents—and our long discussions of Ike or LBJ or Bill Clinton. Ellen and Deborah regularly interrupted their own work—seeing patients and writing books—to ask us the unsettling questions that sent us back to the records for another look. More important, each offered us warmth, friendship, and love—the power of heart.

Finally, the authors are indebted—as is everyone who cares about presidents and politics —to Richard E. Neustadt, who died on October 31, 2003, at age 84, after a lifetime of inspiring the men and women around him.

This book appears at an time that is both thrilling and terrifying. A new leader raises the hope that we may finally find a way through the health care thicket that has grown more gnarled and trackless with every year. At the same time, the economy seems to be falling off a cliff. Our parents' memories of the Great Depression flood back to our minds. Nightmare images of Depression-era breadlines and people huddled around flaming oil cans—long buried as ancient history—suddenly confront a generation that thought that plenty was its birthright. Which way do we go—toward hope, or fear? Perhaps it is a false choice. Fear may, once again, empower hope by enabling a vital president to take action in parlous times. Our fondest wish is that the lessons of this book will guide a new administration, however slightly, toward winning social justice and the people's health.

December, 2008
Brookline, Massachusetts
Lempster, New Hampshire

# Introduction

Tuberculosis tormented the Nixons. When Richard was ten, doctors found a shadow on his lungs and told him to lay off sports while they watched for other symptoms. Then his brother Arthur developed a fever and began to waste away. Doctors, tests, and treatments did not help. Just before dying, the boy drifted back into consciousness and recited a little prayer: "If I should die before I wake, I pray thee, Lord, my soul to take." The boys' tough, abusive father broke down and wept—but not Richard, then twelve years old. He just sat in a big armchair and stared into space, silent and dry-eyed. Two years later, the disease struck still another brother: Harold, the family favorite. After private sanitariums had drained the family savings, the boys' mother moved to Arizona with Harold, hoping the dry climate would save him. To pay the rent, she cared for other boys dying of the disease. Richard stayed behind with his father until Harold died six years later. Memories of hard times and harsh treatment, illness and loss, all stuck to Richard Nixon. They touched the way he thought about politics, bent his lonely personality, and came blurting out when he faced difficulty. In his weepy White House farewell, just before boarding a helicopter and flying away in disgrace, Nixon described his mother, exiled in Arizona and watching the boys in her care die, one after another, while she struggled—helplessly, vainly—to save her son.[1]

Think about the American presidents, and *helpless* is the last word that comes to mind. Arthur Schlesinger had Richard Nixon partially in his sights when he labeled the American presidency "imperial." Presidents travel abroad surrounded by an extraordinary entourage—a flotilla of aircraft, a fleet of cars, a pack of dogs sniffing for bombs, and hundreds of aides, guards, cooks, valets, sharpshooters, and assistants. Once upon a time, Alexander Hamilton assured his countryman that American presidents would never resemble the king of Great Britain, the Grand Seignior, the khan of Tartary, or, as he put it, any other voluptuous potentate. But two hundred years later, the American president commands unrivaled military power and projects influence, for better or for worse, onto every corner of the planet.[2]

The strange truth: American presidents operate between power and frailty, surrounded by soaring ideas and lumbering institutions—atop the world, but just a step from personal and political disaster. *The Heart of Power* explores this difficult, shapeshifting office by following one issue that no modern president can duck—health care reform. Every president from Franklin Roosevelt (who took office in 1933) to George W. Bush (who stepped down in 2009) has grappled with it. Some presidents seize health reform, and others try to shun it—but, willy-nilly, it rises up every president's agenda.

The health reform story illuminates almost every aspect of the presidency. Because health care reform is excruciatingly difficult to win, it tests presidents' ideas, heart, luck, allies, and their skill at running the most complicated government machinery in the world.

The first surprise lies in the sheer impact of the issue. The New Deal coalition consolidated itself (under President Truman), crested (Kennedy, Johnson), and crumbled (Carter, Clinton) partially on health care. The issue proved especially important during the long downward slide. On the other side, clashes over health policy marked the Republican ascendancy from Ronald Reagan through George W. Bush. We get a whole new look at the cycles and eras—what political historians call the periodicity—of American politics when we peer through this lens. Moreover, presidents repeatedly change the way we think and talk about what has become—at $2.2 trillion—America's largest industry.

At the same time, this is an intensely personal story. The person in the Oval Office is a vulnerable human. Presidents get sick, take dubious drugs, get drunk, contemplate suicide, fret about ailing parents, burn with insecurities, and bury people they love. No one escapes the human condition, and nothing reveals the president's humanity like hurt and sickness and death. Health offers a rare opportunity to match the person to the policy. Most presidents never experience hunger or homelessness;

they don't go onto the welfare rolls or end up in jail. But every one of them knows about disease and death. Often, the deep personal hurts are what move these men to commit themselves to a reform that they know is a long shot even in the best of times.

In short, *The Heart of Power* uses health as a lens on the Oval Office. It offers a fresh way to see the men, the presidency, the nation's health care policy, and the great tides of American power. Ultimately, it opens a window on America itself.

### THE MEN IN THE OVAL OFFICE

The delegates to the Constitutional Convention wrangled about almost everything. But when they debated the presidency, their fevers lowered a little. After all, George Washington sat at the front of the room, serenely presiding over the meeting. The delegates knew that when it came time to elect the first president, the reluctant American Cincinnatus would be called back to civic duty. The presidency inevitably begins with biography. Only nineteen men held the office across the entire twentieth century. Their opinions, dreams, and eccentricities shaped their administrations as well as their eras.

The presidents' health offers us a look at the men behind the power. As a group, they have been distinctly unhealthy. Fifteen presidents and former presidents died during the twentieth century—eleven passed away prematurely; eight of them fell more than seven years short of the actuarial tables.[3] The men endured a long litany of hurts and pains. Of course, presidents pose as stoics when it comes to their own strokes or drinking problems, but they often let themselves grow voluble about the illnesses that afflict the people they love.

Dwight Eisenhower suffered heart attacks and a stroke in the White House, but when he talked with his aides about health care, he kept returning to Mamie's mother—Mrs. Doud, as he referred to her. Her death after two hard (and expensive) sick years left his wife disconsolate. Or John Kennedy. Few presidents have been sicker or more heavily medicated. JFK took multiple painkilling injections each day to keep going, and he received the last rites of the Catholic Church four times as an adult. But nothing moved him like his father's stroke. He went before a pro-Medicare rally at Madison Square Garden in 1962—perked up by Marilyn Monroe's melting rendition of "Happy Birthday" the night before—and talked about his dad: "I visited twice, yesterday and today, in hospital, where doctors labor for a long time.... It isn't easy—it isn't easy. He can pay his bills, but otherwise, I would be [paying].... What happens to him and to others when they put their life savings in, in a short time?" Grieving for a crippled father, he took enormous risks to advance the cause of universal health insurance for the aged—and in the process helped redefine the modern presidency. This story ends with a bitter irony: the old patriarch, Joseph Kennedy, would outlive both John and his brother Bobby.[4]

There's more to it than illness, of course. The Oval Office magnifies every quirk. The super-smart, self-righteous Jimmy Carter pored over memo after memo, scribbling esoteric corrections in the margins. George W. Bush, by way of contrast, was all efficiency; he ticked through his health care briefing books, kept his eye on the big picture, remaking Medicare to Republican specifications—but heaven help the subordinate who showed up a minute late to a meeting. In presidential politics, every aspect of the personal is political and helps shape process and outcome, success and failure.

The office, the bureaucracy, the electoral mandate, and the disposition of Congress all matter, of course. But the presidency and its policies always start with a man or a woman sitting in the president's chair.

## THE IDEA MACHINE

The presidency is a great dynamo producing fresh ideas. Each incumbent can inject a small number of deeply felt views into the political process. The force of those ideas as they resonate across the nation (and within Washington) is a pretty safe gauge of an administration's vitality. Forceful presidencies offer an overarching framework—Lyndon Johnson's claim that a great society should be judged by how it treats its weakest citizens or Ronald Reagan's insistence that government is the source of our national problems—and then find policy prescriptions that reach for the vision.

Where do the big ideas come from? Presidents encounter them on the way to the White House. Ideas resonate with a president's personal experience or fire up an important constituency. They bubble up from allies, intellectuals, policy networks, think tanks, and poker buddies. Presidents control one of the world's great megaphones—as Teddy Roosevelt put it, a bully pulpit. Administrations rely on a network of policy entrepreneurs who try to hammer out ideas that connect with the public. Big ideas move political mountains because they inspire followers and sustain movements.

The sure sign of a party in decline is a larder bare of ideas. After Jimmy Carter was elected in 1976, a member of his transition team urged that the new administration assertively educate its appointees in Jimmy Carter's "goals and his philosophy." Strong presidents lead a movement, a party, or even a faction to power, but this one needed to instruct its appointees in what the president stood for. And what was that? An engineer's emphasis on efficiency, detail, and procedure.[5]

Carter's emphasis on efficient management reflects an old political temptation: replace bold ideas with policy technique. Each criticism can be met by a more sophisticated tweak or algorithm. But, as we'll see, technical adjustments never answer political challenges. Clear, bold ideas speak to the public and mobilize allies. In contrast, opponents have a field day caricaturing wonky analytic convolutions. In 1986, for example, Doc Bowen—as President Ronald Reagan affectionately called his wily secretary of Health and Human Services—wanted to expand Medicare. The administration's economists scrambled to float a more market-friendly alternative (with the assistance of the promarket Heritage Foundation). At a Cabinet meeting held to discuss Doc Bowen's proposal, the chairman of the Council of Economic Advisors, Beryl Sprinkel, floated a hastily designed voucher plan that he claimed would be far truer to the administration's emphasis on restoring markets. In response, Secretary Bowen whipped out his pen and drawled, "Now, let me see if I got this right." He began to draw lines reflecting the voucher plan's money trail: from the government to the insurer to the elderly to the provider—line, line, line, line. He kept going—exaggerating a bit, he later confessed—and soon had his paper covered with lines, and the entire room, including the president, chuckling over the whole convoluted voucher thing. A decade later everyone had learned that trick—line, line, line, line—in time to ridicule Bill Clinton's better health care mousetrap.[6]

The urge to build a more efficient, technically correct program has its roots in the Progressive era at the turn of the last century. The Progressives imagined that good technique produced good government—there was no Democratic or Republican way to pave a street, they said; rather, the right way to do a job was to get beyond politics and focus on doing it efficiently. Party politicians developed a derogatory term for the good government dreamers—goo-goos—but the old neoprogressive dream never dies. We'll see the goo-goo illusion alive and well in health care. It inspired Jimmy Carter. And, though politics buried the Carter plan, Bill Clinton cheerfully disinterred the old impulse fifteen years later, linked it to his dream of a third way (neither bleeding-heart liberal nor harsh conservative), and put it at the center of his own run at health reform. Efficiency is a good thing, but it doesn't win political debates or rouse popular support.

As political historian Stephen Skowronek has argued, an emphasis on technique above all else is the sign of a party coalition in decline. Efficient process is no substitute for bold ideas. And it is never a winning strategy in the health care debates.[7]

The mistake is compounded by presidents who are too eager to delve into the details. Throughout the seventy-five-year history detailed in the following pages, there isn't a single example of a president who succeeded by leaping into the wonky debates. "I trust you on the details," said Lyndon Johnson, again and again, as congressional leaders and White House aides hammered out the details of the Medicare program.[8] Johnson knew there was an indispensable role that only he could play: he could best publicize the idea, build support, jawbone interest groups into line, and organize (and lobby) the congressional coalition. When reporters asked Senator George Smathers (D-FL) why he had switched his vote and salvaged the administration's Medicare proposal in 1964, he responded, simply, "Lyndon told me to."[9] Presidents win complicated reforms by doing what the office of the presidency is uniquely designed for—publicizing and persuading. We'll watch more than one president squander that advantage by posing as an expert.

There is, of course, a danger at the other extreme—that of the disengaged executive. The president chooses his analysts, gives them directions, and decides when the debate is over. The staff always knows when the boss has lost interest—and the issue, no matter how well staffed, is probably doomed. During the fading days of George H. W. Bush's presidency, health care aides in the policy boiler room despaired over their inability to turn the boss's attention to an issue that was gripping the American public.

And there is no premium on newness. Many innovations take time to mature and gather popular momentum. The voucher plan that Doc Bowen so neatly dispatched eventually returned. The two Bush presidencies introduced reforms based on the same logic, each one more carefully worked out than the last and tucked into a larger vision that celebrated markets by offering each individual a choice among private insurance plans. A rising Republican coalition, made possible by Reagan's own successes, treated the notion more respectfully than Reagan or his Cabinet had done.

More than any other political office in America, the presidency rises and falls on ideas. Richard Neustadt, the dean of presidential studies, once noted that the power of the presidency is the power to persuade. It is that and more: it is the power to put something new before the public eye, to take a little-known notion and get the whole nation talking about it. And in the debate over health care there is no greater force.

## THE INFERNAL MACHINERY OF GOVERNMENT: THE WHITE HOUSE AS AN INSTITUTION

In the middle of his first foreign policy crisis, Jack Kennedy mused in a late-night telephone call, "It really is true that foreign affairs is the only important issue for a president to handle, isn't it? I mean, who gives a shit if the minimum wage is $1.15 or $1.25 in comparison to something like this?" Most presidents prefer dealing with foreign policy because it offers them the elbow room for bold decisions backed by broad constitutional powers.[10]

By way of contrast, winning that dime on the minimum wage took a knock-down free-for-all with congressional barons. Kennedy had to win a cliffhanger vote to reconstruct the House Rules Committee, which he then stocked with allies who in turn voted to permit his minimum wage proposal to reach the floor of Congress, where, with hard work and a bit of luck, he cobbled together a majority made up of liberal Democrats from the North, conservative Democrats from Dixie, and the occasional Republican. Moreover, threading that political needle took a savvy congressional liaison office that knew which arms to twist and what promises to make.

All of which raises the essential point: there is no owner's manual for running the White House. The Constitution barely defines the job: it gives Congress a detailed role and specific powers but leaves the president brief instructions dominated by an enigmatic phrase: "The executive power shall be vested in a President." What exactly does that mean? The founders did not say, for the most part. The presidency has to be defined through action. As we follow the health care issue from Franklin D. Roosevelt to George W. Bush, we will see four powerful institutional trends shaping and reshaping the presidency.

### Rising Economists

The most dramatic development is the growing economic infrastructure that advises, empowers, and profoundly limits the president. From the

Council of Economic Advisors (established in 1946) to the Office of Management and Budget (established in 1970), the presidents' fiscal tools have grown deeper and ever more sophisticated. In theory, this gives the White House greater control over the federal leviathan. But in practice something quite different is also happening. The presidents' ability to introduce bold health reforms is increasingly constrained by economists buzzing in their ears.

The result is a tension between visionary social reform and economic policy. Dreams of universal coverage—whether Democratic or Republican—face off against the green-eye-shaded battalions whose influence grows from one administration to the next. The entire presidency has been reshaped by this powerful trend.

We can mark the contrast by observing Lyndon Johnson's cavalier attitude toward finance during the Medicare debate in 1964: "Don't ever argue with me ... on health or education," he hectored Vice President Hubert Humphrey (this from a marvelous trove of recently released White House tapes). "I'll go a hundred million or a billion on health or education. I don't argue about that any more than I argue about Lady Bird buying flour. You got to have flour and coffee in your house and education and health. I'll spend the goddamn money." Down-home domestic metaphors took the place of economic models.[11]

Johnson drove his fuzzy economics lesson home when he gave a newly elected Senator from Massachusetts named Ted Kennedy (D-MA), pointers on pushing a bill through Congress without getting tangled up in the finances. Johnson cited Medicare as an example: "The fools had to go to projecting it down the road five or six years, and when you project it, the first year it runs 900 million." The long-term projections, complained Johnson, meant nothing but political headaches for him. "The first thing, Senator Dick Russell (D-GA) comes running in, says, 'My God, you've got a one billion dollar [estimate] for next year on health. Therefore I'm against any of it now.'"[12]

Medicare's soaring costs would soon make Johnson's blithe attitude seem reckless, but his comments signal a hard reality worth pondering: Johnson, like Kennedy before him, low-balled the numbers and evaded economic projections to smooth the passage of his program. An honest economic forecast would very likely have sunk Medicare.

The heretical lesson is one that we will encounter in every administration, with few exceptions to the rule: expanding health insurance never fits the budget, and it never squares with the economic program. For more than sixty years, from Harry Truman's administration in 1945 to George W. Bush's in 2003, not a single economic team signed on happily to an extension of health care benefits. The lesson is simple: presidents who wish to expand health insurance have to hush their economists. Over the years, we'll see each man react in a different way when the economics team troops into the Oval Office and says "No, you can't, Mr. President."

But hushing the economists gets more difficult as time goes on. The economic regime is more and more firmly entrenched in the Oval Office. The rules grow more stringent and the tools more effective. Presidents can still overrule their dismal scientists—as both Ronald Reagan and George W. Bush did. But, for good or ill, doing so grows harder and harder, requiring more nerve and more political capital.

*Power Flows to the Center*

The economists' growing clout reflects another trend: power flows from the Cabinet Agencies to the White House. In the 1950s, President Eisenhower penned courteous letters to his Cabinet members—weighing their opinions, waiting on their consensus, and carefully justifying decisions to the losing secretary. Ten years later, President Lyndon Johnson pushed the Cabinet aside in his voracious quest for social policy breakthroughs. White House staff members, led by Joseph Califano, designed the Model Cities program without even informing Luther Hodges, the secretary of Housing and Urban Development, until the last minute. When Califano finally briefed the secretary, Hodges enthusiastically promised to analyze the program and return with suggestions—only to learn that the president was unveiling the plan that very afternoon. The secretary had no knowledge of a program constructed on his own organizational turf. "Lyndon Johnson's cabinet meetings," quipped Califano to us in an interview, "were just tea parties."[13]

The tide of political power continued to flow to the White House during the administrations that followed. Richard Nixon fiercely upped the ante: "If we don't get rid of these people," he said, speaking of the liberals populating the Cabinet Agencies, "they will sit back on their well-paid asses and wait for the next election to bring back their old bosses." The solution? More power and control to the White House. Nixon injected something new—the permanent campaign. The distinction between political staff and nonpartisan experts began to evaporate and the White House turned all political all the time. The number of White House staff peaked under Nixon, who employed over six hundred officials. President Carter, who won the next election in the backlash against Nixon, moved to reestablish Cabinet government—but that didn't keep him from sacking five Cabinet members in a single week when the going got hard. Joseph Califano, the secretary of Health, Education, and Welfare—and the most prominent liberal head to roll—wryly amended his observation about the declining Cabinet: "Now," he told us, "the Cabinet meetings became tea parties without the tea."[14]

Each president comes to office with a different idea about the role of the Cabinet and exactly how much authority should rest there. Watching the health care debate illuminates the underlying trend: increasing control from the White House. Occasional attempts at restoring the balance of power have done little to arrest the centralization of executive power around the president.[15]

## Organizing the White House

But just what does the White House look like in action? The political parties differ dramatically. Franklin Roosevelt left the modern Democrats an ambiguous legacy when he surrounded himself with gifted intellectuals, assigned overlapping tasks, and gave them license to move from issue to issue. In theory, the loose organization stimulated creativity and bold new ideas—in stark contrast (as the Democrats see it) to the stifling, unimaginative conformity of Republican administrations. President Bill Clinton, the latest heir of FDR's free-form organization, imagined that he might resolve disputes about his health plan by sponsoring formal debates. A skeptical press was soon jeering this as Clinton's Oxford on the Potomac. In sharp contrast, Republicans hew to the solid, unambiguous organizational design of a traditional B-school primer—no ambiguous dotted lines or overlapping functions on their personnel charts.

Each style has advantages and drawbacks—the many subtle trade-offs between careful control and creative chaos. But across the eleven administrations we follow, there is one hubristic reflex (typical of Democrats) that always leads to trouble. No modern president has successfully acted as his own chief of staff. There is no getting around the need for a strong, talented, competent administrator familiar with the levers of power. The chief of staff is indispensable for directing traffic, overseeing process, and following decisions to ensure that they are understood and implemented.

Jimmy Carter's effort to abolish the role—he did not want a functionary between him and his subordinates—illustrated the many pitfalls in the practice. For example, participants at the same health meeting often disagreed on what had been decided. Without a chief of staff, no one was on hand to sort out rival interpretations. The matter had to sit and wait until the president had time to revisit it. The stuffed inbox kept the president focused on day-to-day management—and exacerbated his own predisposition to neglect the big picture. To rephrase the old saw, a president who acts as his own chief of staff has a fool for a boss.

*Leadership*

As presidents struggle with the health care octopus—highly personal, politically perilous, technically complicated—they cast light on that most elusive of things: the nature of leadership. Two skills are especially important—going public and playing the insider game.

Roosevelt understood the power of going public. When members of his staff pushed for Social Security amendments that would guarantee health insurance in 1943, he stopped them. "The only person who can explain this health thing to the people," he said "is me." He did not have the breathing space in the middle of World War II, but he promised his staff that he'd go public for health insurance in his fourth term—although with the cagey Roosevelt nothing was ever certain. Roosevelt had put his finger on the big job: explaining "this health insurance thing to the people." A president advocating a big and complicated change such as health reform must generate a wave of telegrams, letters, and phone calls (and, nowadays, e-mails, text messages, blogs, and tweets).[16]

Until the 1960s, no president took Roosevelt's advice. FDR himself never committed. One of the great mysteries about Harry Truman was why he never threw himself wholeheartedly into the national health insurance battle that he cared so much about. On his whistle-stop train tour during the 1948 election campaign, he developed a short, tough, choppy, extemporaneous, effective speaking style that he honed in speech after speech, hour after exhausting hour. When he introduced national health care after his surprise victory, he told the press that if opponents blocked his bill, he was going to get back on the train and take the case to the people. Advocates pleaded, allies waited, and the press asked about it at every opportunity. But Truman, despite coy hints, remained mysteriously silent about this signature program. Health insurance—always a very long shot—had no chance without vigorous White House leadership.

John F. Kennedy finally took the issue public. Just days after his inauguration, the charismatic Kennedy held the first televised press conference, and it was a smash—an estimated 65 million people tuned in. His approval ratings went through the roof—up to 75 percent—and barely budged for sixteen months. The presidency would never be the same. When it came to health care, Kennedy used the same skills and all the media power of the presidency—campaign-style—on a single policy. He rolled out this strategy for Medicare. "Presidents have tried to marshal public opinion before this for a favored and politically potent bill," commented the *New York Times,* "but probably never on such a scale as has Mr. Kennedy for health insurance."[17]

President Kennedy set the pattern. Building support for a policy is something presidents are uniquely positioned to do. Kennedy did it brilliantly, Ronald Reagan almost without effort. Others—such as Richard Nixon—recoiled at the idea. Still others—for example, George Herbert Walker Bush—proved stone-deaf to the chords that moved the public. Going public is a major weapon in the policy process and a significant test of presidential skill and leadership.

But then there is the inside game—running the complicated machinery of American government. There's nothing like health care to illustrate just how hard it is to drive action through the system, and nothing differentiates the presidents more dramatically than their skill at managing government—especially Congress. Lyndon Johnson was the master of the process in his triumphant first two years. In chapter 5, we retell the story of Medicare's passage, relying on recently released tapes and documents. Our revision offers a daunting example of the skills this president employed to win reform.

The traditional Medicare story turns on Representative Wilbur Mills (D-AR). Mills, the powerful chairman of the House Ways and Means Committee, had long bottled up the Medicare proposal. The 1964 landslide, however, swept more than forty liberal Democrats into Congress—and pushed out three veteran Ways and Means naysayers. Now, concluded Theodore Marmor, Medicare's backers enjoyed "the politics of legislative certainty." Representative Mills, continues the standard story, faced up to the inevitable and adroitly switched sides. He took the administration bill (which covered hospital costs for the elderly), attached it to a rival Republican bill (which covered health care costs for poor people, now called Medicaid) and, on top of that, included the American Medical Association bill (which covered physician costs for the elderly). No one but the brilliant Wilbur Mills had imagined that the three rival bills might be combined. Even President Lyndon Johnson could only stand on the sideline and admire the master legislator as Mills took a modest proposal and built the Medicare and Medicaid programs out of it.[18]

Lyndon Johnson himself repeated this minimalist story in his own autobiography and spiced it up with a tangy Texas anecdote. After Mills had stunned the closed session of Ways and Means with his "bombshell," the chief White House health aide, Wilbur Cohen, rushed back to get President Johnson's reaction. The new proposal would cost an additional $500 million in the first year. What should the administration do? Johnson replied, "Well, I guess I'll run and get my brother." Seeing that his aide was bewildered, the president elaborated:

> Well, I remember one time they were giving a test to a fellow who was going to be a switchman on the railroad, giving him an intelligence test, and they said, "What would you do if a train was coming east going sixty miles per hour, and you looked over your shoulder and another one was coming from the west going sixty miles an hour?" And the fellow said, "I'd go get my brother." And they said, "Why would you get your brother?" And he said, "Because he hasn't ever seen a train wreck."[19]

Thus instructed to accept Mills's bold proposal—and damn the costs—Wilbur Cohen returned to Capitol Hill and gave the chairman the green light. Medicare and Medicaid were soon born. President Johnson, the cheering bystander, summed up the story himself: "Chairman Wilbur Mills, so long the villain of the act, was now a hero to the old folks."[20]

Except it did not exactly happen that way. We now know—through extensive White House telephone tapes and memos—that LBJ cooked up the entire coup with Mills. For fourteen months, Johnson harassed Mills about expanding Medicare—calling him in his office and even catching him with a phone call as he was walking onto the House floor. Lyndon constantly repeated his message: pass Medicare (which he called the Mills Bill), make it bigger and more ambitious, and—always the same promise—all the praise and honor would go to the ambitious Mills. Johnson and Mills had repeatedly discussed versions of the "three-layer cake" that Mills dramatically sprang on the committee—knowing full well that LBJ would back it.

Nor did it end there. "Johnson always acted," Wilbur Cohen later testified, "like he was still running the Congress."[21] He was like a super-majority leader, unabashedly instructing the legislators on the best way to do their jobs. For example, after Mills maneuvered the newly expanded Medicare package through Ways and Means, he gathered with House leaders to call Johnson with the good news. Johnson was already looking to the next potential trap. He wanted them to move fast. The Rules committee might bottle up the bill and give opponents a chance to mobilize. LBJ gave them a memorable talking to, as he asked to speak first to one, then the other: "For God sakes, don't let dead cats stand on your porch. Mr. Rayburn [Sam Rayburn (D-TX), former House speaker and Johnson mentor] used to say: 'they stunk and they stunk and they stunk.' When you get one [of your bills] out of your committee, you call that son of a bitch up before they [the opposition] can get their letters written."[22]

Days after this call, Johnson cleared another hurdle for Medicare in the Senate, where the chairman of the Senate Finance Committee, Senator Harry Byrd (D-VA), remained a firm opponent who might try to bottle Medicare in his own committee. In a legendary ambush, Johnson invited Byrd to the White House for an "extremely important" and sensitive meeting and then, after talking to House and Senate leaders behind closed doors, ushered them all into an unexpected press conference. With TV cameras rolling, Johnson talked about the successful movement of Medicare through the House Ways and Means committee, then turned to Byrd and asked the surprised senator whether there was anything preventing the Senate Finance Committee from quickly holding hearings on Medicare. Byrd tried to evade a direct answer, but Johnson pinned him down, squeezed his arm, and not so gently pressured him before the rolling cameras. Byrd, who was more at home in the Senate hallways than before a national audience, reluctantly stammered that there would be no delay in acting on the bill. Afterward, the hijacked senator commented ruefully, "If I had known what you had in mind, I would have dressed more formally."[23]

Years later, an interviewer asked Representative Mills whether another president—say, Kennedy—could have gotten LBJ's Great Society through Congress. Mills was unambiguous: "No. No, and that's where Johnson doesn't get the credit [he deserves]. He had the greatest ability of any president to get things done."[24]

From an insider such as Wilbur Mills, that was the highest praise. Within a decade, presidential candidates would base their campaigns on the boast that they were outsiders, uncorrupted by Washington's ways. But that shift in the path to the White House does not diminish Wilbur Mills's metric for weighing administrations: the president's ability "to get things done."

## AMERICAN PATHS TO HEALTH SECURITY

Health care and old-age pensions lie at the heart of every welfare state. They touch more of the population than perhaps any other aspect of government. In the United States, old-age benefits—Social Security— have been remarkably stable, but health care changes constantly— always an issue marked by boisterous arguments, surprising twists, and unexpected turns.

On the surface, the question is simple—even boring: how do we get health insurance to those who don't have it? How do we protect it for those who do? The debate has always been about how to do the job best. Beneath the consensus, however, lies the most enduring divide in American social policy: how do we balance markets and governments to achieve a common good? The presidents' health policies have repeatedly engaged this contentious dialogue.

The long health care debate breaks down into three eras, each with its own model of health care rooted in a different vision of politics and market. Naturally, the concepts overlap. But each is analytically distinctive, each rests on a different philosophy, and each reflects the spirit of its time. We might summarize the three approaches as robust government, a mix of government and market, and robust markets.

### Social Security

In the 1930s, liberals imagined a universal right to health care secured by a national, compulsory insurance plan—Social Security extended to medical care. President Roosevelt tapped experts who enthusiastically staffed committees, studied the issue, and devised plans. Three different rounds (1934–35, 1938–39, and 1944–45) each produced a vague draft of three national health proposals. An enigmatic president organized the studies, encouraged the advocates and, in the end, always put the health care battle off for another day. The final commission, hard at work when FDR died, delivered its report to Harry Truman, who plucked up Roosevelt's standard and made the reform, by his own admission, the great lost cause of his life. Liberal Democrats turned national health insurance into the New Deal's unfinished legacy. They would fervently pursue it for the next thirty years; some pursue it to this day.

Conservative southern Democrats were less enthusiastic and quietly demurred when it came to the Social Security model for health care. Part of the problem lay in the threat to southern segregation. What would a universal, federal program mean for southern hospitals? The idea reverberated with black entitlement and even racial integration. Better, they argued, to target government health insurance (and, for that matter, any welfare program) at poor people, and to put the reliable (meaning segregationist) state governments in charge. That more minimal approach might even attract Republican votes.

Through the 1940s, 1950s, and early 1960s, Democrats pushed their government health insurance. Liberals lined up behind Social Security entitlements—first for everyone, later for the elderly—and conservative Democrats touted welfare programs. Critics denounced it all as un-American and socialistic: big government run amuck. By the Kennedy administration, however, the liberals had worked out an effective countercharge: their opponents had fought against the now-beloved Social Security Program.

From the 1940s through the mid-1960s, Americans debated the issue in a distinctly New Deal frame—the language of rights and robust government sound quite foreign to the contemporary ear. Defensive Republicans sometimes acknowledged the liberal spirit of the age. "We know that the American people will not long be denied access to adequate medical facilities," warned the lone Republican President of the era, Dwight D. Eisenhower, as he scrambled to find "a logical alternative to socialized medicine."[25]

The Social Security model lingers among liberals—known, today, by the tone-deaf label "*single-payer model*" or the wistful "*Medicare for all.*" As a real force in the Potomac debates, however, the Social Security model was last seen in the 1970s—when it was eclipsed by a mixed approach sold as the American Way.

*The American Way*

Americans eventually hashed out an alternative to direct government action: public policies operating through private institutions. The Eisenhower administration made the crucial breakthrough—barely noticed at the time—when it waived the income tax on employer-sponsored health insurance premiums. This created a clear incentive to provide health insurance—higher salaries mean more taxes, but higher insurance premiums are tax-free (the change locked in place an increasingly shaky IRS ruling from the previous decade). An enormous federal government tax expenditure, which today totals over $200 billion dollars a year, shifted the main burden of health insurance from the shoulders of the government (where Truman thought it belonged) to the backs of business (where the Eisenhower administration pushed it).

Social scientists call the result a shadow welfare state. Obscure government regulations (buried in the tax code) nudge private organizations (such as employers) to take over social welfare functions (most notably, health insurance). In the traditional welfare state, government offers benefits directly to the citizens—the Social Security approach, which remains the European model to this day. In the United States, government tries to achieve the same goals while operating in the shadows, inducing private institutions such as employers and insurance companies to provide social welfare benefits.[26] Of course, that's not the language that ushered in this innovation. In the great health insurance debates of the 1950s, the proponents simply tagged it *the American Way.*

Eisenhower thought the approach could be extended beyond full-time workers. Why not use government dollars to induce private insurance companies to cover the poor and the old? That, however, was pushing the shadow welfare state a bit too far for the Republicans of the 1950s. As Eisenhower had warned his party, in the next decade the Social Security model won the contest to cover the elderly (through Medicare), and the conservative Democratic variation, a welfare-style program, insured the poor (through Medicaid). These popular but shockingly expensive policies proved to be the crest of the Social Security model.

Richard Nixon—often invoking the brothers he lost to tuberculosis—fixed the public–private alternative firmly into place. As vice president (1953–61), he helped lead the Eisenhower administration's charge toward Republican-style insurance programs. As president (1969–74), he proposed national health insurance constructed around employers; government would simply fill in the gaps. The Nixon administration also introduced and popularized HMOs as a way to inject efficiency and cost control into American health care. Nixon himself always seemed as enthusiastic demolishing the Social Security approach—synonymous, in his mind, with Senator Ted Kennedy of Massachusetts—as he was about achieving his own reform. He was the first Republican president to accept the premise that all Americans should have health insurance, but he ridiculed the liberal folly of wrecking the entire private insurance system merely to cover the minority of Americans who lived without insurance. In this he succeeded. No administration—in fact, no presidential nominee from either party—would again propose national health insurance provided directly by the government.

Nixon's plan came close. Even as the Watergate scandal engulfed him, his administration negotiated furiously with the Democrats in an effort to win his national health insurance program. The chief Democratic staffer on Ways and Means would always recall the last gasp of the effort. He was standing in the urinal outside the conference room of the Ways and Means Committee on the day of the big vote. Chairman Wilbur Mills pulled up in the adjacent urinal, turned to his aide, and said, with a sigh, "Bill, we don't have the votes. Maybe next year." In fact, the committee approved the Nixon–Mills proposal by a 16–15 vote—the first time that the Committee on Ways and Means of the U.S. House of Representatives had ever approved a comprehensive health insurance program.[27]

The failed Nixon plan would become nothing less than the official Democratic policy wish. Every subsequent Democratic presidential nominee would offer variations of Richard Nixon's plan—filling in the gaps around employer-provided health insurance. Only two Democrats, Carter and Clinton, actually won the Oval Office in the thirty-four years after Nixon's administration fell in the summer of 1974. Each embraced national health insurance, each sponsored a variation of the Nixon plan, and each lavished as much attention on cost control and systems efficiency as on expanding health care coverage. When Barak Obama won the White House in 2008, his health plan offered another variation of the Nixon idea.

Why have Democrats wandered so far from their New Deal roots in Social Security? In part, they have been responding to the brute pressure of rising health care costs. In part, they have been handcuffed by economists' mental models and scoring algorithms. In part, they have been hamstrung by shifting political conditions. By the end of the Nixon administration, the New Deal and its coalition had vanished into history. A rising Republican era—signaled, perhaps, by California's Proposition 13 in 1978 (the start of the antitax rebellion) and solidified by Ronald Reagan's reelection landslide in 1984—rewrote American politics. Democrats now touted what had once been a Republican perspective. And the Republicans themselves moved on to a still more forceful embrace of individual choice and private markets.

## The Market Unleashed

Republicans finally shook off the New Deal and began to forge their own governing philosophy with the rise of Ronald Reagan in the 1980s.

There is a common view that they rode a backlash against the welfare state into power and have simply tried to slash all programs ever since. A close look at the presidents, as they grapple with health care, gives rise to a more subtle perspective. With time, the Republicans have aimed not merely to demolish social welfare benefits, but to reconstruct them so that they reflect essential Republican principles. This means withdrawing support for the Eisenhower and Nixon era compromises, which accepted a forceful role for government in promoting security— the ultimate New Deal goal. Instead, the rising Republicans believe in something entirely different: the power of individuals taking risks in an open market.

The first efforts, during the Reagan administration, were marked by enthusiastic pratfalls. David Stockman got the old man's blessing to carve billions out of Social Security—the "original sin" of big government—and watched the president's approval rating plunge 16 percentage points in the ensuing outcry. Conservative economists in the Cabinet had no better luck floating their health care voucher plan to head off Doc Bowen.

Over time, however, the advocates refined their promarket approach. They aimed to drag Medicare out of the Social Security mindset— according to which government simply doles out the payments to health providers. Their alternative, enthusiastically supported by George W. Bush, sought to force the old program into the new age of economic competition: beneficiaries would choose among different plans that—in good market fashion—prospered or perished by how well they served their customers. Thus President George W. Bush managed the single largest expansion in Medicare history, hoping to use the new benefits to win market reforms.

The same market logic pushes Republicans, such as President George W. Bush and Republican nominee John McCain, to try to repeal the Eisenhower tax break. Give individuals their own personal tax credits and let them go to market and make their own insurance purchases (with limits on the tax break so people don't spend too much on health insurance). From this perspective, the market will wring out the excesses that have so long bedeviled health care. The new Republican idea, encapsulated in the Bush concept of the "ownership society," envisions a world in which individuals take responsibility for all the critical choices that shape their fate, including the generosity of their health benefits and their retirement security. Government, and even private intermediaries such as employers, should get out of the way.

*Peering Ahead*

Today, health care policy offers quite a dramatic choice. Republicans strive—at least until the market meltdown of 2008, with great verve and self-confidence—to remake government programs, employer benefits, and personal health care options. They challenge the logic of shared risk and long-term security. Instead, they want to push us all into the competitive marketplace.

Democrats resist. They know what they oppose: the race toward markets, the destruction of social solidarity, the loss of shared risk. But what, exactly, are they for? Democrats have yet to coalesce around a clear alternative to the call for markets. If there is one irresistible lesson that emerges from the chapters that follow, it is this: no one can introduce a fresh vision like the person in the Oval Office.

Every president changes the conversation about health care in America. Presidents can snatch an idea—from interest groups, from advocates, from business leaders, from some faceless technocrat in a distant state—and inject it into the bloodstream of national debate. Some presidents manage to make minor adjustments to the way we think about the issue; others shift the entire paradigm. As we haunted the archives, we were often surprised to see which presidents made the greatest impact. But every one of them, from FDR to W., had some effect, whether large or small.

We follow the health care presidency across seventy years, from Franklin D. Roosevelt to George W. Bush. In each chapter, we investigate a major health policy episode in the context of the man, the times, and the administration. We pose the same questions about each administration: What are the secrets of success? What snares await the presidents as, inevitably, they confront this issue? The answers are embedded in every page that follows. We summarize the most important dos and don'ts—our recommendations for presidents pursuing health reform—in the final chapter.

But, most of all, we come away impressed with the drama: every president has a health story. Every president has felt the power of illness to inflict pain and suffering on those he loves. In the Oval Office, the presidents' personal health care experiences have become entangled with the great ideological and political currents of their times. And there, at the heart of power, health and politics mix, shaping the future of our health care system and of our nation itself.

# Franklin Delano Roosevelt

*The Enigmatic Angler*

After four ballots, the Democratic Party Convention of 1932 finally brushed aside Governor Al Smith and nominated Franklin Delano Roosevelt for president. Tradition dictated that a committee would travel—not too quickly—to New York and proffer the nomination to Governor Roosevelt. But with the country in the grip of the Great Depression, this nominee chose something more dramatic. As soon as the California delegation put him over the top, Roosevelt chartered a small trimotor airplane from American Airlines and made the rough nine-hour flight to the convention in Chicago, battling strong head winds all the way. He landed in the midst of a brawl between advisors about the speech that Columbia professor Samuel Rosenman had helped write for him. Serene and unflappable, Roosevelt took the hasty edits and electrified the convention—and the country. "This appearance before a National Convention," he told the delegates, "is unprecedented and unusual, but these are unprecedented and unusual times.... I broke traditions," he continued. "Let it be from now on the task of our party to break foolish traditions." And break tradition they did.[1]

More than eight months later, on Saturday March 4, 1933, Roosevelt took the oath of office. The entire banking system teetered on the edge of complete collapse—four thousand banks had already gone under. On Sunday, Roosevelt called Congress into extraordinary session. On Monday, he snatched up a World War I measure, the Trading with the Enemy Act, and used its (questionable) authority to shut the nation's banks. On Wednesday he held his first press conference and promised "delightful family conferences" without the old stuffiness or written questions—the press loved it and the transcript, even in that parlous moment, repeatedly notes *laughter*. On Thursday, the Emergency Banking Bill, which put all the resources of the Federal Reserve behind the nation's banks, flashed through a frightened Congress in eight hours—the president signed it forty-five minutes later before a phalanx of news cameras. On Sunday, FDR went on the radio and gave a warm, calm talk—the first Fireside Chat—explaining in plain language why the system had failed and what he had done to fix it. "Let me make clear that the banks will take care of all needs," he assured the nation, smoothly adding, "[I]t is my belief that hoarding during the past week has become an exceedingly unfashionable pasttime." When the banks opened the next day, a reassured nation poured its cash back into the institutions—$1.25 billion went back into American banks in March alone. The first 100 days of the Roosevelt administration had begun with a bang. The inspired, frantic, chaotic jumble of proclamations, programs, and public statements (stretching from March 9 to June 15, 1933) would become the unreachable star of every subsequent administration.[2]

In the pantheon of American presidents, Franklin Roosevelt ranks alongside George Washington and Abraham Lincoln. Each of these greats redefined the relationship between government and the people. Franklin Roosevelt described his own contribution as "a long overdue political and economic reconstruction" that took the Constitution's negative rights—government may not interfere with the people's rights to speak freely, practice religion, own guns, or enjoy equal protection under the laws—and appended positive economic rights. Government would now guarantee the people's basic economic needs. "Necessitous men," said Roosevelt in a speech, paying homage to Abraham Lincoln, "are not free men." The government must "benefit the great mass of our farmers, workers, and businessmen." His philosophy, Roosevelt would say at different times, could be summed up as "human security," "social justice," or—when talking to church groups—"Christianity." By the time Roosevelt was through, the government's role extended to protecting economic security. FDR repeatedly cast his innovation in the resonant tones of the American founding: the "four freedoms" and the new "economic bill of rights."[3]

Taking responsibility for the economy was part of an even larger political project. The presidency replaced the parties, the Congress, and the states at the heart of American politics. From now on, the person in the Oval Office would represent the people and their aspirations. In negotiating this change, Franklin Roosevelt birthed the modern presidency and transformed American government. Throughout his tempestuous thirteen years in the White House, he relished his role—perhaps more than any other president. Roosevelt had a love affair with power in that place, wrote political scientist Richard Neustadt: "It was an early romance and it lasted all his life."[4]

Beneath the great transformation of national government lay the famous multitude of New Deal promises and programs. None had a more curious passage through Roosevelt's three-plus terms than national health insurance—the New Deal's lost reform. Health care dropped out of the Social Security package (in 1935), almost became an issue in the 1938 midterm campaign, and seemed to gather momentum again in 1944, when Roosevelt tasked a trusted advisor—the same Samuel Rosenman who had drafted his dramatic acceptance speech twelve years earlier—to prepare a health plan and a strategy for winning it. But by the time the plan was ready, President Roosevelt had died. The elusive reform passed into Harry Truman's hands and, from him, down through the decades, tantalizing generation after generation of Democrats who would chase Roosevelt's great unfulfilled social policy.

It is an odd legacy. President Roosevelt not only failed to win health insurance but also barely tried. And therein lies one of the great mysteries in the history of American health care policy. At its center sits a man of extraordinary power and political skill, deeply familiar with illness. He was a president during extraordinary times, with extraordinary opportunities. But when it came to health care, Roosevelt always disappointed his liberal advisors and chose not to fight. Why did he keep ducking? Understanding those choices illuminates FDR's persona and administration, as well as the health care experiences of every modern president.

There are many metaphors for Roosevelt's management style, but the one that best captures his health care policies is that of the expert angler. Roosevelt loved to fish, and according to his Labor Secretary and admirer, Frances Perkins, he had an almost "childish vanity about his skill." Fishing was one sport that FDR could master with his powerful upper torso and atrophied legs. Early in his presidency, FDR took long cruises during which he would angle for big game in warm Caribbean waters.[5] (Once, when Roosevelt docked in Galveston, a young Congressman named Lyndon Johnson clambered aboard and charmed the president with a heavy load of bull about fishing and boating.) FDR's management style reflected his passion for fishing. He

skillfully let out many lines, pulling in some, lengthening others, constantly changing lures, sometimes sitting patiently, and always knowing
instinctively when to set the hook and when to cut bait. Naturally, all
the lines led right back to Roosevelt.

## MISTREATED AND OVERCHARGED

Roosevelt grew up gifted and charmed. He was handsome, wealthy, well
educated (Groton, Harvard, Columbia Law), well traveled (he always
had that vaguely European accent), and much fussed over, especially by
his mother. He also enjoyed the most famous family name in politics.
Franklin knew and admired his distant cousin, Theodore Roosevelt; he
adopted Theodore's pince-nez spectacles as well as his habit of calling
things "bully"—as in the "bully pulpit" that they would both so effectively stand on. In 1905, President Roosevelt became "Uncle Ted" when
Franklin married the president's niece, Eleanor Roosevelt.[6]

Franklin entered politics in 1910 and glided into a seat in the New
York state Senate. Three years later, when Democrat Woodrow Wilson
won the White House—thanks to a split in the Republican ranks between
President William Howard Taft and Uncle Ted—Franklin became assistant secretary of the Navy. He served until the end of the Wilson administration (with time out for a failed run for the U.S. Senate in 1914) and
became the Democratic nominee for vice president in 1920. He was only
thirty-eight years old when he ran with Governor James Cox of Ohio
and got thumped. The Republican candidate, Warren G. Harding, didn't
even bother to campaign—and crushed the Democrats, 16 million (and
404 electoral votes) to 9 million (and 127). But Franklin cut a fine figure
on the campaign trail and the political wreckage did not seem to mar
his own image. Franklin Roosevelt faced a bright, and apparently easy,
future.

### Polio

The following August, the charmed life came to a terrible end. While
the family was vacationing at its retreat on Campobello, an island off
Northern Maine, Franklin began to complain about feeling tired and
"logy." That did not change his robust exercise routine; Franklin and
two sons went sailing, leaped ashore to stamp out a brush fire, jogged to
a favorite swimming lake, jogged back, and plunged into the icy ocean
water. Franklin returned to the house, exhausted and chilled. By the

next morning, he felt sharp pains in one leg. Over the next three days, an acute paralysis spread over his entire lower body all the way up his chest. Roosevelt had contracted poliomyelitis—polio.[7]

Medical follies came next. The local GP arrived and declared the problem a heavy cold. As Roosevelt's condition deteriorated, family friends called up and down the Maine coast before locating Dr. W. W. Keen, a celebrated physician—now in his eighties—who had performed one of the most dramatic operations in presidential history when he removed a cancer from Grover Cleveland's upper mouth (secretly, on the presidential yacht) in 1893. Now Keen arrived, misdiagnosed a blood clot in the spinal column, later changing that misdiagnosis into another—an intractable spinal lesion—and charged the family the astounding sum of $8,000 for the less-than-helpful consultation.

Finally, the family located an expert in "infantile paralysis," Dr. Robert Lovett of Children's Hospital in Boston, to become Roosevelt's physician. Lovett gloomily insisted that there was nothing anyone could do to improve Franklin's muscular control, a judgment Roosevelt rejected. After that, Roosevelt directed his own rehabilitation with a vigorous exercise program. He grittily stuck to his routine and cheerfully minimized the problem. Almost everyone around him commented on his sheer determination. Eventually, Roosevelt bought and managed a hotel in Warm Springs, Georgia, where geothermal waters enabled him and other people with polio to exercise in a warm pool. "The water put me where I am," said Roosevelt, "[and] the water will bring me back."[8]

The hotel became the 1920s equivalent of a modern rehabilitation hospital, where FDR designed exercise regimens for the polio victims who flocked to the facility. He wrote a letter describing how he managed his own rehabilitation from polio and his observations on how to treat the effects of the illness, "judging from my own experience and that of hundreds of other cases which I have studied." It was published in the *Journal of the South Carolina Medical Association*. Roosevelt asked to present his work at a meeting of the American Orthopedic Association in 1926. When the Association refused, he and Eleanor crashed the meeting and secured a commitment from the orthopedists to evaluate the Warm Springs program. The association made good on its promise and confirmed the program's positive effects. Speaking to his fellow Warm Springs patients at a 1934 reunion in the White House, FDR said: "During that first year, I was doctor and physiotherapist rolled into one." Roosevelt's work at Warm Springs is now the province of an entire medical specialty called physiatry. No president has ever come closer to practicing medicine without a license than Franklin Delano Roosevelt did in the 1920s in rural Georgia.[9]

Frances Perkins claimed that the illness remade the man. "The pain and suffering had purged the slightly arrogant attitude" of the young Roosevelt. Now, she wrote, the "lack of humility" and "the streak of self righteousness" were replaced by a more serious, more warm-hearted, more deeply empathetic man. "He had a firmer grip on life and ... he had become conscious of other people, of weak people, of human frailty." Not everyone agreed with Perkins; Franklin's son James claimed that his father remained his father and would have been a great man, polio or no. But every observer was impressed at Roosevelt's courage, grit, and spirit in the face of the illness.[10]

### Political Comeback

Eleanor kept Franklin in the public eye—giving talks and meeting public officials. Although their marriage had foundered in 1918 when she discovered a stash of love letters between her husband and his elegant secretary, Lucy Mercer, Franklin and Eleanor stuck together and forged an extraordinary political partnership. In 1924, Franklin resumed his public role. He addressed the Democratic national convention and, in 1928, was elected governor of New York.

It was not easy for a man in a wheelchair to negotiate the political trail—especially in the 1920s, long before anything was "handicapped accessible." Franklin would arrive at the national convention and be lifted out of his car, dropped into a wheelchair, and wheeled down the service corridors of the convention hall. When he arrived near the stage, he would need help standing up, and someone would lock his stiff metal braces into place. Then, gripping his son James with one arm and his cane with the other, he would "walk" by swinging himself forward—always distracting observers with smiles, charm, and wit—until he reached a podium he could grip for support. He took some spectacular spills when his braces failed or a podium collapsed—but the falls never seemed to rattle him. Throughout, Roosevelt forbade any pictures of himself in a wheelchair or with his leg braces showing. The media conspired to keep the secret. Running for governor in 1928, FDR stopped just short of a brazen lie: "Seven years ago ... I came down with infant paralysis, a perfectly normal attack.... By personal good fortune, I was able to get the very best of care and the result of having the best of care is that today I am on my feet." On his feet, perhaps, but gripping the railing, the podium, or his son to keep from crashing down.[11]

As governor, Roosevelt took an immediate and strong interest in health care. In his first annual message to the legislature, he declared it "the duty of the state to give the same care to removing physical handicaps of its citizens that it now gives to their mental development." Restoring to health those "who have the misfortune to be crippled" was "as important in a modern state as universal education." He made the same comparison to the *New York Times:* "Public health ... is a responsibility of the state.... The state educates its children. Why not also keep them well?" He formed a special committee of citizens and experts to "study a new health program for the state" and then tangled with the legislature when it "absolutely declined to pass the bill." In 1931, speaking at a governors' conference, Roosevelt pointed to health insurance, along with a more progressive tax system and unemployment insurance, as part of the remedy for the growing economic crisis.[12]

Prepared by personal life to understand the consequences of illness, and by professional experience to understand its policy implications, FDR stepped into the White House with a brief but unparalleled freedom to act. But the story of President Roosevelt's health care policy is a story of baiting hook and encouraging supporters, then always pulling back.

### Health and Politics in the Oval Office

Did Roosevelt's illness sensitize him to the illness of others? Search as one might for evidence of this, very little emerges. He rarely spoke about health care during his presidency—only two speeches focused on it during his entire tenure. Indeed, FDR's public life after polio focused on denying his illness.

A second question turns on Roosevelt's reaction to the profession that so abused him. Physicians misdiagnosed, overbilled, discouraged, and rebuffed him. He pursued his vigorous and largely self-designed rehabilitation program in the face of naysaying physicians who told him, between 1921 and 1924, that medicine had nothing to offer him. Nor did he find the exercise specialists or their regimens particularly helpful. Roosevelt might easily have entered the Oval Office with a big chip on his shoulder where doctors were concerned. And yet, just the opposite seems to have been the case during most of his administration. He deferred to, flattered, and retreated before organized medicine. He seriously weighed the views of the few medical professionals to whom he turned for advice about health policy. On the other hand, Roosevelt constantly stirred his liberal advisors—renewing their hopes for a good brawl with organized medicine. His last word on the subject seemed to promise—yet again—a battle with the American Medical Association once World War II had been won.

Among the many enigmas that surround Franklin Delano Roosevelt, few are more intriguing than the relationship between his own illness and his health care politics. Perhaps the angler valued political mastery too much to be distracted by his personal traumas.

After meeting with the newly inaugurated Roosevelt in March 1932, the great retired Supreme Court justice, Oliver Wendell Holmes, then ninety-two, is said to have remarked of the fifty-year-old president: "A second-class intellect but a first-class temperament."[13] Whether Holmes was correct about the intellect (indeed, whether he was referring to Franklin Roosevelt instead of Teddy, who appointed him to the Supreme Court) is open to debate. But Holmes was right about FDR's tempera-ment—a constellation of personal attributes and styles that, according to some scholars, virtually defines the effective president.[14] Perhaps it was that first-class temperament that enabled Roosevelt to toss off his own hurts when he pondered health care policy.

## CREATIVE CHAOS: ROOSEVELT'S MANAGERIAL STYLE

Roosevelt was a complex man. He had few intimates but could inspire loyalty, affection, love and enmity from both close associates and distant masses. He drew intelligent people to him, used them for his purposes, and not infrequently tossed them overboard when he no longer needed them. Roosevelt was enormously persuasive—opponents sometimes emerged from sessions in the Oval Office lauding the man in the wheelchair with that signature cigarette holder. He was manipulative: fully capable of telling people (even the same person) diametrically opposite things at different times on the very same day; when confronted, he laughed off the contradictions. He could be vindictive: long before Richard Nixon took the heat for it, FDR used the Internal Revenue Service to harass his opponents.[15] He had extraordinary political intuitions and was the first great presidential communicator to speak directly to the public, thanks to the exciting medium that had developed in the previous decade—radio. Roosevelt touched individual citizens in a way that only John F. Kennedy and Ronald Reagan have equaled since.

Roosevelt's managed by controlled chaos—both within the White House and through the executive branch—always keeping things loose through misdirection, competition, and ad hoc processes. Future Democratic presidents would often try to emulate FDR's three-ring administrative circus—as he called it—but none pulled it off successfully. In part, this reflects the nature of the presidency when Roosevelt took office. The White House staff in 1932 consisted of four personal secretaries and one executive secretary; by the time he died, a formally organized Executive Office of the President had a staff of over 1,000. Today, it is closer to 2,000. It was easier to play the master of ceremonies with a staff of five than with a cast of thousands.[16]

And play the master of ceremonies he did. "He saw the job of being President as being FDR," commented Richard Neustadt. One way he kept control was by assigning multiple aides and groups the same task— and keeping them in the dark about one another. He once told his secretary of the treasury, Henry Morgenthau, "Never let your left hand know what your right hand is doing."[17]

Roosevelt used competition as a means of keeping himself informed and of pushing his aides. Assistants charged with some task would report what they had found, only to discover that FDR, having been briefed earlier by another capable assistant with the same assignment, knew everything the aide had to report—and more.[18] Roosevelt used the competition and confusion as a way to keep his options open, to discover different perspectives, and to keep everyone on their toes. He kept issues alive by commissioning studies, talking, arguing, listening, waiting, floating plans, changing direction, and finally deciding—"only," as Schlesinger put it, "at the long frazzled end."[19]

## FDR: THE TIMES

There was plenty of action to challenge FDR during his long presidency. The major events and trends are well known, but we recall a few points because they frame his health care presidency.

Roosevelt took office in March 1933 with one overwhelming task: saving the nation from economic collapse. His first year focused on the crisis and solidified the unlikely coalition of liberals, urban ethnics, African Americans, and southern segregationists that kept the Democrats in office for all but eight of the next thirty-five years. He began with his brilliant inaugural address, continued with radio broadcasts, and mastered the press with informal Oval Office press conferences twice a week. He was the first president to speak so directly to the American people, and he used his public support to threaten and cajole resistant congressmen (of whom there were many) into supporting his legislative program. Indeed, his inaugural address laid down a gauntlet, now largely forgotten: if Congress did not grant him the authority he needed, he would ask for "broad executive power to wage a war against the emergency, as great as the power that would be given to me if we were in fact invaded by a foreign foe."[20] At a time when Hitler had just become chancellor of Germany and Mussolini ruled Italy, the idea that desperate democracies might grant their leaders extraordinary powers did not seem far fetched. Roosevelt got his way and generated the famous frenzy of alphabet agencies and programs. "Take a method and try it," said the president. If it fails, try another. Above all, "try something."[21]

During its second year, the Roosevelt administration turned from immediate recovery efforts to long-term economic security. FDR sent one of his most trusted domestic policy aides, Harry Hopkins, to Europe in June 1934 to study the social security programs pioneered in Germany and the United Kingdom; at the same time—typically, Roosevelt wanted action in all three rings of his circus—he commissioned a new Committee on Economic Security (CES) to "explore thoroughly the possibilities of a unified social insurance system affording protection [against] all major personal hazards which lead to poverty and dependency."[22]

The CES plays a critical role in our story, for it offered FDR his best opportunity to address health care security during his first term, when his political influence was at its height.

In January 1935, the CES recommended the creation of what is now known as the Social Security Program, which FDR signed into law—after a considerable legislative battle—in August of that year. This 1935 achievement is in some ways the capstone of FDR's domestic presidency—and arguably the most important piece of social policy in the twentieth century. In November 1936 he was resoundingly reelected, carrying 46 states and 523 electoral votes.

But after 1936, the politics turned more difficult. The Supreme Court had begun overturning New Deal measures in 1935, and in response, Roosevelt proposed legislation expanding the size of the court (the constitution does not specify the number of justices) so that he could inject fresh (and sympathetic) blood. The legislation failed in 1938, although two members of the Court got the message and swung their votes. The

New Deal was safe from judicial review after that (a switch in time, quipped the political wags, saved nine). Roosevelt also tried to remake the legislature by "purging" conservative Democrats. That plan failed miserably, and in contrast to the court, the members who beat FDR's electoral threat felt no urge to back off from their confrontations. In the 1938 midterm election, the Democrats suffered serious legislative losses (inevitably, since their majority had been so lopsided —331 to 89 in the House). A new coalition of conservative southern Democrats and Republicans came to dominate the Congress. By the last two years of his second term, FDR was weakened at home and was turning his attentions toward the crisis in Europe—especially after Germany attacked Poland in September 1939.

Reelected in 1940, Roosevelt regained his dominance on the American political scene as a war president during the great conflict. His leadership secured reelection to a fourth term in 1944, but the war left him scant time, energy, or resources for domestic innovation. In 1944, as he began to contemplate the shape of postwar America, his health and energy were failing. Domestic advisors expected a great push for health reforms—inspired by the new programs in Great Britain—as part of the return to domestic politics. But in April 1945, less than a month before victory in Europe, Roosevelt died.

## SOCIAL SECURITY AND HEALTH (1934–1935)

The angler-in-chief trolled the troubled waters of health care coverage three times during his long presidency (although the issue occasionally broke the surface between these episodes). In the first two instances, which occurred in 1934–35 and 1936–39, FDR played with the idea of universal health insurance but never set the hook. The third time, in 1944–45, Roosevelt's early death leaves us uncertain about what he might have done to shape a postwar nation. This last turn to health care produced the plan that Roosevelt's advisors passed on to Harry Truman—FDR's most enduring and underappreciated health care legacy.

### The Committee on Economic Security

The Committee on Economic Security (or CES) may have offered the United States its best hope of achieving universal access to health insurance. Certainly, the political prospects have rarely seemed better: a powerful president with an ambitious reform agenda, an economically devastated nation, and lopsided Congressional margins of 219 in the House (322–103) and 44 in the Senate (69–25).

It may seem odd that FDR entrusted health care to a committee on *economic* security, whose focus and expertise lay elsewhere. President Bill Clinton had a health care task force of 500 that labored for months on health care alone. Other presidents have relied on domestic policy councils and on aides with deep health care expertise. Why the Committee on Economic Security?

This banal historical footnote illuminates FDR's attitude toward health care: in the early part of his administration, he regarded it as part of the economic challenge that confronted workers. Illness and its attendant costs were on a long a list of economic troubles —including money for retirement, disability, unemployment, and dependent children. One important advisor later explained that Roosevelt had an intuitive understanding of how Social Security would work, but no comparable feel for health care insurance.[23]

Right from the start, President Roosevelt established a pattern that he would maintain throughout his administration: he stirred the health care waters and watched to see what might surface—and despite plenty of hints and feints, he never committed himself.

The CES consisted of five Cabinet secretaries and delegated most of its work to a technical committee chaired by Perkins's deputy, the assistant secretary of labor Arthur J. Altmeyer; Altmeyer was a progressive from Wisconsin who powerfully shaped the administration's Social Security legislation. A colleague from Wisconsin, Edwin Witte, directed the staff. At a meeting in August 1934, Roosevelt charged the committee with finding ways to alleviate the economic plight of the American worker. He did not mention health care one way or the other. Witte came away with the impression that protection against the costs of illness was clearly within the CES mandate, though not as important as the other issues. Old-age pensions and unemployment insurance topped the list, but "hardly less important were deemed health insurance, public employment and relief." Anxious for more direction, Witte consulted with eight other senior administration officials but got no more insight into FDR's wishes. Witte later wrote that he never got any guidance from FDR on health care issues.[24] For his part, Altmeyer believed that "the President ... felt that unemployment insurance should have top priority," and that health insurance was third on the list, at best—not surprising in a nation where a quarter of the workforce was out of work.[25]

The CES formally announced its plans in September 1934 and suggested that it would consider a long list of programs: unemployment insurance, old age insurance, retirement annuities, family endowments, crop insurance, invalidity insurance, and health insurance. It also announced that one of its five technical subcommittees would tackle medical care. The mere mention of health insurance—much less an entire committee devoted to it—prompted a vigorous response from the ever-vigilant American Medical Association. It pushed Secretary Perkins to include physicians on any committee considering health care.[26] And the AMA also went directly to the top.

### The Profession Strikes Back

Organized medicine had two direct routes to the president: his personal physician, Ross McIntire (an ear, nose, and throat specialist who had been chosen for this responsibility because Roosevelt suffered from chronic sinus problems), and the eminent New England neurosurgeon, Dr. Harvey Cushing, whose daughter—whom one historian describes as "beautiful, vivacious and rich"—had married Eleanor and Franklin's son James (the first of four marriages for James). McIntire checked in on Roosevelt every morning at 8:30 while the president took breakfast in bed and every evening when he exercised his legs in the newly constructed White House pool. Dr. Cushing was one of the few people in the United States who continued to address Roosevelt not as "Mr. President" but as "Franklin." Cushing's correspondence with FDR before his death in 1939 is full of proud references to shared grandchildren, jocular exchanges about family events, and quotations from classical Roman historians.[27]

Both McIntire and Cushing gave FDR an earful of the AMA's strong opposition to any governmentally sponsored insurance. Harvey Cushing dismissed European social insurance programs—irrelevant to America—and warned Franklin not to force health insurance on American physicians[28]

Roosevelt made at least two decisions in response to the AMA's protests. First, he decided in the fall of 1934 to create a Medical Advisory Committee (MAC) to the Committee on Economic Security, and designated Dr. McIntire his liaison. Ross McIntire became Witte's chief link to FDR, and Witte vetted CES health initiatives with McIntire before moving forward with them. McIntire also became Roosevelt's link to the leadership of the AMA. Thus, an ENT physician chosen because of the president's sinus problems, with no policy credentials or training, became a key link between the president, his health care policy process, and organized medicine at one of the most critical moments in the history of the American health care system.

Roosevelt chose the members of the Medical Advisory Committee, which included leaders of organized medicine as well as his inlaw, Harvey Cushing. In a letter accepting the invitation to join the MAC, dated October 8, 1934, Cushing wrote Frances Perkins: "I am glad the Committee has thought of establishing such an advisory group, particularly since most of the agitation regarding the high cost of medical care has been voiced by public health officials and members of foundations most of whom do not have a medical degree, much less any first-hand experience with what the practice of medicine and the relation of doctor to patient means."[29]

In these views, Cushing voiced the suspicion of physicians through the ages that reformers were charging like bulls through medicine's china shop. In this case, his reference to "foundations" also reflects the fact that two CES staff members responsible for medical issues, Edgar Sydenstricker and Isidore Falk, came from the Milbank Fund, a New York philanthropy (still in existence) whose members advocated universal health care coverage.[30] Dr. Cushing found Mr. Sydenstricker especially irritating and eventually complained about him to Roosevelt.

The Committee on Economic Security was operating on a tight timeframe. FDR understood the importance of striking fast. He chartered the CES in June and asked for its report by December 1, 1934. Because it was not fully staffed until September 1, the CES had three months to design a national program of economic protection for working and elderly Americans. The decision to organize a Medical Advisory Committee inevitably pushed health care issues behind in the crowded queue at the Committee on Economic Security. The AMA bluster also discouraged Social Security advocates on the committee, who feared that the medical profession might delay or even kill the entire Social Security package. "It was my original belief," recalled Witte, "that it would probably be impossible to do anything about health insurance in a legislative way, due to the expected strong opposition of the medical profession. I found that this was also the view of Secretary Perkins and Dr. Altmeyer, whose primary interest was in unemployment insurance." Harry Hopkins, a member of the CES who grew so close to FDR that he eventually won the sobriquet of deputy president, was more interested in health insurance than in any other phase of social insurance, but he knew that this subject would have to be handled "very gingerly."[31]

The effects of delay and political controversy soon became clear. On November 13, Cushing lunched with FDR in the White House. The surgeon was in town for the first meeting of the Medical Advisory Committee, scheduled for November 15. Dr. Cushing complained about the strident advocacy for governmental "sickness insurance" among the MAC staff. Roosevelt reassured him that the administration would proceed slowly and give the medical profession plenty of time to study any proposals and weigh in with its opinion. He also promised to separate the health bill from the rest of the Social Security Program.[32]

Of course, FDR routinely said different things to different people. But not this time. The next day, November 14, Roosevelt addressed the National Conference on Economic Security. Drafts of his talk show that he penned most of the following words himself, inserting them into a draft written by Arthur Altmeyer: "There is also the problem of economic loss due to sickness—a very serious matter for many families with and without incomes, and therefore an unfair burden upon the medical profession. Whether we come to this form of insurance soon or later on I am confident that we can devise a system which will enhance and not hinder the remarkable progress which has been made and is being made in the practice of the professions of medicine and surgery in the United States."[33]

Roosevelt saw the problem but was making no commitments—all options were open, including indefinite delay. But when families could not afford health care, the burden fell on both the sick and the doctor (who would offer care without payment). FDR did make one promise that every health reformer would repeat for the next half century: no one would hinder the "remarkable progress" of the profession. It all certainly sounded deferential to the white coats.

### "Grand Times" and "Foul Means"

Advocates for health insurance on the CES and its staff continued to press for inclusion of health care coverage within the emerging social insurance package. In addition to Sydensticker and Falk, its chief proponents included Harry Hopkins, who had directed public health programs for FDR in the New York state government. Relieved by Roosevelt's words, the AMA became less truculent during the next two months, which led Witte to muse briefly that it might still be possible to work out a health insurance plan that the Medical Advisory Committee and AMA would support.[34]

But advocates ran up against the caution of other senior aides, including Perkins, Altmeyer, and Witte himself.[35] Eleanor Roosevelt was also said to have concerns about the effect of sickness insurance on the quality of medical care.[36] And now FDR had clearly indicated his own intention to delay. At a final decisive meeting at Perkins's home on December 23, 1934, the leaders of the CES, approved a final report that included recommendations for increased expenditures on public health measures, but none on health insurance. FDR accepted the report the next day.

On January 6, 1935, Cushing sent Roosevelt a handwritten "Dear Franklin" note, thanking him for a Christmas box of preserved fruit, gushing that "the children had a grand time at the White House parties," and then going on to praise FDR's decision to hold off on health insurance: "I'm glad you did not stress immediate sickness insurance—though friend Witte seems to be doing so. We need more time, and more local experiments with the various plans proposed if the backing of the profession is to be secured. This will be necessary for the success of any plan though public health officials backed by the Milbank Fund don't seem quite to realize this."[37]

Roosevelt, however, had not pulled in all his lines. Perhaps an agreement with the AMA could be worked out. They had been relatively quiet since his November 14 talk, so he granted the Committee on Economic Security a three-month extension to consider health insurance. The January report included language suggesting that the committee would make recommendations regarding coverage at a later time.[38]

The AMA responded with a roar. At an emergency meeting of its House of Delegates in February, it made a tactical change designed to unify opposition to any CES intimations of government health care. It accepted the idea of voluntary health insurance coverage (which it had previously opposed) as long as it remained in the hands of the medical societies (the Blue Cross and Blue Shield Plans); it also supported the increased expenditures for public health activities that were part of the original CES report. These moves were enough to bring several wayward medical groups, including the American College of Surgeons, which had supported government health insurance, back into the medical fold.[39]

The AMA generated a storm of protesting letters, telegrams and editorials criticizing the president. FDR's personal files from the period contain newspaper clippings reporting the ferocious attacks. A rather plaintive memo from Steven Early, one of FDR's personal secretaries, to Ross McIntire on January 21, 1935, cried foul: "Dear Doc: I wonder if there is an indirect method of reaching the responsible officers of the American Medical Association and advising them that the editor of their journal is resorting to foul means of attacking the President of the United States."[40]

In Congress, which had by then received the president's Economic Security Program, members of the House Ways and Means Committee announced that they would not even hold hearings on any package that contained a health insurance program—or even a mention of further studies of a health insurance program. The White House gave back-channel approval to cut any mention.[41] The entire economic program faced tough going, especially in the Ways and Means Committee. Many Republicans opposed the measure, and southern Democrats fretted about the implications for segregation. Senator Thomas Gore peered at Secretary Frances Perkins during Senate hearings and mocked, "Isn't this a teeny-weeny bit of socialism?"[42]

Meanwhile, populist Huey Long thundered on the left with something that was more than a teeny bit like socialism: a 100 percent tax rate on any income over $1 million and on any estate over $8 million, all redistributed to the common folk—making, in his words, "every man a king." A California physician named Francis Townsend advocated another popular scheme: pay everyone over sixty years old a monthly stipend with just one condition—they had to spend every penny. Long and Townsend could be heard in the background as the administration and Congress negotiated the far more moderate Social Security package.[43]

## The Debate Goes On

Within the Committee on Economic Security and its Medical Advisory Commission, the debate over health insurance continued. Cushing clashed heatedly with Sydenstricker. In March, Stydenstricker and Falk proposed a package that, according to Witte, seemed to gain some traction with CES members. In a striking preview of proposals gaining favor in many states today, the two CES staff proposed levying a tax on employers to support federally approved state health insurance programs for the non-poor and drawing funds from general revenues to support state-run health insurance programs for low-income Americans. This proposal could be piggybacked on the Economic Security Program making its bumpy way through Congress.

Witte was concerned that this plan could jeopardize the entire economic program. "At this stage, I indirectly consulted the President,
through Dr. McIntire," he wrote, "and was advised that it was his view
that it would be very unwise to throw health insurance into the hopper
while the rest of the program was still before Congress. I then strongly
urged that the committee ... [consult] the President in advance of any
filing of any formal recommendations."[44]

Perkins and Josephine Roche, assistant secretary of the treasury and
a member of the CES technical committee, duly trooped over to the
White House, where FDR responded with his special brand of ambigu-
ity: the committee could "file a report in favor of compulsory health
insurance which the committee had in mind," but he himself would
"decide what should be done with it."[45] The CES obediently delivered
its final recommendations on June 1, 1935. In a side letter accompanying the report, Perkins wrote FDR: "In view of the controversial character of certain phases of the subject, I suggest the report not be made
public until the Social Security Bill, now pending before the Congress,
has been enacted into law."[46]

On July 1, 1935, FDR received a letter from his childhood friend
and Hyde Park neighbor Gerald Morgan, who had written a book on
social insurance. Referring to a previous conversation with FDR about
the opposition of the AMA to health insurance, Morgan proposed providing Americans cash benefits with which they could purchase health
care—another idea that would return, generations later, as health care
vouchers.[47]

On July 26, 1935, FDR replied: "Dear Gerald: Many thanks for your
note. Your suggestion is one way out which may be the best we can do.
However, I doubt if this highly controversial subject will come up even
at the next session of Congress. The latter is exhausted by my suggestions! Love to Mary and boys, Affectionately."[48] The Social Security
Bill was signed into law on August 14, 1935. The CES report on health
insurance—which never saw the light of day—did release one residual
spore that might just have bloomed into something big. The Social Security Act contained a little-noticed clause giving its governing commission,
the Social Security Board, the charge to study new ways to provide health
insurance to Americans and to report back to Congress on the subject.
Altmeyer dismissed this mandate. The Social Security Board was busy
and the AMA aroused. "If the President had indicated that he wanted
to press for a health insurance program, there is no doubt that the Social
Security Board would have given the subject more attention."[49]

In the event, FDR met with Perkins in September 1935 and informed her that he wanted the Social Security Board to take no action on health insurance until after the 1936 election at the earliest.[50] At the same time—here's that characteristic misdirection again—Roosevelt had the CES report forwarded to the Social Security Board in January 1936 with the instruction that the board undertake "further research" on health insurance. As always, Roosevelt sent different instructions in different directions while keeping his own options open.[51]

The election campaign further clarified Roosevelt's public views on universal health care coverage—at least for the time being. Campaigning in New Jersey on October 2, 1936, Roosevelt spoke at the dedication of a new medical center in Jersey City. He faced a swelling volume of inquiries from physicians and journalists on his attitudes toward what the doctors called "socialized medicine." Roosevelt put all those nettlesome questions to rest.

> Let me tell you with great sincerity of the great praise which is due to the Doctors and the Nurses of the Nation for all they have done during those difficult years that lie behind us, often at great sacrifice.... And these professions can rest assured that the Federal Administration contemplates action only in their interest. I mention, just in passing, the splendid Social Security Act recently enacted by the Congress. That action taken in the field of health is clear.... For that Act ... contains four provisions that are very often forgotten, especially in the heat of a political campaign. Those four provisions have to do with health, and those provisions received the support of outstanding Doctors during the hearings before the Congress.... This in itself assures the Nation that the health plans will be carried out in a manner compatible with our traditional social and political institutions.... Let me add that the Act contains every precaution for insuring the support and cooperation of the Medical and Nursing profession.... The overwhelming majority of the Doctors of the Nation want medicine kept out of politics. On occasions in the past attempts have been made to put medicine into politics. Such attempts have always failed and always will fail.[52]

Not surprisingly, the president's talk—one of the only speeches he would make during his presidency that was devoted entirely to health care—received thunderous applause from the AMA, which printed a glowing editorial about the speech in the *Journal of the American Medical Association.*

The political usefulness of the speech became clear immediately. On October 7, 1936, reacting to a letter from Dr. L. D. Redway, the chairman of the Public Relations Committee of the Medical Society of the County of Westchester, Stephen Early, sent a note to McIntire:

"Doctor McIntire: Here is the Westchester letter with a copy of the Jersey City address.... Do you want to fix up an answer for us—or shall we do it?" McIntire replied in handwriting: "Suggest you write a letter quoting paragraph marked # and stating this should be an answer to anyone for no legislation is contemplated."[53]

Indeed, for the rest of Roosevelt's presidency, whenever he received an inquiry from physicians about his attitude toward "socialized medicine," "state medicine," or any similar hot-button term, his staff would reply by citing the 1936 assurance that physicians "can rest assured that the Federal Administration contemplates action only in their interest." Certainly, this meant the end of universal health insurance under Roosevelt's tenure in the Oval Office—at least for now.

## AMAZING PUBLIC SUPPORT—TECHNICIANS
## WORKING WITH ALL SPEED: 1937–1940

In a Roosevelt presidency nothing was ever quite as it appeared. This was a president who kept his options open. And so he let the issue of health insurance stay alive but deep beneath the surface, with no presidential commitment to bringing it into view. The result was a second go-around on universal coverage that, even as the CES initiative was fading, started to rise under the auspices of an entity with the numbingly bureaucratic title of the Interdepartmental Committee to Coordinate Health and Welfare Activities.

The Interdepartmental Committee's health care initiative had its origin, somewhat improbably, in a letter from Cushing to Roosevelt written on November 10, 1934, as the neurosurgeon was preparing to leave New Haven for Washington to lunch with the president. The letter contained a suggestion that seemed intended to rescue (or divert) the MAC from an anticipated clash over sickness insurance: "Before Mr. Witte's Medical Advisory Committee gets deep in this tangled subject [of sickness insurance], would it not be a good move just at this time to take into consideration the establishment—if not of a governmental department—at least of a super-bureau of public health to coordinate a number of welfare agencies? ... There will be difficulties about such a concentration, but you are accustomed to overcoming difficulties, and such a favourable opportunity as the present may not occur again."[54]

As he wrote back on November 13—and probably told Cushing at lunch the same day—Roosevelt said that he liked the idea but doubted that the time was wholly ripe. "The difficulty," said the rueful bureaucrat in chief, is that "shuffling bureaus between existing departments raises much ruction." However, he forwarded the letter to Perkins the same day, asking whether they should "set up an interdepartmental committee of coordination of the existing health and welfare activities."[55] Perkins replied dutifully that she would discuss the matter with her colleagues, but it was not until May 2, 1935, that she responded: there was no need for a "super-bureau" of the type Cushing suggested, but it would be useful to have a committee coordinating federal health and welfare agencies. The committee should consist of "technically trained persons, to study and make recommendations concerning specific aspects of the government's health activities." Wary, like FDR, of provoking physicians, Perkins added that the committee would "recognize professional interests."[56]

In a first rush of enthusiasm, Roosevelt scribbled on Perkins's memo: "I hope you will issue this at once."[57] But then he thought better of throwing another issue—however tangential—into the Social Security maelstrom. On May 8, he wrote Perkins more formally: "I think this is a good idea to be developed during the summer (read: once Social Security is safely home). Will you let me have the kind of endorsement which I can send to the other Departments?"[58] When Perkins responded, Roosevelt told her to wait until after the signing of the Social Security Act.[59] The day after the Social Security Bill was signed, Perkins nudged Roosevelt, who issued an order creating the Interdepartmental Committee.

That presidential statement—Roosevelt edited it himself—implied that the committee's activities would consist chiefly of bureaucratic housekeeping, including "a complete coordination of the government's activities in the health field."[60] But the committee soon emerged as something very different. It became a haven for advocates of comprehensive health insurance, who, with FDR's apparent acquiescence, used it to push the coverage issue back onto the national agenda.

The committee was chaired by Josephine Roche, a strong advocate of universal insurance. Roche, Altmeyer, and national health insurance advocates drew a now-familiar lesson: national health insurance had gone down in 1934–35 because the public did not support or understand it. Without a strong campaign to mobilize support for the policy, most Americans did not see it as a social problem. The Interdepartmental Committee set out to awaken the public to what its members thought was a national health care crisis.[61]

External events assisted them. As the economic condition of the country improved, the residual threat associated with uncovered medical expenses became clearer, and a number of private groups organized to press for universal coverage. The first national survey of American health care, conducted in 1935–36, found large gaps between the rich and poor in terms of their access to basic medical services.[62] National public opinion polls began including questions on health care, revealing (as they so often did in subsequent decades) popular support for government assistance with the costs of paying for medical services.[63] Inevitably, when it came down to specific policies, differences of opinion emerged. Perhaps intrigued by this evolving political climate, FDR's thoughts seem to have turned back to health care coverage, especially for the poor. The successful implementation of Social Security and his landslide reelection in November 1936 may have convinced him that he could start trolling for new social initiatives. On January 21, 1937, he received an invitation from the AMA to address its annual meeting the coming June. In his February 3 reply declining the offer, he abandoned the elaborate deference he had shown organized medicine in past communications and instead threw out a modest challenge: "As you remember in my [second] Inaugural Address, I stated that one-third of the people in our country are lacking in the bare necessities of life.... I might have added that this one-third of our people is unable to secure adequate medical and hospital care. It would seem to me that there is no better time for the American Medical Association to give careful consideration to this vital problem. I assure you in this connection that the Federal Government will welcome the cooperation of the American Medical Association and will be glad to receive any suggestions which the Association may make."[64]

Concurrently, Altmeyer and Roche suggested to FDR doing another survey of the health needs of Americans, which he approved.[65] Roosevelt also approved, in March 1937, the chartering of the Technical Committee on Medical Care under the aegis of the interdepartmental body to conduct the survey and make recommendations based on its findings. Isidore Falk, who had been one of the key drafters of the CES report on compulsory health insurance (and one of the Milbank liberals who had so gotten under Dr. Cushing's skin) joined the Technical Committee.

In the summer of 1937, a few key senior administration officials—including Roche, Altmeyer, Hopkins, and Surgeon General Thomas Parran (a former Roosevelt aide from the New York state government days)—met at the Brookings Institution and decided the time was right to formulate a National Health Program. They charged the Technical Committee with the task.[66] Health care was stirring again.

The president, however, still did not relish head-on confrontation with organized medicine. After his mildly provocative letter of February 1937, he and his staff expended enormous energy on avoiding an almost comical collision with the AMA. Senator James Hamilton Lewis (D-IL)—a colorful, spats-wearing member of the Democratic leadership known as "Pink-Whiskers"—went before the AMA annual meeting in early June, gave them the president's regards and then lobbed a bomb: if doctors did not rise to the challenge of addressing the health care needs of the indigent, the government would take over the health care system, and that doctors might then be treated as though they were "an office of the army." Lewis insinuated that he was speaking for FDR—some press accounts have him flatly saying so—and the AMA leadership quickly wrote the president on June 10, agreeing to cooperate with the administration in getting care to the indigent but pointedly asked him to clarify his views on the subject of government-run medicine. FDR referred the letter to one of his secretaries, Marvin McIntyre, who in turn wrote a sheepish, "strictly personal" letter to Lewis asking for his help in making the issue go away: "[I find myself] in a bit of an embarrassing situation with respect to a letter from the American Medical Association to the President.... I do not see how I can properly acknowledge it without committing the President definitely to statements made by you to the Association. As a matter of fact, I do not know just exactly what you said to the Association and, as you know, the whole subject is rather a delicate one.... Would it, in your opinion, be all right if I just let the matter slide." *Time,* a distinctly Republican publication in this era, heated up the matter with a cover story on June 21, 1937, entitled "Nationalized Doctors." The very first sentence told the sensational story: "Only a handful of the 9,200 Doctors who attended the convention of the American Medical Association last week ... knew before hand that President Roosevelt had been discussing a plan to federalize their entire profession."[67]

In reply to *Time,* Lewis made it clear that he was not going to help FDR with this problem—he cheered the American Medical Association for "expressing their desire to ... cooperate with the president ... in serving with medicine and hospitalization [of] the poor and those unable to protect themselves." He made more mischief by telling the AMA leaders that they would be hearing shortly from the president—and then decamped to Europe, where he ignored repeated entreaties from both FDR's staff and the AMA. The matter dragged on into the fall and the winter, with Lewis stoutly refusing to help get Roosevelt off the hook onto which he had stuck him.[68] The president was exquisitely sensitive to any public perception that he supported compulsory health insurance, any state intrusion on the prerogatives of physicians, or any open conflict with the nation's doctors. And yet, there was the issue—promoted by a member of the Senate leadership and blaring from the cover of *Time*.

The White House could not control Lewis. But it did allow the potentially explosive work of the Technical Committee to proceed—albeit always under Roosevelt's cautious control. On February 11, 1938, Josephine Roche sent the Technical Committee's final report to the president. Noting that the report had been unanimously adopted by the Technical Committee, she gushed, "The Interdepartmental Committee feels that this report and its recommendations are the most important result of its three years of work ... because it represents the first complete agreement as to method and program for meeting health needs ever reached by all the Federal agencies working in health and welfare fields." She then asked permission to call a conference of "interested groups" to discuss the document in the near future.[69] The conference was part of the committee's strategy to make health care issues more visible, attracting public support.

The program set out by the report contained five major elements, which would be repeated by health insurance bills for the next decade. It included expansions of the maternal and child health program, federal grants for hospital construction, grants to the states to pay for the medical care of the "medically indigent" (those too poor to pay medical bills), a voluntary program of grants to states that wanted to set up statewide health insurance programs for the general public, and a disability program. Some members of the committee argued against creating separate programs for the indigent and the rest of the population. They feared that Congress would address the problem of the poor and take pressure off health insurance for everyone else.[70] This concern would prove justified, both in 1938 and in the years ahead, when programs such as Medicare and Medicaid would extend coverage to the most needy—and sap support from more comprehensive health insurance legislation.

Three days later, in a meeting with Roche and Altmeyer, FDR sanctioned the release of the report and approved the idea of the national conference. When the report hit the press in late February, it attracted widespread attention, including prominent coverage in the *New York Times* that emphasized data on the burden of illness afflicting the Americans, the unmet costs of care, and the need for programs to address these issues. At the same time, the president cagily instructed Roche to schedule the meeting for June 1938—after Congress had adjourned—and suggested that it be announced by Roche's office, not the White House. In other words, he encouraged the project—nudging it along at every step of the way—while keeping a safe distance from it himself.[71]

In the meantime, Eleanor Roosevelt had changed her views on health insurance. In June 1938, she encouraged a gathering of 4-H club members to try "socialized medicine" in their communities. "Don't hang back from new things," she told a group of rural boys and girls, according to the *Washington Post*.[72]

On July 17, 1938, the Interdepartmental Committee for the Coordination of Health and Welfare Activities (evidently unburdened by its numbing and now anachronistic title) convened a three-day National Health Conference that was attended by a wide array of groups—ranging from organized medicine to labor unions and agriculture interests. The conference enthusiastically cheered the Technical Committee's National Health Program.[73] The president, however, did not attend. He was fishing aboard the Navy cruiser USS *Houston*—and in the middle of a fateful voyage with lasting implications for health reform.

The conference was the high point of this second New Deal venture into health care reform. On July 23, Roche eagerly telegrammed the president: "CANNOT RESIST SENDING YOU WORD AMAZING PUBLIC SUPPORT AT NATIONAL HEALTH CONFERENCE FOR NATIONAL HEALTH PROGRAM. AND [SIC] WHICH IS MOUNTING DAILY AS EVIDENCED BY PRESS COMMENT TELEGRAMS, AND LETTERS. OUR TECHNICIANS ARE WORKING WITH ALL SPEED TO DEVELOP SPECIFIC PROPOSALS WHICH WE EXPECT TO HAVE READY FOR YOU ON YOUR RETURN. MEANWHILE WE ARE FOLLOWING YOUR INSTRUCTIONS TO MAKE NO PUBLIC COMMITMENTS AS TO FUTURE PROGRAM."[74]

Another telegram from one of Roosevelt's secretaries reached the *Houston* about the same time. This one reported that the AMA's president had pledged "QUOTE WHOLEHEARTED COOPERATION IN ANY EFFORTS WHICH YOU MAKE FOR BETTERMENT IN THE HEALTH CARE OF THE PEOPLE OF THIS COUNTRY UNQUOTE," and went on to note that this was a "WELCOME SURPRISE BECAUSE CONFERENCE EXPECTED DETERMINED OPPOSITON FROM MEDICAL ASSOCIATION."[75] The AMA had decided on a new strategy of give-and-take instead of outright opposition.[76]

The advocates of universal coverage were now in full-throated charge, so confident that they turned down an offer from the AMA leadership to embrace the other four elements of the national program (including state programs to support care of the indigent) if the administration would abandon the proposal to create state-based health insurance programs.[77]

President Roosevelt had his hands full in the summer of 1938. Although he enjoyed enormous majorities in both the House (where Democrats outnumbered Republicans almost 4–1) and Senate (almost 5–1), the conservative Democrats—especially from the South—had turned decisively against the New Deal. In July, just before the national health conference, FDR took to the hustings and crossed the country trying to knock off some of the conservative members of his own party. In August, after the month-long recreational cruise from California to Florida on the USS *Houston*, he picked up the campaign again in the South. In Georgia, which he considered a second home thanks to the spa at Warm Springs, Roosevelt took on the courtly, mild-mannered, and formidable (not to mention formidably conservative) Senator Walter George.

The whole effort was a bust. Senator George and most of the other conservative Democrats easily won reelection. Although the Democrats still held a big majority (ninety-seven seats in the House), a coalition of southern Democrats and northern Republicans would now block New Deal reforms. And there was still another problem in the electoral wreck: Two years after beating back the Roosevelt challenge, Walter George took the gavel of the powerful Senate Finance Committee. The "amazing public support" stirred up by the health care conference had advocates all excited. But if and when FDR decided to go for national health insurance, he would have to figure out a way to get it through Walter George's committee. And in this era, committee chairmen were not easy to get around. The national health insurance debates would continue—but the Congressional politics would be out of joint for the rest of the Roosevelt administration—and beyond.

Meeting with Roche and Altmeyer on return from his cruise and campaign swing, FDR found their enthusiasm briefly infectious. Altmeyer later recalled: "He was so impressed that I remember very distinctly. He said: 'We'll make this an issue this fall in the campaign.'" But then, he immediately reversed course. "No," Altmeyer recalled him saying in his next breath, "I think it would be better to wait for a presidential year."[78]

FDR then began pulling the rug out from under the health care reform movement—perhaps simply calculating the legislative odds. In

September 1938, the AMA, which had been steadily strengthening its Washington presence, issued a statement expressing its opposition to any form of governmentally sponsored insurance. That same month, the president instructed Roche, Altmeyer, and the Technical Committee to take no further action with regard to the National Health Program.[79] Perhaps in response to this directive, on October 12, 1938, the committee sent the president a long, unsigned memorandum, drafted, presumably by Roche: "Following the National Health Conference, the recent recommendations of the Technical Committee ... have become of such potential importance as a basis for development of a national health program that I am prompted to present [them] to you in brief review."

The memo went on to recount in detail the response to the July conference, the committee's consultation with all the major interest groups, and the agreement during the conference itself on the need for a "well integrated health program." The memo continued that "the influence of the conference has already found expression in numerous significant developments," noting that the AMA in a recent meeting of its House of Delegates had "endorsed the principles included in the Committee's recommendations of expansion of public health and hospital facilities, medical care for the medically needy and disability insurance." Although the memo pointedly omitted discussion of the AMA's reaction to the idea of state/federal program of health insurance, it contended that the states were actively discussing the issue.[80] But by now, the midterm election results were in. In November 1938, FDR told Roche and Altmeyer at another White House meeting that he would forward the committee's report to the Congress with a message saying only that it merited further study.[81] Another memo followed from the committee on December 15, 1938, contending that "[i]n ... recent discussions, the committee has been impressed anew with the general recognition of the need for a national health program and the unquestioning assumption that action will be taken." The memo laid out the five-point program for the president's review still one more time.[82]

Roosevelt did not evidently share this "unquestioning assumption" about further action. He repeated his decision to forward the report to the Congress with no endorsement and instructed Roche, Altmeyer, and the committee to place no pressure on legislators to consider it.[83]

On January 23, 1939, the president sent the Interdepartmental Committee's report to Capitol Hill as part of a presidential health message, with no recommendation for action. At this point, the *New York Times* could already see the handwriting on the wall: "Mr. Roosevelt's health program has been caught in a legislative draft.... The chill imposed upon it will undoubtedly give it a cold which will incapacitate it for this session of Congress—and possibly permanently."[84]

Senator Robert Wagner (D-NY), dutifully announced that he would introduce legislation containing the report's main recommendation, which he did on February 28, 1939. Altmeyer contends that he personally arranged with Wagner to develop the legislation[85] (perhaps the wily Roosevelt had approved Wagner's action, keeping the issue alive but free of presidential fingerprints).

When hearings were held on Wagner's bill the following April before the Senate Committee on Education and Labor, the American Medical Association opposed it in its entirety, backing away from its previous endorsement of sections of the National Health Program. The Public Health Service also opposed some of its public health provisions, revealing a brewing turf war within the administration's own health care bureaucracy. Without backing from the administration, the legislation died in committee.[86]

On September 1, 1939, the world changed. Germany invaded Poland, and France and Britain responded with declarations of war against the Third Reich. The president's attention turned from domestic programs to defense and industrial mobilization for war. In mid-December, however, he acceded to a request from his surgeon general and former New York state health director, Dr. Thomas Parran, to support a program of hospital construction in poor communities.[87] The proposal would cost only $50 million a year rather than the hundreds of millions required for the Interdepartmental Committee's full program. (Anticipated defense expenditures by then constricted budgetary options.) It would make the Public Health Service and some advocates of health care programs happy. And, by covering only the costs of construction (not of operation), it avoided even the appearance of governmental support for health services, thus avoiding a fight with the doctors. Hospital construction offered the president a dignified exit from troubled health care arena—for now.[88]

The president told Altmeyer and Roche about this decision when they met again with FDR in late December to discuss what to do about the failing National Health Program. "He said," Altmeyer recounted, "he wanted to have only a hospital construction bill, which indicated that he had changed his mind about making a national health program an issue in the 1940 presidential campaign."[89] Hoping to push the president, however gingerly, toward more aggressive health care action, the

Interdepartmental Committee voted on January 9, 1940, to recommend that the hospital program not only include funds for maintenance of the newly constructed hospitals but also support the building of outpatient diagnostic centers. The AMA and the American Hospital Association promptly opposed the idea, and the president rejected the recommendation on January 10. The committee requested a meeting with the president. At the January 16 gathering, the president gave his obstreperous health care reformers more bad news: not only would there be no maintenance funds and no diagnostic centers, but he was also reducing their request for construction funds from $50 million to $10 million. He told them that Dr. Parran would administer the program.[90] Hirschfeld contends that early on in the evolution of the National Health Program the Public Health Service and the Maternal and Child Health Bureau had bolted. Rather than support the reformers' five-part program, the bureaucrats in these agencies fought to preserve their own programs. Parran, a Roosevelt intimate, had succeeded in protecting what his agency cared about: hospital construction.

Ever the master of spin, the president showed the value of keeping some glimmer the National Health Program alive when he replied on January 17, 1940, to a letter from Mary Dublin, secretary of the National Consumers League, inquiring about the president's health care plans. Roosevelt answered that his proposed hospital construction program "may be considered at least a beginning toward strengthening and increasing the health security of the Nation."[91] Roosevelt was, after all, running for reelection in November 1940, and he could not ignore the liberals in his New Deal coalition.

On January 30, 1940, the president forwarded legislation to Congress proposing $10 million dollars for hospital construction in poor communities. Patronizingly dubbed the "Forty Little Hospitals Bill," the legislation passed the Senate but died in the House. Roosevelt's second battle for national health insurance ended not with a bang, but a whimper. But by now the president and much of America were watching Europe to see what the Nazis would do now that they had conquered Poland.

FROM CRADLE TO GRAVE?

Universal health coverage disappeared from the public agenda during America's struggle with fascism. Nevertheless, the Social Security Board kept the issue warm behind the scenes. The board's authorizing legislation gave it a mandate to study the issue; and the board was home to advocates of health care coverage, including I. S. Falk and the irrepressible Wilbur Cohen, a social insurance expert who would have an enduring imprint on national health policy. Eventually, Washington insiders would quip that a health expert was someone who had Wilbur Cohen's phone number.

Starting in 1939, the annual reports of the board began discussing health issues, and in 1942 it endorsed comprehensive health and social welfare insurance for all Americans.[92] In 1943, as the tide of war began turning toward the allies, the British published the Beveridge report, a comprehensive social welfare plan for postwar Britain that included health insurance. The Beveridge plan famously called for social insurance "from cradle to grave"—a phrase Roosevelt insisted that he himself had coined. "Why does Beveridge get his name on this?" he joked to Frances Perkins. "[I]t's not the Beveridge plan, it is the Roosevelt plan." Roosevelt was not entirely joking: he began to turn back to the idea of comprehensive health insurance.[93]

In his January 1943 State of the Union address, FDR reflected on postwar American society. He took back his tag line and called for social insurance that would extend from "cradle to grave."[94]

Public support was also increasing. The labor movement began to seriously engage the issue of comprehensive health care coverage. Polls showed growing public support for governmental health care coverage.[95] And it was now clear that the Supreme Court would not strike down the administration's progressive legislation. On June 3, 1943, Senators Robert Wagner and James E. Murray (D-MT) and Representative John Dingell (D-MI) introduced the Wagner–Murray–Dingell Bill—a national health plan that would be placed in the Congressional hopper, in one form or another, for at least the next decade. The bill left the old National Health Program behind and advocated comprehensive national health coverage for all Americans, financed by employer and employee contributions.

When Cohen and Falk, who wrote the bill, went to brief Senator Wagner he listened politely for five minutes and gave his okay. He didn't need to worry over details—the bill wasn't going to pass. This would just put the issue on the table.[96] The *New York Daily News* underscored the point: "It looks to us in this instance as if Senators Wagner and Murray have been sold a bale of extremely dangerous goods by some fanatic or others. It is to be hoped that Congress will scrutinize this bill from the ground up before it lifts a finger toward passing it or anything like it."[97]

Nothing was going to happen until the president put his shoulder to the wheel and pushed. The liberals around Roosevelt kept urging and hoping. Secretary of the Treasury Henry Morgenthau decided in mid-1943 that his department would propose an expansion of Social Security to cover health care. Sir William Beveridge, who had designed the newly proposed British system, made a successful American speaking tour in May 1943. The social reformers from the two sides of the Atlantic engaged one another. In what might have been seen as a prophetic exchange, Beveridge found his English tweeds too heavy for the American weather and borrowed clothes from Arthur Altmeyer, the chair of the Social Security Board. Their ideas about social insurance, thought an enthusiastic Morgenthau, could be pressed into service as easily a gentleman's suit.

"Now what they are proposing in England is not only good for today, it's good for the post war [period]," wrote Morgenthau in his diary. "[T]hey are going to get unemployment insurance; they are going to get sickness insurance and the whole business." And Americans already had the machinery in place and set to go. "Now the beauty of the study of the social insurance over something else is … you have got the mechanics.… It wouldn't be an additional burden from the standpoint of machinery. We will just extend it."[98]

Morgenthau thought he had persuaded FDR to endorse his plan in September 1943. Other advisors warned that this would "stir up more than a hornet's nest" (the very words Truman would hear when his turn came). Roosevelt first said that he'd do it and then, on reflection, that it would have to wait. His analysis would prove prophetic: "The people are unprepared [for a health plan]," the president told Morgenthau on September 27. "The only person who can explain this medical thing is myself." Roosevelt had precisely fingered the problem: the people had not been prepared. And he was going to need their help—a popular groundswell—to get a national health program through the reluctant Congress.[99]

Even while Morgenthau was lobbying for health insurance, Roosevelt was meeting with Senator Walter George (D-GA). FDR had tried and failed to purge George in 1938; now, the conservative Georgian chaired the powerful Senate Finance Committee. Any bill with financial provisions—like health care insurance—would have to go through him. Morgenthau heard Roosevelt say exactly what George wanted to hear: "You don't want, I'm sure, to have anybody come up and present a social security [based health care] plan at this time.… I know you don't want it.... We can't go up against the State medical societies; we just can't do it."[100]

Roosevelt's advisors all got the point: Congress was not going to pass a national health insurance bill until FDR himself explained the "medical thing to the people"—until, that is, the president rallied enough popular support to push Congress. Gingerly, the president seemed to lay the groundwork for just that.

In January 1944, Roosevelt returned to health care coverage. His "economic bill of rights" included "the right to adequate medical care" and "the opportunity to achieve and enjoy good health" as well as the "right to adequate protection from the economic fears of old age, sickness, accident and unemployment."[101] That same month, the Social Security Board's annual report again endorsed compulsory national health coverage as part of social insurance. Roosevelt campaigned for a fourth term on his economic bill of rights platform, including its call for adequate medical care, and after he won the 1944 election, he signaled a new activism on health care. The president's State of the Union address in January 1945 again included reference to "adequate medical care" but he did not go into details.

But the details were being worked out behind the scenes. Sam Rosenman, who had been with FDR from the start, began to put together a plan, an address, and a set of tactics. This time, the people putting the plan together were operating, not in the thickets of the bureaucracy, but in the White House and under the direction of one of FDR's most trusted advisors. One member of the group predicted, in 1944, that FDR "was clearly looking forward to doing battle with those fellows in Chicago"—referring to the American Medical Association, headquartered in Chicago.[102] Many future Democratic presidents would face this battle—though not all of them relished the prospect.

Working with a colleague at Columbia university, Milton Handler, Rosenman produced an early draft in January 1944. Handler attached a plaintive note to his version of the draft: "I find it difficult to write on social security problems in colorful terms. The subject, though an intriguing one, is quite technical and my writing on it tends to bog down." But both sides—especially opponents of the idea—would soon find a way to make the technical details catchy, even dramatic.[103]

That first draft laid out the logic of the argument: the war had exposed terrible health problems: "[W]e are reaping today in wartime the consequences of our past neglect. Between forty and fifty percent of those called in the military draft have been rejected on grounds of health." The solution: health insurance, disability protection, and hospital construction.[104]

On April 12, 1945, less than a month before victory in Europe, the Rosenman team was putting the finishing touches on FDR's national health insurance speech when the incredible news hit: FDR was dead. The national health insurance plan would now have to be routed to a new man, Harry S. Truman.

## FDR AND HEALTH CARE

Historians have largely granted FDR a bye on universal health coverage. They have traced his repeated decisions not to engage the issue (until, perhaps the end) as the results of the tangled politics of Depression-era America, the press of other issues, his waning political fortunes during the late 1930s, the war, and finally, his ill health. All these factors are relevant. But they are not enough to explain why one of the most effective domestic presidents in American history made the decisions he did—decisions that repeatedly led him to hold back proposals to extend health care coverage to vulnerable Americans.

Certainly, it would have been difficult for him in 1934–35 to pass both Social Security and health care coverage. And he had no choice but to put Social Security first. But he might have pushed for a health care program immediately afterward; and he might even have decided to use his connection with the American public to fight for both programs (as Harry Hopkins urged him to do). This was, after all, a leader who did not shrink from a good brawl, and who won more than he lost.

Why did he duck? Several factors appear to have shaped his behavior; we will see them all again in future presidents.

First, FDR did not appear to be comfortable with the issue. In contrast, to his firm grasp of Social Security, he did not intuitively understand how health insurance would work. This is a problem that would bedevil health care advisors seeking to engage future presidents. The issue is complex, and the policies are peripheral to the experience of most politicians. It is, as Professor Handler lamented, "quite technical"; the entire thing "tends to bog down."

Second, other issues—unemployment insurance, Social Security, aid to families with children—mattered more, especially in the early years of the New Deal. Roosevelt was content—at least until 1944—to delegate health care to a largely apolitical group dominated by economists and labor experts. FDR was the first president to face the familiar health care conundrum: Americans favor government guarantees of access to health care, but they don't generally value it nearly as highly as they do a host of other topics that rise and fall on the national agenda: war, terrorism, defense, the economy, political corruption, crime. Health care is technically complicated and politically undervalued.

Historians attribute Roosevelt's decision to abandon the fight the second time, in 1938, to his waning political influence after the midterm election. His purge campaign flopped—worse, it was counterproductive, for it empowered the conservatives who had run against the president and won. But the blunt fact remains: he seems to have been unwilling to take risks for health care that he took for other programs.

His tendency to avoid political risk for health care issues may have been explained in part by a third consideration. Roosevelt seemed to show timidity in the face of the American Medical Association. Alone among modern Democratic presidents (and among some Republicans as well), FDR avoided confrontation with organized medicine. Some historians explain FDR's posture by citing the AMA's tremendous influence with the Congress at this time—but it was in fact their victory over FDR that made the doctor's reputation for invincibility. FDR took on other interests that were every bit as formidable, but the few times he spoke publicly on health care during the 1930s he talked as much about the prerogatives and burdens of the profession as he did about the health care needs of the public. Indeed, during the 1936 campaign, he even seemed to promise the doctors a veto over federal health care policy. FDR's deference to physicians' knowledge and their economic interests are all the more surprising because of his own experience with physicians who misdiagnosed him, overbilled him, and then quite wrongly dismissed the efficacy of his own treatment for polio.

Why was he so deferential? We can only speculate. Perhaps it was because of his close personal relationships with physicians whom he trusted—McIntire and Cushing—and who presented the American Medical Association's views in a sympathetic light. Cushing, in particular, was a giant of American medicine during the 1930s. Revered then—and now—as an extraordinary surgical innovator, he did not hold any AMA office (although some speculated that he wanted one), but he espoused its views on universal coverage and he had unparalleled access to FDR. His influence may have been all the greater because he did not abuse it. In fact, he only rarely visited the White House.

McIntire was far less charismatic and renowned, but he saw the president twice a day, and FDR clearly relied on him for policy advice as well as for medical treatment. Roosevelt would not prove unique among modern presidents in using personal physicians as health care sounding boards. Presidents, like everyone else, develop emotional relationships with caretakers. These relationships, as we shall see, have mattered frequently in presidential health care policymaking, and they may have mattered here as well. Any abstract distrust or skepticism about the medical profession could recede in the very intimate relationship that evolves between a man and his doctors.

Moreover, in the 1930s and 1940s, physicians had a far more powerful monopoly over medical information than they have today. There was no academic field of health policy in the 1930s. There were no legions of health economists, sociologists, or former public health care officials who stood ready to draw on research to rebut the self-interested claims of organized medicine. Roosevelt's advisors on health care were predominantly labor economists without much knowledge of health care delivery. Cushing's warnings to FDR about letting "public health officials" and foundation staffers tell doctors how to practice would likely have given any responsible policymakers pause at the time. The proliferation of health care experts and the mistakes of organized medicine would give future presidents more freedom to challenge the medical profession, although that same abundance of health care expertise could prove paralyzing, as the Carter and Clinton administrations discovered.

Some historians dismiss the importance of the doctors—even the fabled Harvey Cushing. They point back to FDR's inevitable bottom line: politics. Health insurance, as Monte Poen puts it, was political dynamite from the start. And, crucially, there was no popular uprising for health care like the ones that Huey Long and Francis Townsend were leading for pensions.[105] After the 1938 purge debacle, the legislative deck was even further stacked against health insurance. Congressional scholars call this period the era of the committee chairs for good reason—barons such as Walter George dominated the legislature.

How could FDR win health insurance? He himself put his finger on what may have been the only way: it was going to take a public uprising to get this through Congress, and no one could lead that charge more effectively than the president. But the reality remains: he never did.

Commentators so respect Roosevelt's temperament that they tend to treat his repeated decisions to equivocate, defer, and then bypass health care issues as correct almost by definition. Surely, had it been possible to push universal health insurance to fruition, this titan of liberalism would have done so. But when FDR's actions are compared to those of later presidents—another explanation emerges. The issue did not really grab him. To him, it wasn't worth the risks. He didn't have the confidence that the policy would work, or that the benefits would be worth the costs—politically, personally, economically, or socially. He wasn't passionate about it. His personal experience makes this fact the ultimate enigma. But, as we'll see again and again, presidential passion may be the crucial factor in determining whether the health care fight takes place. It may seem like the simplest possible lesson, but FDR shows how crucial it is. The first question of health reform is how badly the president wants it.

The final irony lies in the legacy. Generation after generation of Democrats would look at health care as the New Deal's unfinished task, FDR's lost reform. Roosevelt repeatedly put off the fight that future generations would see as his liberal dream deferred.

# CHAPTER 2

# Harry S. Truman

*We'll Take the Starch Out of Them—Eventually*

Vice President Harry Truman was up on Capitol Hill discussing stalled bills with congressional leaders. As Sam Rayburn (D-TX), the speaker of the house, mixed their drinks, he remembered that the White House press secretary had called for Harry. "I didn't think it was anything important," recalled Truman. He returned the call and a short while later Eleanor Roosevelt was putting her hand on his shoulder and telling him, "Harry, the president is dead." Stunned, Truman responded, "Is there anything I can do for you?" "Is there anything I can do for *you?*" answered Eleanor. "You're the one in trouble now."[1]

"Boys, if you ever pray, pray for me now," President Harry Truman told the press the next day. "I don't know whether you fellows ever had a load of hay fall on you, but when they told me yesterday what had happened, I felt like the moon, the stars, and all the planets had fallen on me."[2]

Only a year earlier, Truman had been a relatively low-ranking senator from Missouri—he had barely even spoken to Franklin Roosevelt. *Newsweek* summed up the astonishing rise: "Harry S. Truman—the man who wanted to be a Representative, not a Senator, a Senator, not a Vice President, a Vice President and not President"—now stepped into the Oval Office.[3]

People liked Harry. "In his first few months in the White House" reported *Time,* "Harry Truman ... enjoyed a personal popularity—it was almost indistinguishable from sympathy—that few presidents had ever achieved." His Gallup Poll numbers reached higher than Roosevelt's. "The plain people had cottoned to the plain Missourian who seemed so eager to admit his inadequacy, but ... willing to take on burdens and make quick decisions."[4] Four bruising years later, the line on Harry had not changed: "Nothing had altered the president's Missouri flavor, his small town neighborliness or his appetite for homely jollity."[5]

But the press invariably added a hard twist to this plain-folks picture—"Harry Truman was a sincere, hard working man who unfortunately had to step into a job that was too big for him. A great many of the American people feel sorry for him."[6] A great many underestimated Harry Truman.

This chapter tells the story of Truman and his greatest frustration. "I have had some stormy times as president," he wrote in his memoirs. "I have had some bitter disappointments ... , but the one that has troubled me most, in a personal way, has been the failure to defeat the organized opposition to a national, compulsory, health insurance program."[7] President Truman would come to stand as the hero of the great struggle for health reform.

His status as the icon of that lost cause shines a light on what Americans admire in a president. Truman inherited the issue—the idea, the plan, and the strategy—from the Roosevelt administration. He did not design a national health program, he did little to lobby it through Congress, he never took the cause directly to the American people (though his allies begged him to do so), and he never came close to winning. But he believed in the reform, stated it clearly, and clung to it doggedly. Few people have ever been more passionate about a government program than Harry Truman was about national health insurance. For the next quarter-century, Americans would debate health care within the framework he established.

## HARRY TRUMAN

Truman liked to tell childhood stories. A lot of them turned on health. For example, one summer morning, when he was about six, young Harry walked out into the field to get an armful of green corn for pudding. As he went by, Uncle Harrison—the two-hundred-pound poker-playing bachelor after whom Harry had been named—called him over for a tall tale.

*That Personality*

"Do you know," asked Harrison, "what was the most corn a man ever ate at one sitting?" Harry didn't, so Uncle Harrison told him about an old pal who ate thirteen ears on a bet and got so sick they had to call for the doctor. Well, the doctor worked him over most of the night and when there was nothing more that medicine could do they sent for the parson. The poor fellow told the preacher he was not much of a praying man, but the extremity was so terrible, he'd give it a try. So he fell to his knees and petitioned the Almighty: "O Lord, I am in great pain and misery. I have eaten thirteen roasting ears, and I don't seem to be able to take care of them. I am praying to you for help, and Lord, I'm not like the damned howling church members in the amen corner; if you'll relieve me of seven of these damned ears of corn, I'll try to wrestle around the other six."[8]

Vintage Harry: feisty, irreverent, cheerful, and down to earth. This is the story of a self-reliant fellow—he'll even meet the Almighty halfway. Note how the childhood memory holds a skeptical place for the medical profession. And finally, there's his most familiar characteristic, peeking out from the tall tale: in vivid contrast to the presidential giants on either side of him—the aristocrat and the five-star general—Truman always struck contemporaries as an average American, "a Missouri farm boy who grew up to be president of the United States," as the *New York Times* put it.[9] Or perhaps his celebrated traits were what his countrymen wanted to believe were typical in the agitated world that emerged from the Great Depression and World War II.

What Truman himself valued most in a leader was decisiveness. Roosevelt juggled political possibilities and always held his options open; Eisenhower, as we'll see, agonized between contending choices. Truman decided, announced his judgment, and plowed ahead. When Truman wrote an essay on outstanding presidents, he put his first measure of greatness right in the title: "Making Up Your Mind."[10] Harry himself was nothing if not decisive. In his autobiographical writing, he has so many people calling him "cussed," "stubborn," "contrary," and "Missourian" (all synonyms in the Truman lexicon) that it is clear he relished the trait in himself. His mother liked to tell reporters that Harry plowed "the straightest furrow in all Missouri."[11]

*Early Years*

Truman was the last American president without a college degree. He had intended to go, but when hard times fell on his parents, he took a job with a railroad construction outfit alongside grizzled hobos who worked two weeks until payday, drank their entire paycheck over a weekend, and then slouched back for another round of work. Truman made up for his lack of a college education by reading voraciously. When schoolchildren later asked him which library books he'd read, he replied "all of them." "Not all readers become leaders," wrote Harry. "But all leaders must be readers."[12]

Truman got his first taste of leadership during World War I, when he commanded an artillery unit. (To get into the military, he had to cheat on the eye exam by memorizing the chart.) Captain Truman had a narrow miss—he got up at 4:30 one morning and watched a German shell blast the spot where he'd just been sleeping. But Harry was never more frightened than the morning of July 11, 1918, when he took command of Battery D, 129th—an obstreperous unit of "wild Irish and German Catholics" that had already run through four commanders. To his relief, Harry hit it off with his men. They would become his first and most ardent political constituents: his army buddies would push him into politics.[13]

Truman's time in France offered another hint of things to come. Captain Truman was responsible for his unit's canteen. He proposed a way to organize things and after six months was running such an efficient operation (with "bedrock prices" and "no credit accounts") that the canteen had paid out $10,000 in dividends. For the rest of his life, Truman proudly rattled off the numbers on his canteen balance sheets. Truman would make his political reputation, both local and national, by efficiently overseeing accounts.[14]

After the war, Truman started a clothing store—he called it "the shirt store"—with Eddie Jacobson, who had helped him run the camp canteen. They did fine until a postwar recession swamped the business. Another army companion, Jim Prendergast, came to Harry's rescue. Jim's uncle, Tom J. Pendergast, was the formidable boss of the Kansas City political machine and needed a clean, popular veteran to put up for county judge (as they called their commissioners). Harry's introduction to the 10th Ward Democratic Club was a machine classic—clear, brief and autocratic: "Now I'm going to tell you who you are going to be for for county judge," puffed the machine enforcer, Mike Prendergast. "It's Harry Truman. He's got a fine war record. He comes from a fine family. He'll make a fine judge."[15]

Truman soon proved a most unorthodox machine politician. As judge, and then presiding judge, he set out "to clean up the county's financial condition," organized a good government group, and started constructing roads, hospitals, and public buildings. Truman insisted on letting the contracts to the lowest bidders—a gross violation of machine practice. Well-connected contractors came in to complain and when Harry refused to budge, Big Boss Pendergast (who was delighted to have this fresh face in his organization) cheerfully backed him up: "I told you he's the contrariest man in the country," he told the unhappy insiders. "Now get out of here."[16]

Truman floated bonds for his building projects. The party men growled that voters always rejected bonds. "I responded," recalled Truman, that "if I could go to the voters and assure them that ... able engineers and architects would have control of the construction ... the bonds would carry." Sure enough, the bonds carried; Truman easily won another term, and the county got handsome new roads and public buildings. They became a source of local pride—the county published a handsome book of photos featuring the Truman public works.[17] "Doggone it, Harry," gushed a local Ford dealer twenty years later (in a letter criticizing Truman's national health insurance plan), "every time I write that 'President Harry Truman' I can see the old book the county put out with the roads you built." Of course, Truman shrugged off the cheerful memories and went straight to the greater cause: "I'm glad you wrote me because there are a lot of people like you who need straightening out on the subject [of my national health program]."[18]

In 1934, Harry wanted to run in a safe House district, but Tom Pendergast had other plans. The St. Louis and Kansas City machines had each controlled a Senate seat. Now, the St. Louis Democratic organization violated the unwritten rule and tried to grab the second seat. Pendergast tapped Harry to go up against the St. Louis encroachment, and they squeaked out a narrow victory. Senator Truman arrived in Washington under the cloud of machine politics—a tag that insinuated vassalage, corruption, and tainted urban power. The earnest New Dealers ignored the new machine guy from Kansas City.

Harry never entirely escaped the shadow of the machine, but he never apologized for his past. On the contrary, he kept a picture of Tom Pendergast in his Senate office—even after the big boss landed in jail. "I never deserted [Tom Pendergast] when he needed friends," Truman later recalled. "I never ran out on him when the going was rough."[19] Truman's contemporaries generally saw Harry as an independent straight-shooter who had climbed through the tough and venal world of machine politics—honest, steady, and small.

*Into the White House*

Truman faced a long-shot Senate reelection in 1940—the *St. Louis Post Dispatch* pegged his chances at "nil."[20] But he eked out a narrow win and then made his reputation in the Senate the same way he had made it in the army and on the county board. Truman proposed a defense subcommittee of the Committee on Audit and Control to investigate waste and corruption in government war contracts. Under Truman's leadership, the committee produced some thirty bipartisan reports—and not one contained a dissenting opinion. As with the army canteen and the county's public works, Truman made his name as Mr. Efficiency. And in every case he always got along with his colleagues.

Harry Truman's next step up seemed even more accidental than the rest of his career. He had promised to support James Byrnes for vice president in 1944. When a member of the Missouri delegation to the Democratic national convention suggested that they put Harry up for VP, Truman flatly ruled the suggestion out of order. When a knot of Democratic leaders called him into their hotel room to offer him the post, Harry told them he was not a candidate. Meanwhile, President Roosevelt was up to his old tricks, scribbling last-minute notes announcing a choice or two: It's Wallace or Douglas. It's Douglas or Truman. And, finally: It's Truman. Up in the hotel room, the party leaders told Harry that the president had settled on him for VP. Nothing doing, responded a skeptical Truman.

Finally, Roosevelt himself called. Roosevelt famously shouted into telephones so that everyone in the room heard both sides of the conversation. Truman later recalled the conversation:

> "Have you got that fellow lined up yet?" bellowed FDR.
> "No, he is the contrariest Missouri mule I've ever dealt with," responded Robert Hannigan, the chairman of the Democratic Party.
> "You tell him," responded FDR, "if he wants to break up the Democratic party in the middle of a war, that's his responsibility." Then he banged down the phone.
> To say I was stunned is to put it mildly. I sat for a minute or two.... Finally I said, "Well if that is the situation, I'll have to say yes, but why the hell didn't he tell me in the first place?"[21]

One reporter from the *St Louis Post Dispatch* commented that Truman looked "scared to death."[22] Less than nine months later, he was the president.

## HARRY'S HEALTH

When Harry was in second grade, a bad bout of diphtheria left him paralyzed for six months, unable to use his arms or legs. His mother, Mattie, wheeled him around in a baby buggy. They gave me ipecac and whisky and "I've hated the smell of both ever since," reported Truman, who would later make do with bourbon.[23]

### An Ounce of Bourbon

Harry recovered and grew up to be extremely hale—perhaps the most robust modern president—except for agonizing stress headaches. And heavy drinking. When he was county judge, working up to fifteen hours a day, he'd get so keyed up, as he wrote to Bess, "that I either had to run away or go on a big drunk." He took off on long trips to survey public buildings across the country.

By the time he got to the Senate, the recurring headaches had grown savage. His congressional aide and friend Vick Messal wondered whether maybe Harry was drinking too much. William Helm, the Washington Correspondent for the *Kansas City Journal Post* later wrote that he never knew anyone who could hold his liquor as well as Senator Truman; he once saw Harry down five drinks with no visible effect.[24]

Stress or drink, Harry suffered from the political rough and tumble— and Missouri politics got plenty rough. During his difficult 1940 Senate reelection campaign, the Republicans who now controlled the County Court charged that Truman had fiddled with the county school fund when he had served as Judge. They foreclosed on his mother's farm—the county held the mortgage—and put everything up for auction. Harry, who was off at the Democratic convention, always thought this a bare-knuckle political jab. He did not have the money or the political clout with the rival party to save the family farm. The stress and humiliation took their toll. Later during the convention, Truman felt so weak and dizzy that he thought he was having heart attack and clung to a railing until bystanders came to his assistance.

The following year, after a gall bladder attack, headaches, nausea, and fatigue, Truman checked into Bethesda Naval Hospital. The examining physician's notes echo Harry's agitation: "Last year he ran for reelection and had a particularly fatiguing campaign ... in which a great deal of vilification was hurled at him.... The attack on him affected him and caused him much mental anguish. His symptoms increased more than ever from this time on. In the last few months there has been an increased amount of activity in the Senate.... He felt he would be unable to continue his present pace."[25]

However, as Truman rose through the Senate and into the White House, the stress attacks abated. President Truman enjoyed terrific health. He checked into the new presidential suite at Walter Reed Medical Center only once in almost eight years. And he seemed to grow more hearty and vigorous as time went on. By the end of his second term, visitors were marveling at the sixty-eight-year-old president's appearance. Cabell Phillips summed up the popular wisdom when he reported in the *New York Times* that the president was "blessed with a tough hide and a secure conscience so that he could roll with the punches." As David McCullough concluded, Truman relished the office at the pinnacle of his profession.[26]

Harry also became increasingly vocal about staying fit. "I've learned what to do to take care of myself physically," he told a health assembly meeting in 1948. Sounding every bit the modern fitness coach, he dispensed lifestyle exhortations: "You know, the most of us, the reason we are not physically fit is because we are too lazy to take care of ourselves. We sit down and wait until this paunch comes on, and when we get bent over, then we try to correct it by heroic methods."[27]

"I eat no bread but one piece of toast at breakfast, no butter, no sugar, no sweets," boasted Truman in his diary during his last year in office (1952), "so I maintain my waistline and can wear suits bought in 1935!" The president carefully minded his weight—*obsession* is only a little too strong a word—and the issue invariably appears in press stories about him. If the president was on vacation, reports noted that "he kept his weight level by frequent swims" (sidestroke to keep his glasses dry); if a reporter met him for his early morning walk, he'd allow that although Truman had gained fifteen pounds around Christmas, he'd quickly lost five of them already.[28]

The routine that kept the president trim had him rising every morning at 5:30. He walked a brisk two miles at the old army pace of 120 steps a minute—he was especially proud of his fast pace and often bragged about it—then ate his frugal breakfast and downed an ounce of bourbon—his personal prescription for sound health and good circulation.[29]

In fact, the most dramatic health incident during Truman's presidency was the death of his ninety-four-year-old mother. When she broke her hip in February 1947, Harry flew straight home and then followed up with two more visits—he stayed by her side for twelve days in May. Harry's correspondence shows considerable concern with the complexities of caring for an aging mother. But a condolence telegram from one subordinate after Mattie died in July accurately summed up the situation: "[Y]ou were fortunate in having your mother longer than most [of] us." This was a sad moment, but not one that Harry seemed to connect to his views of health care policy. As her doctors told the press in her last days, "her tired old heart is slowing down.... It's just a case of a fine old machine wearing out."[30]

Harry's own physician, Colonel Wallace Graham, was a young army surgeon whose father doctored Harry's mother. Graham became a poker-playing fixture in the White House. He insisted on answering every single letter about the president's health—no matter how unusual. "Has the president a psychiatrist to watch over his mental health?" wrote one earnest citizen. Graham dutifully wrote back that "the president has available to him ... all types of specialists."[31]

The rest of the staff teased Wallace for his devotion to the task. Once, on a weekend cruise, Harry asked to see some of the letters. As Truman related the story in a letter to his mother, Graham "brought me about two dozen and I gave them a tear across the middle and threw them in the ocean." The president explained that Graham would "constantly tell me to relax"—now the doctor could take his own medicine and enjoy the cruise. Graham's reaction? "He almost wept because he thought I'd lose some prospective votes by [his] not answering those letters."[32]

Truman, one of the hardiest twentieth-century presidents made national health insurance his great personal crusade. Certainly he was proud of his own health—bragging on his walking pace, vain about his weight, sharing his regimen, urging his own health habits on others. Why did the health issue speak to him so? He was often asked the question, and his different answers all point to the same source.

### Truman's Passion

Truman traced his passion for national health insurance not to his own health but to the important episodes of his career: his success in the military, his triumph as county judge, the illnesses he heard about from constituents, and a New Deal prairie populism.

"My special interest in health dates back some 30 odd years," he told a health meeting in 1948. "When World War 1 came on I helped recruit a regiment of Field Artillery for service and I was appalled at the large number of young men who were unfit for Service." This was a Missouri national guard unit, continued Truman, so the men knew one another. "When a man was rejected for a physical disability it was tragic for him and for those of us ... in the outfit. That made me pause and think." Truman was reflecting on what had had been so important to him about the army—the respect of his men, and the camaraderie they shared— and blamed poor health for depriving other men of the experience. The Rosenman Commission that prepared the Roosevelt–Truman health program put particular emphasis on the number of men and women rejected for health reasons during World War II.[33]

A second memory seemed even more important, or at least came up more frequently: his experience as a county judge. "There were derelicts who had lost all they had, and they didn't have any ambition. We took good care of them. And then there were those who were just making a living.... If sickness overtook these families they were sunk. I've seen people turned away from the big hospitals in town to die, just because they did not have the money to get in. I built a hospital to take care of these people." Could there be a better statement of the classic liberal vision? Truman would take care of hard-working people, poor families just getting by, and the losers who "didn't have ambition."

Harry also emphasized the middle class: "I found that the indigent and the very rich were well cared for in the county, but a family on the average income from $1,500 to $3,000 per year just could not afford to get sick or have ill health." Or, as he put the same thought in the letter to Ben Turoff, the Missouri Ford dealer who needed "straightening out" about national health insurance, "I am trying to fix it so the people in the middle income bracket can live as long as the very rich and the very poor.[34]

Once he warmed up on the subject—in talks and letters—a kind of prairie populism burst out: "I'm surely sorry that Nellie has had to go back to the hospital," Harry wrote to a friend in 1952. "What a bunch of robbers they are! How can anyone be against my health program? We'd be able to meet situations such as Nellie's if we had it." Truman remembered, personalized, and repeated the figures that he saw in memos. "In my youth, most doctors charged from $15 to $25 to officiate at a birth—now they want $500 just for prenatal care. Can you imagine a $2,400 a year clerk raising four children?"[35]

Truman always believed his health reform was inevitable—that modernity itself demanded the change. When Representative John Kee (D-WV) forwarded him a constituent letter criticizing the "big, strong, lazy men" who "lay around and let someone else who is working feed them," Harry responded with a full-out blast: "Conditions[,] as you know, have changed very greatly since the pioneer days of West Virginia ... and it is necessary to meet those changed conditions with a modern approach. If we could turn the clock back ... I think all of us would be heartier citizens with shorter lives.... It is interesting, however, to find people who still continue to live in 1890 instead of 1950. I fear some of our Senators and Representatives ... are still living in 1890. Perhaps like Rip Van Winkle they will come out of their slumber and find how the world has progressed." Opponents of national health insurance, he often said, "really want to go back to the horse and buggy days."[36]

In the end, Truman's support for national health insurance reflected a fiercely liberal impulse: "We take care of these people," as he put it, "when they are sick." To Truman, this was a basic right, an essential part of citizenship. It drew on his deep commitment to New Deal principles and his conviction that national health care—and the emerging American social welfare state—was a fundamental feature of both fairness and modernity itself. Americans enjoyed a better life, he said in a 1952 address, "because the national policies of these 20 years have [been] directed to meet human needs, and not just to meet private greed." There would be plenty of people to tell him why he was all wrong—that it was he and his allies who violated American free market values—but Truman never heard them. As he wrote, again and again: "I just don't understand how anyone can be against my health program."[37]

## NATIONAL HEALTH INSURANCE

Truman had been in office four months when Japan surrendered on August 14, 1945. Americans had braced themselves for a longer war—invading Japan would be far more treacherous than the Normandy landing. Then the terrible bombs brought sudden victory.

The abrupt peace forced a different challenge on the new president. A booming economy, organized almost entirely around war production, now had to be converted back to peacetime production. In less than a single month, the Pentagon cancelled $15 billion worth of orders[38]—a full 7 percent of the national GNP. Economic problems piled up—production, inflation, strikes. Social pressures compounded the headache. Millions of veterans came home and found no place to live. The news magazines trumpeted the housing shortage with photos of army men on the street, their furniture stacked up, sometimes a wife and child sitting glumly on the curb alongside them.[39] Truman had blamed the maladroit reconversion following World War I for sinking his own business and was eager to protect the new generation of veterans. Truman thought big.

## I Shall Shortly Communicate with Congress

On September 6, three weeks after VJ day, he astonished Congress with an ambitious Reconversion Program. Truman called it his inaugural address, his State of the Union address, the real start of the Fair Deal, and the date he assumed the office of the president in his own right—all rolled into one. "The sudden surrender of the Japanese has not caught us unawares," began Truman, who then presented a high-flying twenty-one-point plan—each point further broken down into multiple proposals and aspirations. The whole business ran to almost 16,000 words. The president called for unemployment compensation, price controls, government reorganization, full employment legislation (to pursue Roosevelt's economic bill of rights, helpfully restated in the text), price stability for farmers, comprehensive housing legislation, a revised tax code, an extensive program for veterans, fair labor standards—the list went on. Finally, crammed into point number twenty-one, along with plans for stockpiling strategic material, education, and Social Security, Truman promised another blockbuster: "I shall shortly communicate with the Congress recommending a national health program to provide adequate medical care for all Americans and to protect them from financial loss and hardships resulting from illness and accident."[40]

As Harry cheerfully recalled, it was the longest presidential message to Congress since 1901. It was too long to deliver. The president had it printed and sent to Capitol Hill, where all hell immediately broke loose.[41]

Many liberals were thrilled. Months earlier, when Truman first talked to Roosevelt's domestic advisor and legal counsel, Sam Rosenman, about drafting the speech, Rosenman leaned forward and said eagerly, "You know, Mr. President ... this is the most exciting and pleasant surprise I have had in a long time." "How is that?" asked Harry. "Well, your conservative friends ... up on Capitol Hill ... say ... the New Deal is as good as dead—that we are all going back to normalcy." In Truman's own description of the exchange, Rosenman concluded with a pitch-perfect summary of Harry's own view: "This [message] really sets forth a progressive political philosophy and a liberal program of action that will fix the theme for your whole term in office." Some historians question this exchange, suggesting that Rosenman must have already known how Truman felt, but that misses Harry's real point: this message was his great New Deal confession, his liberal testimonial.[42]

On the other hand, Harry's conservative friends were flabbergasted. Republicans and southern Democrats had thought they were finished with the "Roosevelt nonsense." The Harry Truman they knew was a down-to-earth Missouri moderate who focused on waste, fraud, and sound budget practices—and now this! Senate Minority Leader Joe Martin (R-MA) summed up the Republican reaction: "Not even President Roosevelt ever asked for as much in one sitting." Some of Harry's own advisors had firmly warned him against launching such an ambitious and liberal program in one great gulp. The press jumped in and concluded that Truman's "waltz with Congress" had come to an abrupt end—even before it had really begun.[43]

Six weeks later, with the political waters still roiling, Truman sent Congress his comprehensive health program.

## What I Am Recommending Is Not Socialized Medicine

National health insurance had percolated during the Roosevelt years. FDR had encouraged the electric 1938 conference that laid down a five-point national health—the foundation for future liberal thinking. Roosevelt backed off and declined to endorse the resulting legislation that Senator Robert Wagner (D-NY) slipped into Congress in 1939; nor did he back the more ambitious plan submitted by Senators Wagner and James Murray (D-MT) and Representative John Dingell (D-MI) in 1943, or Secretary of the Treasury Henry Morgenthau's plan to Americanize the Beveridge Report in Great Britain. In his third term, Roosevelt had prophetically stated the problem: Congress did not want a health plan; the American people were unprepared for it; "the only person who can explain this medical thing is myself."

As Roosevelt pondered his fourth term, he seemed to be ready to take up the fight—although with FDR, nothing was ever certain. In his 1945 State of the Union address, he promised to return with a health message and gave Sam Rosenman the job of organizing the plan, the strategy, and the address.[44]

When Roosevelt died, Rosenman passed the health insurance material to Truman. In May 1945, a month after Truman took office,
Murray, Wagner, and Dingell once again submitted their legislation.
Rosenman advised Truman—still focused on the war—that any statement he made "should not be directed at any particular piece of legislation but should be general in form—stating objectives and purposes
rather than details." Truman followed the advice and ducked when the
press asked about the bill: "I am not familiar with its details ... but in
principle I am for it."[45]

This Murray, Wagner, and Dingell effort—like its predecessors—went
nowhere. Crusty Georgia Senator Walter George (D-GA) still ruled the
Senate Finance Committee. Over in the House, powerful Robert Lee
Doughton (D-NC) chaired the Ways and Means Committee. Doughton—
eighty-three years old, notoriously hard of hearing, and no friend of the
New Deal—had been in Congress since 1911. Neither even bothered
to schedule hearings. They left the health reformers to ponder the first
hurdle—hostile congressional barons who could simply shrug off health
reform without so much as a vote or a hearing.

During the summer and early fall, as the war finally ended, Rosenman
polished the health message that had emerged from the Roosevelt White
House. Truman enthusiastically put his own stamp on the document.
For example, one issue running through the drafts illuminated a long
philosophical argument among health reformers: what to do about
poor people? Liberals had argued long and hard against health programs directed only at poor patients: they would reduce pressure for
a universal plan; they would turn health care into a form of dole; and
they violated a deep liberal conviction—all citizens had an equal right
to decent care. To FDR the matter was largely a question of tactics,
but to Truman it was a matter of principle. Roosevelt was willing to
separate poor people from everyone else; Truman was not. Between the
second and the third draft of the health plan, a provision for the indigent disappeared. Truman's compulsory health insurance would cover
everyone.[46]

On November 19, 1945, Truman sent Congress his health care message. The message called for five reforms (clearly descended from the
enthusiastic health care conference way back in 1938): hospital construction, expanded maternal and child health services, a broad program
of medical education and research, national health insurance (presented
simply as "prepayment of medical costs"), and disability insurance to
protect workers from sickness or injury.[47]

One line immediately leaped out from the long text: "The American people ... will not be frightened off from health insurance because some people have misnamed it 'socialized medicine.' I repeat—what I am recommending is *not* socialized medicine." The next day, the *New York Times* quoted the line and reported the inevitable rejoinder: "cries of socialized medicine ... were heard from the Republican side of the Senate."[48]

After Truman's message had been read, Senator Wagner and representative Dingell introduced bills "to carry out its objectives." Reformers cheered the great breakthrough—for the first time, a president had endorsed a specific health insurance proposal. Michael Davis, an ardent health insurance advocate and chairman of the Committee for the Nation's Health, put it elegantly: "There are educational hills, organizational swamps, and political rivers to cross. But a presidential message is a milestone."[49]

The new proposal contained a political trick to ease the way through Congress—that mother of all "organizational swamps." The new Murray–Wagner–Dingell legislation skipped the financial details. If Congress liked the idea, explained Senator Wagner mildly, "the method of financing such a plan can be worked out jointly by House and Senate Committees."[50] Without financing provisions, proponents could slip past the finance committees—Senate Finance, House Ways and Means—which were both in enemy hands. Instead, the Senate version went to the friendlier Committee on Education and Labor, chaired by none other than cosponsor James Murray. The House sent the bill to the Interstate and Foreign Commerce Committee.

The press reacted mildly. The American Medical Association emphasized the features it supported (such as building hospitals) as much as the provisions it spurned (federal control of medicine). But the health proposal was almost lost in the big story of the day: screaming headlines reported that 270,000 workers were on strike across the nation. The *New York Times* tucked an unintended irony right next to the report on the Truman health message: hospital maintenance men had struck across New York, and veterans had been called in to operate the elevators. Two days later, a great strike at General Motors sent 180,000 more men to the picket lines while Truman seized the transit lines in Washington, D.C., after bus and trolley operators walked off the job.[51]

Truman sent his great milestone message to a hostile Congress amid roiling national labor crises and then did—nothing. The next day, Truman held a press conference that ranged across all kinds of topics:

the new commander of the U.S. fleet, the labor crisis, world peace. The questions went on: Should Washington, D.C., have the right to vote? (Yes, said Truman) Were we still making atom bombs? (Yes, again). Not a word on health care: not at this press conference, nor at the next, or the one after that. Truman announced his plan—which faced a long uphill battle in both public and congress—and then followed it up with silence.

Reformers fretted about the lack of momentum. The following month, they ran a large advertisement in the *New York Times* and the *Washington Post* signed by 198 opinion leaders—including Eleanor Roosevelt, Mayor Fiorello La Guardia, John Dewey, Aaron Copeland, and Gerard Swope (of GE)—urging Congress to support President Truman's Health Plan. "We agree with [the president's] statement," ran the defensive advertisement, "that the American people ... will not be frightened off from health insurance because opponents have misnamed it socialized medicine." Michael Davis wrote President Truman asking him to at least mention the advertisement in one of his press conferences. Truman wrote gracious and optimistic notes to the sponsors. "I think we are going to get that health program through eventually."[52] But he did not follow up either at his press conferences or—except for a few glancing references—in his speeches.

Roosevelt had hit on the essential wisdom: "The only person who can explain this medical thing is myself." Truman embraced national health insurance with a fervor Roosevelt never showed. Yet, despite increasingly desperate pleas by health care reformers, he never used his bully pulpit to try to rally the public. Scholars focused on national health insurance often wonder why the president did not spend more time pushing his proposal. In the context of the time, his initial reluctance is not surprising. He was surrounded by crises. And compared with his elegant predecessor, he was an awkward speaker who had not yet found an effective voice.

The American Medical Association—or its propaganda arm—was not so reserved. A telegram went out screaming for donations. "OBVIOUSLY THIS IS THE BEGINNING OF THE FINAL SHOWDOWN ON COLLECTIVIST ISSUE. NOT ONE DAY DARE BE LOST.... DO NOT UNDERESTIMATE THE CRISIS.... FIGHT FOR PERSONAL FREEDOM AND PROFESSIONAL INDEPENDENCE."[53]

I. S. Falk, a liberal member of the Social Security Board who had helped craft the Murray–Wagner–Dingell bills, sent the White House a copy of the telegram warning that the organization's budget before this "crisis" had been $200,000—half from physicians, half from drug companies. That would soon seem a piddling amount. While President Truman tossed his plan on the public agenda and turned to other troubles, the American Medical Association organized one of the great public relations campaigns in modern American politics.

Many observers, from Harry Truman to *The New York Times,* would later offer a simple post mortem: the American Medical Association—vociferous, even vicious—killed national health insurance. But did the extraordinary political mobilization really matter? Conservative Democrats, allied with conservative Republicans, dominated Congress. Many wanted to overthrow the New Deal—not extend it. Senator Wagner was not going to fool anyone on the Hill when he tried to sneak a health bill past the southern grandees and their powerful committees.

As *Newsweek* put it after Truman's first year, "The friendly feeling most members have for Mr. Truman proved to be personal, not political—politically he took a beating on virtually every account." National health insurance was just one more fallen liberal idea.[54]

However, the great AMA campaign—and Truman's failure to meet it head-on—mattered in a more subtle way. The Truman plan could win only if a great public uprising pushed Congress—unlikely as it might have been amid labor unrest and a rising red scare. By dominating the public conversation, the AMA cut off even this unlikely long shot. By failing to challenge them, the president passed up the long shot without a contest.

*A Fine Mess*

Before Congress had scheduled hearings, a sprawling bureaucratic turf war erupted across the administration. The weary Truman maxim—scrawled across memos flying up and down the bureaucracy—kept pleading for "united action on the part of those agencies in the executive branch." Nobody complied.[55]

In contrast to FDR, Truman believed in crisp organization and struggled to get his administrative boxes lined up. But imposing order took time, and in its first year, the administration caught a lot of bad press for chaos. "White House aides are grumbling among themselves because of the loose system for getting decisions," reported *Newsweek* in April 1946. The problem seemed to get worse when Sam Rosenman left after the first year (amid Republican insinuations that FDR's favorite advisor now wielded undue power behind the scenes in this unexpectedly liberal administration).[56]

The health plan provoked a bureaucratic free-for-all. Truman had assigned Watson Miller, the head of the Federal Security Administration (FSA) to direct the national health program; the FSA, a sub–Cabinet Agency formed in 1939, would eventually become the Department of Health, Education, and Welfare. It did not have the clout of a full Cabinet Agency, and Miller quickly found himself battling the Children's Bureau, the Department of Veterans Affairs, the Public Health Service, the Department of Agriculture, and the Department of Labor.

Officials in the Children's Bureau were eager to extend their own health program designed to cover the wives and children of service men. They did not want to compromise their agenda by endorsing the controversial Murray–Wagner–Dingell Bill—which offered less coverage to their beneficiaries. Instead, the Children's Bureau bucked Truman to back a bill introduced by Senator Claude Pepper (D-FL).

The conflict ran deeper than the clash over competing proposals. The Children's Bureau, formed in 1912 and lodged in the Department of Labor, had been the brainchild of Progressive women's groups. The agency retained the intense allegiance of liberals focused on children's causes but reflected the ethos of a different era. The old Progressive reformers had been comfortable working through the states and targeting programs to the needy; in contrast, the FSA embodied a New Deal philosophy focused on federal action and universal programs.

To make matters worse, officials in the Federal Security Administration surveyed the bureaucratic terrain and concluded that they ought to manage (opponents would say snatch) the Children's Bureau along with the Social Security Board and the Public Health Service. Meanwhile, Secretary of Labor Lewis Schwellenbach (a former senator from Washington whom Truman thought "a real guy" and "a wheel horse")[57] felt that his department should hang onto the Children's Bureau, at least until his bit of turf could be tucked safely into another Cabinet Agency—perhaps a new Department of Public Welfare.

After long rounds of negotiation, a cheerful memo in March announced that "the differences have now been largely reconciled"— the Children's Bureau would (grudgingly) support Murray–Wagner–Dingell. And everyone would kick the long-term organizational matter down the road. When asked about it, all hands were instructed to respond: "the matter of a federal organization to handle the [health] program is presently under review by the White House."[58] Despite the bureaucratic minuet, children's advocates and women's groups would drain energy from the health insurance battle, fighting instead to keep their bureau from sinking into an unsympathetic sub–Cabinet Agency.[59]

Administrator of Veterans Affairs General Omar Bradley also vexed the administration. Truman sent him a memo stating that the Federal Security Administration had "primary responsibility" for the health effort and asking the administrator of Veterans Affairs "to assist in every way possible." General Bradley immediately shot back a crisp Yes, sir—"You may be assured that I will be pleased to cooperate with Mr. Watson B. Miller, Federal Security Administrator, whom you have asked to assume primary responsibility for organizing the administration's efforts for successful action on S. 1606 [Murray–Wagner–Dingell]." The very model of a responsive bureaucrat.[60] Except that six weeks later, Senator James Murray had a complaint for the president. In testifying before the Senate Committee on Education and Labor, "General Bradley did not commit himself to support of the Administration's health program, nor did he point out how important it is to the health of our veterans and their families."[61]

Why was the general balking? The usual reason. Bradley worried that the proposal would interfere with his VA health programs. Before he went up to the Hill to testify, he had drafted a memo, circulated with Truman's signature, announcing that the proposed national health plan would in no way "supplant," "change," or "impair" existing Veterans Affairs programs. This, apparently, had not been enough.[62] Truman, his patience stretched thin, shot back a letter to Senator Murray: "I think you will find General Bradley is One Hundred Percent for the Administration's measure."[63]

The Office of War Mobilization and Reconversion, which oversaw the entire legislative program, came into the act and sprayed memos and phone calls to these and other players—FSA, Veterans, Agriculture, Labor—trying to organize the administration's legions around Warren Miller's health care leadership. President Truman, who had a low tolerance for bureaucratic scuffling, tried to sort things out in a Cabinet meeting.

But even his faithful doctor blundered into the maelstrom. In April, precisely as the president was trying to get "a unified front" in pushing for Murray- Wagner- Dingell, Colonel Graham dropped a note into the bureaucratic scrum. Writing on White House stationary, Graham warned, "Should the President endorse the Wagner, Murray[,] Dingell coalition or their bill it will automatically light the torch of antagonism of the great percentage of the medical profession who in turn will respond quite lustily by their own reactions and by their influence through thousands of their patients. The Wagner, Murray, Dingell combination do not have the answer to the President's health message." Perhaps worrying that he had not been clear, Graham scrawled a postscript in longhand— "I would highly suggest that the President not take any stand regarding pending legislation on this issue."[64]

Eventually, Truman would get his staff properly lined up. Three years later, health reform would be scrupulously coordinated; when one enthusiastic administrator talked to the press before getting clearance, he got a sharp reminder from the president: "May I again call your attention to my desire that legislative proposals be coordinated and cleared within the executive branch in coordination in accordance with established procedures." Truman did not share the Democratic penchant—evinced by Roosevelt, Kennedy, Johnson, and Clinton—for overlapping advisors and spontaneous innovations. FDR's habit of discussing the same thing with multiple Cabinet members "even though they were not responsible personally [for the issue]," wrote Truman, "engendered rivalry and conflict."[65]

As time went on, Truman relied increasingly on his Cabinet officers, the Council of Economic Advisors (organized under Truman in 1946), the National Security Council (1947), the Bureau of the Budget, and various formal commissions. Budget Director Frank Pace later suggested that it was Truman who "created the institution of the presidency." Historian Donald McCoy put it a bit more carefully: Truman finished the transition that FDR had begun—the presidency became as much an institution as a personal office.[66]

However, neither the chaos of the early years nor the cleaner organizational charts that came later touched Truman's real problem: Congress. National health insurance always got a cold reception when it went to Capitol Hill.

## I Call It Socialism

On April 2, 1946, Senator James Murray opened hearings on the bill he had cosponsored, S. 1606. In his opening remarks, Murray asked that out of respect for the president, critics refrain from calling the legislation "socialistic" or "communistic."

Senator Robert Taft (R-OH), the ranking Republican on the committee, sat and fidgeted. Taft was a conservative anti–New Dealer who hoped to be the Republican presidential candidate in 1948. He was famously brusque and cold, a man with weak people skills. "Bob is not austere," reported his wife; "he is just departmentalized."[67] Now, Senator Taft interrupted the chair:

> "I think it is very socialistic.... It is, to my mind, the most socialistic measure that this Congress has ever had before it, seriously." Referring to the end run around Senate Finance, Taft added, gratuitously, "This committee is being run as a propaganda machine."
>
> "That's a slander and a falsehood," returned Murray, losing his cool. "You had so much gall and so much nerve that you would not let me complete my statement. I would have been glad to give you an opportunity to express yourself ... but you are very impolite, you are very sarcastic ... you think you are pretty smart, a good bluffer, and a bulldozer, but you cannot get away with it...."
>
> Taft announced that he had to leave for another committee and asked the chairman's permission to announce his own intention of submitting an opposition health bill.
>
> Murray had not finished his opening statement and had slated Senator Wagner for the first formal statement. He asked Taft to "subside." Taft tried to plough on, and Murray, shouting, talked over him. "I will have to demand that you subside.... You've been impertinent and insulting...."
>
> Taft—needling Murray—again interrupted. "I intend to offer a complete bill...."
>
> Now Murray was good and hot. He put the discussion off the official record, but reporters gleefully filled in the blanks. "You can shut your mouth up and get out. You're so self-opinionated and ... so self-important."
>
> Taft countered that the committee ought to adjourn until the chair could regain his temper. Murray countered: "I'm the chairman of this committee, and I want you to subside. If you don't shut up, I'll get these officers in here to have you thrown out."
>
> Taft announced his intention to boycott the committee and—back on record—announced, "Everyone will know that the report of this committee ... will be a partisan report which can command ... no respect."[68]

The departmentalized Senator Taft walked out, and things went downhill for health reformers from that rocky start. A long line of groups—the American Bar Association, the National Grange, the Protestant and Catholic Hospital Associations (the last despite long negotiations with the administration)—all condemned Murray–Wagner–Dingell. They joined the medical and hospital associations in warning against compulsory medicine, against socialism, against the destruction of American medicine, against the threat to the American way of life. To accommodate all the groups in this unhappy chorus, Murray scheduled an additional two weeks for the hearings.

Even worse, many of the administration's allies—such as the Department of Veterans Affairs and the Children's Bureau—were tepid at best.
The annual meeting of the League of Women Voters, which was already
on record as supporting national health insurance, now refused to reaffirm its support. By the time the hearings were over, the bill was sunk in
the Senate. Senator Murray admitted defeat and promised to try again
after the November midterm elections.[69]

Over on the House side, the end run around Ways and Means
accomplished nothing. Representative Clarence F. Lea (CA) chaired the
House Committee on Interstate and Foreign Commerce; he had been in
Congress for twenty-nine years—first as a Democrat, then representing
both parties. Lea took a more direct route to the same outcome and
simply declined to hold hearings on Dingell's bill.

As promised, Senator Taft submitted his own health legislation. The
Taft–Smith Act would authorize $200 million in federal matching grants
for states to subsidize private health insurance coverage for the poor. The
administration summarily rejected Taft's approach: it was a piddling
sum, it would undermine a universal program, it offered a boondoggle
to the insurance industry, and it eviscerated a right to health by forcing
people to prove their poverty in order to qualify for aid (a "means test"
as the health wonks call it). William Green, the president of the AFL,
put it pungently at the hearings on Taft's bill: "The Workers of this
country are not prepared to accept the pauper oath as the approach to
better health."[70] For the duration of the Truman administration, Robert
Taft's "pauper bill" offered (from the liberal perspective) a meager and
infuriating counterpoint to Truman's great aspiration.

## Meanwhile

The health insurance hearings offered drama, but nothing to match the
great wave of strikes rolling across America. Even as Murray and Taft
tangled at the start of the hearings, the United Mine Workers began a
nationwide coal strike—on top of the GM strike that had now dragged
on for over a hundred days. In May, as the health insurance hearings ground to an end, the railroads began the most crippling strike of
all—300,000 workers walked out, shutting down the transportation
system.

On May 24, Truman delivered a national radio address and the next
day went before Congress and asked for emergency legislation to draft

the railroad workers into the army. In the middle of his speech, the secretary of the Senate handed him a slip of red paper with good news— the strikers had settled. The president awkwardly finished his address anyway, and the House, caught up in the drama of the moment, voted him the powers. "Harry Truman had shown," reported the *New York Times,* "that he could be tough—plenty tough."

Most liberals, on the other hand, were furious at the idea of using a military draft to break strikes. "Is this Russia or Germany?" asked the *New Republic.* The Senate stoutly resisted Truman's emergency measure. Claude Pepper declared that he would give up his Senate seat before voting for such a measure. Wayne Morse (R-OR) called the interrupted speech a staged "ham act." Union leaders tagged Truman the "number one strike breaker." Senator Taft echoed his liberal colleagues and charged Truman with violating "every principle of American jurisprudence." The emergency authority was no longer needed, but the Senate aired its disdain by burying the measure, 70–13.[71]

National health insurance went down this first time with little notice. In August, far removed from the political pyrotechnics, Congress lifted the first provision out of Truman's health proposal and quietly enacted it. The Hill–Burton hospital construction program would soon be building hospitals around the nation. Here was the sort of program Congress liked best: it offered well-organized, prestigious local institutions concrete (literally) benefits that, in turn, gave individual members of Congress plenty of opportunities to pose for pictures and soak up local gratitude. The program modernized the infrastructure of American medicine, funding almost one out of every three hospital construction projects in the United States over the next two decades.[72]

KEEPING THE ISSUE WARM

Three months later, in the midterm elections of November 1946, the Republicans won both houses in Congress for the first time since 1928. The GOP picked up fifty-five seats in the House and thirteen in the Senate. National health insurance—along with the rest of the Truman program—went from long-shot to impossible.

Under the circumstances, Truman's advisors warned him to stay clear of health insurance. Clark Clifford, who had taken over from Sam Rosenman as White House Counsel, wrote that "the time was not right" for a health message.[73] Truman brushed off the advice. As he later told an interviewer,

"half the members of my Cabinet suggested that I never mention the subject. Several members said 'you are going to stir up a hornet's nest.' So
did Civil Rights, but both were right!"[74] On May 19, 1947, Truman sent
a brief health message to congress. He was pleased, he wrote, that some
measures (such as hospital construction) had passed, but "we must not
rest until we have protected our working people from sickness."[75]

But everything was different now—Truman was simply keeping
the issue warm. After sixteen years in the New Deal wilderness, the
new Republican majority began lobbing explosive charges against
the Democratic establishment. The new Speaker of the House, Joseph
Martin, warned about "subversionists high up in the government." The
House Un-American Activities Committee now moved to Washington's
center stage and began its high-octane attack on communist "sympa-
thizers," "fellow travelers," and "stooges."[76]

The political agenda—the media, the issues, the national debate—
shifted dramatically. Earnest news articles explained how to distin-
guish "honest liberals" from "communist dupes." Whether people are
"innocent, gullible or willful makes little difference," wrote FBI director
J. Edgar Hoover in a long *Newsweek* special on "How to Fight Communism," "because they further the cause of communism and weaken
our American democracy."[77] News stories were full of ominous alarms.
The communists (or their gullible dupes) were seeping into the NAACP,
they controlled fifteen CIO unions, they infected the Protestant churches
(some theologians at Union Theological foolishly defended "the rights
of a very unpopular minority").[78] *Newsweek* ignored Truman's 1947
health message and featured, instead, another story explaining how
Hollywood writers were "the real reds and parlor pinks."[79] All in all,
summed up FBI director J. Edgar Hoover, at least a million Americans
were, one way or another, assisting the communists.[80]

In this context, health reformers made irresistible targets. Opponents
had long scored national health insurance as "socialized medicine."
Now the familiar critique turned treacherous. Republicans (along with
conservative Democrats) used the *House Committee on Expenditures
in the Executive Department* to search for the communists behind the
push for national health care. Senator Homer Ferguson (R-MI) charged
that the Social Security Board employed a communist staff member (the
FBI investigated and cleared the staff).

Ferguson's committee trained "the white light of investigation"
on the Public Health Service, the Department of Agriculture, and the
Office of Education. "The medical profession and all our hospitals can

be taken over by the federal government and forged into a new and gigantic health bureaucracy," warned Republican Representative Forest Harness (R-IN). "It would only be a matter of time until Washington likewise moved into the field of education, religion, the press, the radio. Freedom soon would be in total eclipse."[81]

The fight spilled into all kinds of health policy crannies. When the administration moved to join the World Health Organization, for example, Congress approved the measure but added a stipulation that "[t]he United States is in no way to be committed to any legislative program approved by WHO." Representative Harness explained, "We're in there with Great Britain, Russia, Yugoslavia, Rumania and Hungary. All have some form of socialized medicine or compulsory health insurance." He knew the public health careerists would stop at nothing to press "socialized medicine on America by use of federal employees and Government money."[82]

Harry Truman faced up to the roiling Congress. "It is one of the tragedies of our time," responded Truman, "that the security program of the United States has been widely used by demagogues and sensational newspapers ... to undermine the Bill of Rights, ... to frighten and mislead.... The sacred rights of individuals ... [are] in continuous jeopardy." And, speaking to our own day: "If the government cannot produce witnesses in court, then it cannot prosecute."[83]

Truman's 1948 State of the Union address—perhaps his most ardent and eloquent—almost brazenly touted the administration's least popular agenda items. First, civil rights which incensed the southern Democrats: "Some of our citizens are still denied equal opportunity.... Most serious of all, some are denied equal protection under laws."

Next, national health insurance—and, again, no throttling back: "The greatest gap in our social security structure is the lack of adequate provision for the Nation's health.... This great Nation cannot afford to allow its citizens to suffer needlessly from the lack of proper medical care."[84]

There was not the slightest chance of winning on either issue. Truman used the 1948 State of the Union address to restate his most ambitious views—and fire the first shots of the most famous presidential election of the twentieth century. National health insurance would play a major role in the president's campaign.

This time, Truman got his health care program neatly lined up. In January 1948 Truman commissioned a report on the nation's health. The job went to Oscar Ewing, a savvy liberal and former chair of the Democratic National Committee who had became federal security administrator five months earlier. Ewing delivered his report, *The Nation's Health—A Ten Year Program*, in September 1948—right on time for the traditional start of the election campaign.

The report was meticulous in its portrayal of the American health care system. In only two states did more than half the people have health insurance; less than 10 percent were insured in twenty states. The poorer the state, the lower the insurance rates. Private health insurance, concluded the committee, covered a fraction of the population, offered them inadequate coverage, and was hardest to get where the need was greatest. Private health insurance had failed.[85]

In fact, a robust system of private health insurance—like the one which grew in the next decade—would meet many of the aspirations in the Ewing report. Private insurance would fall short mainly on fairness, on the liberal vision of a right to health care.

The commission, operating by consensus, did not formally endorse a government health program. But in the preface to the report, Oscar Ewing pointed Truman to the path: "I have reexamined the whole matter [of national health insurance] as objectively as possible.... The arguments that have been made against national health insurance have been carefully weighed and I still find myself compelled to recommend it." He then shifted to language that would soon be coming directly from the president. "After all, we are dealing with human lives and human suffering and anguish. Every year, over 300,000 people die whom we have the knowledge and skill to save.... By and large, only the well to do and, to a certain extent, charity patients get satisfactory medical care. The in-between groups ... are the ones desperately in need of better care. I see no possible way to provide funds needed for adequate medical services ... except through a system of national health insurance."[86]

Ewing sounded for all the world like Harry Truman. And Truman, for his part, began to slip data from the report into his familiar arguments for national health care. The report gave Truman new talking points—he'd repeat them in speeches, letters, and interviews for the rest of his life. The new facts and figures first sprang to Harry's lips during the great election campaign of 1948.

GIVE 'EM HELL, HARRY

The campaign of 1948 turned Harry into the perpetual saint of lost political causes. No one thought he had a chance. Democratic leaders scratched desperately for alternative candidates. Supreme Court

Justice William Douglas turned them down. So did General Dwight Eisenhower. Truman's approval ratings plummeted all the way down to 29 percent while the Democrats brawled among themselves. The reliable big-city machine leaders abandoned Truman and tried to save their own clout. (When Eisenhower refused to run, Boss Frank Hague of Jersey City crushed out his cigar and faced the political facts: "Truman, Harry Truman, oh my God.)" Southerners, the staunchest Democrats of all, bolted over civil rights and nominated Governor Strom Thurmond of South Carolina on a platform of racial segregation. Roosevelt had occasionally made noises about civil rights, acknowledged Thurmond, but "Truman really means it." The left turned to Henry Wallace and nominated him at a large, enthusiastic convention in Philadelphia. Wallace and the Progressive Citizens of America scorched Truman's harsh stance toward the Soviet Union, demanded the destruction of nuclear weapons, and embraced a "pink Communism" that would change America through evolution.[87]

The fractured Democrats were up against smooth Tom Dewey, governor of New York, who had given Roosevelt himself a run for his money (winning 46 percent of the popular vote in 1944). Before the campaign, Senator Taft scornfully challenged the Democrats to go ahead and run on Truman's compulsory health insurance, but most Democrats preferred to run away from it instead (the tumultuous Democratic Convention would endorse civil rights and ignore health care).

Less than a month before election day, *Newsweek* ran its regular poll of fifty newspaper correspondents. The group had never failed to pick the political winner. The startling result: all fifty writers chose Dewey. Only seven thought Truman's reelection would be "in the best interest of the country." Truman saw the magazine on his campaign train and cracked, "I know every one of these fifty fellows. There isn't one of them has enough sense to pound sand in a rat hole."[88]

Instead, Truman pounded sand into the Republicans. His speechwriters hit upon a new style. They gave him raw material—no finished drafts, no rhetorical flourishes. Harry unleashed his new approach during a fiery speech that woke up the dreary (they expected to lose) and weary (he didn't speak until late at night) Democratic convention. Speaking without notes in a fierce, hand-chopping, short-sentence style, Truman shouted his defiance: "[We are] going to win this election and make these Republicans like it—and don't you forget that." He refused to run away from national health insurance: flinging the Taft gauntlet right back at the Republicans, he announced plans to call the do-nothing Congress back into special session and challenged them to go ahead and pass their own (Taft–Smith) health plan.

Then Truman "set out on a campaign itinerary that would have killed a less sturdy fighter," as *Newsweek* put it.[89] "It almost killed me," recalled Clark Clifford. "They were long, long days. I was young and strong and in perfect health. From time to time I wasn't sure I was going to make it." But Truman kept it up through his grueling whistle-stop tours—fifteen speeches in fifteen towns over fifteen hours a day. Chopping the air and spitting out his familiar indictments: "Your typical Republican reactionary is a very shrewd man with a calculating machine where his heart ought to be." "These Republican gluttons of privilege are cold men. They are cunning men....They want a return of the Wall Street economic dictatorship." "GOP means just one thing these days: Grand Old Platitudes." He wasn't afraid to take down the local power brokers: "Ole Man Moore [retiring Senator Edward H. Moore (R-OK)] never was any good anyway." They "are a bunch of old mossbacks.... They are living back in 1890."[90]

Through it all, national health insurance remained one of his trusty themes. In Indianapolis—hooked up to the radio—Truman blasted the critics in his short-sentence staccato:

> What did the Republicans do with my proposal for health insurance? You can guess that one. They did nothing. All they said was—"Sorry. We can't do that. The medical lobby says it's un-American." And they listened to the medical lobbies in Congress.
>
> I put it to you. Is it un-American to visit the sick, aid the afflicted, or comfort the dying? I thought that was simple Christianity. Does cancer care about political parties? Does infantile paralysis concern itself with income?[91]

As the campaign went along, excitement built. Little knots of rural people waved flags and signs as Truman's train went by. Small farm communities turned out en masse to cheer. The crowds gathered and grew. They took up the famous shout: "Give 'em hell, Harry." By the time the campaign reached Boston, a quarter of a million people stood along the tracks; in New York, a million people lined his route.

Truman ended his final campaign speech—back home in Missouri (after a day that included speeches in Ohio, Indiana, and Illinois) with national health insurance. The notes—the "raw material"—banged out by the staff on the fly—illustrate the Truman treatment.

Each year more than three hundred and twenty five thousand Americans die, whose lives could have been saved if they had had proper medical care we know how to provide.

*This is greater number of Americans than were killed throughout World War II.*

I have been urging the adoption of a national system of health insurance so that the heavy medical expenses of the average family could be paid for out of an insurance fund.

This is not socialized medicine. It is plain American common sense!

The Republican Congress *flatly refused* to act.

We must have a Congress that will consider the health of our people *more* important than the health of the livestock of our farms.

We must have a Democratic Congress.[92]

On election day, Truman made up for his low margins in eastern cities (Wallace cut into his vote and threw the Northeast to Dewey) by rolling up a big vote in the Republican heartlands. Truman won by 2 million popular votes (4 percent) and 114 electoral votes; the Democrats took back both chambers of Congress. The results even seemed to thrill some opponents. The reliably Republican *Time* Magazine gushed that this was a wonderful lesson in American democracy for the world to see. *Newsweek* cheered "the greatest upset in American political history."[93]

Truman had begun and ended his extraordinary campaign with national health insurance. The idea was back in political play.

### TRUMAN TRIES AGAIN

After his extraordinary victory, Truman delivered an eloquent inaugural vision of spreading freedom: "As more and more nations come to know the benefits of democracy and to participate in growing abundance, I believe that those countries which now oppose it will abandon their delusions and join with the free nations of the world."[94]

However, as he turned back to domestic politics and faced the familiar skeptics, a touch of exasperation crept into Truman's speeches. The 1949 State of the Union address is famous for coining the Truman tag line, a "Fair Deal." But compared to the bold speech of the previous year, it was short and almost grumpy. Health care was buried below a complaint about the St. Lawrence Seaway: "This is about the fifth time I have recommended [a health plan].... We need—and we must have without further delay—a system of prepaid medical insurance which will enable every American to afford good medical care."[95]

Six weeks later, Truman addressed the Democrats' traditional Jefferson–Jackson Day dinner. This was, he began, a happy time for the Democratic party. He reminded the party faithful how they had won the unexpected victory: "The central issue of the campaign last fall was the welfare of all the people against special privilege for the few." And then Truman got down to the problem at hand:

> We are meeting determined opposition. The special interests are fighting us just as if they had never heard of November the 2d....
> The special interests are on the job year in and year out—7 days a week, 24 hours a day. They work through their lobbies and pressure groups, through the editorial pages and the columnists and commentators they control. They twist and misrepresent the measures the people voted for. They are again trying to frighten the people with the old, worn-out bugaboo that socialism is taking over Washington.

The speech surveyed a host of issues—labor unions, minimum wage, housing programs, river basins, agricultural price supports, full employment. In each, the same forces that slammed his health proposals—selfish lobbies, powerful pressure groups and the bugaboo of socialism—were at work.

At the very end of the speech, Truman mused about a new strategy. "I did a lot of traveling around the country last fall, and I found that the people were vitally interested in what their Government was doing. In fact, I may even get on the train again and make another tour around the country. If I get on that train, I am going to tell the people how their Government is getting along. And I know how to tell them."[96]

For six exhilarating weeks, this beleaguered and often maladroit politician had whipped up crowds across the heartland. He had found his voice. Could that magic somehow be recaptured and applied to the political debates in Washington? Might another campaign rouse the nation and prod a recalcitrant Congress toward national health insurance? Harry Truman seemed to be on the verge of a bold innovation—"getting back on that train" and taking his issues directly to the people. Since he cared about health so intensely, why not give the AMA the same hell he had dished out to the Republicans? In effect, Truman was groping toward a new—a modern and media-savvy—presidency.

His allies tried to push the president along. They announced that the president "would do everything possible" (Federal Security Administrator Oscar Ewing), that he would probably go on the radio (AFL President

William Green), and that he would "go all out" (Senator James Murray) to rally the public for national health insurance.[97]

But Truman never did leap into the fray. On the contrary, he practically refused to talk about his health plan. A reporter asked in March when the president was going to send his national health bill to Congress. Truman said only, "It isn't ready. Whenever it's ready. I will let you know." At the same press conference another reporter asked, "Are there any further plans for getting on the train and telling the people about your program?" Truman said only they'd have plenty of time to pack their bags. In April, after Truman had submitted his plan, reporters tried again, "Do you plan a radio speech to go with your national health program?" Harry answered mildly, "We have had it under consideration, and it is still under consideration. I will announce it in plenty of time so that all of you will know."[98]

Reporters were still waiting for the old campaign lightning to strike again at the first press conference in May: "Mr. President, is it getting near train time for a speaking tour on the health program?" Harry joked the question aside:

The President: No. No. I will give you plenty of notice so that you can pack your trunk.

Q: Will we need a trunk?

The President: You needed one last fall. [laughter]

Q: Mr. President, do you mean to infer that we might need it again?

The President: Well, I can't tell you that. It's a little too early.

Truman still basked in his election triumph. But he surprised the press and disappointed his friends by doggedly staying out of the fight. The odd bobbing and weaving continued in one press conference after another: On May 12: how does your personal physician feel about national health insurance? Truman's answer: ask him. Two weeks later, a reporter pressed him about health care again and got the oddest answer of all. "I am not answering any questions—specific questions—about specific bills. My program is before the Congress, and I am for … all of them."[99]

Why did Harry keep ducking? Some historians suggest the answer lies in Truman's deep concern for careful process. The president had asserted tight control over his administration—no more feuding agencies touting competing plans—and his very success hamstrung both him and his health reform: all legislative proposals had to be cleared with the Bureau of the Budget. The green eyeshades at the bureau measured proposals against the administration's fiscal and budgetary policy—if legislation did not fit, it could not be designated an "official" administration bill. Throughout the winter and spring, Oscar Ewing worked with congressional allies to get their legislation in line with the 1948 report on the nation's health. Despite the effort, the results failed to clear the bureau's macroeconomic bar. The health bill got only the vague stamp of approval—the president was "generally in accord" with its goals but did not submit it to Congress as an "administration bill."

The administration's friends on Capitol Hill wanted to surge ahead—expand hospital construction, grow public health, and win national health insurance. Truman ardently supported the measures. But these were all budget-busters, and they all got stamped with the weaker "generally in accord" label. The distinction mattered to Harry. Some historians surmise that Truman grew so cautious in talking about his health proposals because he did not want to expose the difference between being "in accord with" and formally endorsing legislation.[100]

If so, neither the press nor the public grasped the fine distinction. On the contrary, news accounts jumped right past it, linked the president directly to the Murray–Dingell bill, and speculated about why Truman was not putting more muscle into his cause. The president had formally submitted his latest health care message on April 22, 1949, and three days later Senators Elbert Thomas (D-UT), Claude Pepper (D-FL), Hubert Humphrey (D-MN), and James Murray and Representative John Dingell (D-MI) filed their legislation. (Senator Wagner had retired in ill health).

This time, Truman's health message got right to the main event: "a nationwide system of national health insurance." Truman drew on the Ewing report to describe the limits of private health insurance—"those who need protection most cannot afford to join." And he seemed to plead with the southern legislators by emphasizing that "the administration of the program should, of course, be decentralized to the greatest possible extent"—winking away his civil rights agenda in the medical sphere.[101]

The press coverage was withering. "With disarming casualness," wrote *Time* Magazine, "President Truman sent up to Capitol Hill one day last week what was potentially one of the hottest political and economic issues Congress has ever had to handle.... Harry Truman had asked for the moon and left Congress in the position of having to haggle over the 6 pence [the financing provisions]. He had kept his campaign promise by submitting the bill. But as he well knew, his compulsory insurance proposal—the only real issue in the bill—had little chance of passing in this session of congress."[102]

*Newsweek* put it even more bluntly: "Truman's compulsory health insurance program has no chance for approval at this session of Congress. Its authors in the administration privately admit this." The real goal, concluded the authors, was to kindle enough enthusiasm to "force it through in some future session."[103]

The *New York Times* offered a stuffier version of precisely the same points. Mr. Truman "gave no detail on the cost or the methods of financing the program" (opponents would rush to fill in the gap with eye-popping numbers) and concluded that the highly controversial proposal "is believed by competent Congressional observers to have little chance of approval, at least in this session."[104]

The *Times* went on to note that the debate was complicated by two other proposals already sitting in the hopper. Senator Taft had again submitted his bill to provide federal funds for the poor. And now Senator Lister Hill (D-AL)—something of a health hero for negotiating the hospital construction bill—joined George Aiken (R-VT) in a bipartisan group blessed by the American Hospital Association; the Hill–Aiken bill provided federal funds to states that subsidized premiums on private insurance plans for the poor. Senator Hill was a liberal southerner and an old Truman pal, but relations had frosted over civil rights. Truman was never inclined to trim his policies; the rising tension over civil rights made negotiation between health bills even more unlikely.

In May, another Republican health bill appeared. Sponsored by Senators Ralph Flanders (R-VT), Irving Ives (R-NY), and Representatives Jacob Javits (R-NY) and Richard Nixon (R-CA), the proposal would establish a private insurance system and—in contrast to the other conservative congressional proposals—included no means test. The proposal offers our first glimmer of future President Nixon. Here was a young politician—in his second term—making his name as a fierce anti-communist (liberals would say *a witch-hunter*) signing onto a liberal Republican bill that emphasized private markets and paid attention to poor people's dignity. This was the first intimation that the ambiguous Nixon would eventually stand alongside Harry Truman—two presidents who cared about health care, failed to win their own signature program, and yet decisively shaped the policy debates long after their troubled days in the White House.

The great question remains: why didn't Truman fight for a plan he cared about? He had discovered his voice and won people over with his feisty "give 'em hell." He was surrounded by allies begging him to take up the fight and tantalized them with hints of another whistle-stop tour.

Surely, the distinction between an official bill (which fit the administration's budget guidelines) and a recommended bill (which did not) was too subtle for the press and the public—and did not preclude a public campaign in any case. Perhaps the president did not want to spend political capital on what was (the media all agreed) an almost certain loser. Still, the writers had all said the same thing about him six months earlier during the election; he had scoffed at them—not enough sense to pound sand in a rat hole—and proved them wrong. Or perhaps it was the sheer mass of favored programs—civil rights, health care, fair housing, reversing the antiunion Taft–Hartley legislation, and the rest of the Fair Deal—that faced fierce opposition? Where to begin the fight—over what issue, and against which enemy?

A final explanation puts all the others in context. Truman was inventing the modern presidency as he went along. He was the first peacetime president to inherit a government that sat at the middle of the national economy (spending roughly 15 percent of GDP, five times the level of the last Republican administration). He was the first to have a council of economic advisors, a national security council, and an enemy with an atomic bomb. He was first to confront the perilous Cold War. He followed Roosevelt—a classic charismatic leader who left behind the task of rationalizing the chaotic, newly nationalized political system. And, despite the skillful reelection campaign that left him and his staff exhausted, nothing in his life had prepared him for talking to the nation. What, exactly, should he say? How partisan could he be in a national address during the Cold War? What, in short, should a president's role look like? These were fresh questions in the Truman years.

The Truman story also introduces the daunting new checklist for bold innovations: coordinate the executive agencies who prepare the reform, gather enough (but not too much) detail from the specialists, overrule the economists who counsel against domestic programs (they are always budget-busters), rouse the public, and negotiate the change through Congress—the "graveyard of health reforms."[105]

## The Keystone to the Socialist Arch

If the proposal had no chance, no one had told the American Medical Association. The AMA mobilized for this campaign as if Armageddon were at hand.

The association retained Whitaker and Baxter, a savvy husband and wife public relations firm that assigned thirty-seven assistants to the national campaign against Truman's proposal. Their central theme contrasted state compulsion (cue ugly images of bureaucracy, socialism, and degenerate European ways) with the "voluntary American way" (sunny pictures of democracy, free enterprise, and small-town doctors).

Whitaker and Baxter shrewdly warned AMA leaders that "you can't beat something with nothing" and pushed them into supporting private health insurance plans (beyond the physician-run Blue Shield plans). In 1949, the AMA reversed its longstanding position and claimed that it had been for private insurance all along. The great American health alternatives—a universal government program versus private insurance markets—were now both before the public.[106]

The campaign against Truman's program included all kinds of inspired moves. The agency reproduced *"The Doctor,"* a nineteenth-century painting by Sir Luke Fildes (see figure 4): a country doctor sits in a dark cottage, head in hand, watching over a sick child as the frightened father hovers near the doorway and the mother rests her head on a nearby table—exhausted, perhaps weeping. Through the window, dawn is breaking, signifying that the young patient has pulled through the night and will recover—because of the work of this wise, caring doctor. Whitaker and Baxter printed 70,000 copies and added a celebrated caption— "KEEP POLITICS OUT OF THIS PICTURE … Compulsory medicine is political medicine…. It would bind up your family's health in red tape. It would result in heavy payroll taxes—and inferior medical care for you and your family. Don't let that happen here."[107]

The campaign's real brilliance, however, lay not in its sometimes overheated imagery but in its extraordinary organization of organizations. The American Medical Association framed arguments and then lined up hundreds of groups (by one count, 1,829 of them) to echo their indignation over socialized medicine. The campaign, in turn, appears to have inspired still other groups to join the AMA's army and proclaim their own all-American opposition. Letters, memorials, memos, and petitions expressing outrage flowed into Washington.[108]

The campaign's arguments filtered deep into the national conscious. We can trace its reach by following one rhetorical flourish as it rippled into the culture. Whitaker and Baxter published a fifteen-page pamphlet of questions and answers entitled *The Voluntary Way is the American Way*, which, deep in the Q&A, concocted a quotation from Lenin:

> *Q:* Would socialized medicine lead to socialization of other phases of American life?
>
> *A:* Lenin thought so. He declared: Socialized medicine is the keystone to the arch of the Socialist State.

Senator Murray asked the Library of Congress to track down the quote and, as expected, they found nothing like it—most scholars assume Whitaker and Baxter dreamed it up. But that did not diminish its effect.

The quotation first found its way into newspaper editorials across the nation. An editorial in the *Chicago Herald America* put it this way: "Lenin—the god of the communists is quoted as saying: 'Socialized medicine is the keystone to the arch of the socialist state.'"[109]

By March 1951, Lenin's judgment had radiated beyond the usual suspects. Oscar Ewing received a committee report on socialized medicine from the New York State Bar (he was a member) with a note reporting that the document was approved "not only unanimously but with great applause." Deep in the report—on page twelve—the committee noted: "On the highest socialistic authority, socialized medicine is considered a real major step in the direction of the socialist state. Said Lenin: 'socialized medicine is the keystone to the arch of the socialist state.'"[110]

The line—and others like it—slipped into the American rhetorical ether, recycled from generation to generation even to our own day. During the 2000 election campaign, for example, the president of the conservative Association of American Physicians and Surgeons published an essay in the association's publication, *The Medical Sentinel,* that ends by unwittingly dredging up Whitaker and Baxter's 1949 handiwork: "Lenin once said that 'medicine is the keystone in the arch of socialism' and I believe those who are promoting 'universal coverage' via government run and government controlled medicine know this."[111]

The administration and its allies struggled against the barrage. But it was a complete mismatch. Oscar Ewing gave speeches, engaged in formal debates, and furiously wrote letters to individual organizations restating Truman's original disclaimer: no one is proposing socialized anything. But the angry buzz only grew louder and the enemies multiplied. The AMA had thrown millions into the campaign. The entire budget of the Committee for the Nation's Health—the best-known group pushing Truman's plan—was just over $100,000. And all this over a plan that was unlikely to pass in any case.

Representative John Dingell sent a final, desperate plea to the president that summarizes the entire battle from the reform perspective:

> The campaign of misrepresentation directed against Health Insurance by the American Medical Association, with an expenditure within the fortnight of $1,110,000 for advertising ... indicates that this plan of slander and untruth will reach proportions which may well prove dangerous not only to the cause of health insurance, but to every liberal committed to the idea....
>
> Therefore I want to appeal to you as President of the United States.... I feel that you are the only one who can effectively nullify this pernicious AMA campaign and can actually turn the tables upon the reactionaries. There is not another force in the Nation that equals that of the presidency when it comes to disseminating the truth.... Your voice and your voice alone can and should nullify the effect of the $20 million slush fund and the thousands of comments and editorials either written by the "presstitutes" or reproduced from boiler plate sent out from a central advertising agency.
>
> ... You should take to the air.... There is no one else in the nation today who can do it. We have no substitute for you. While I realize that your burdens are great, for the good of the cause I entreat you to enter this fight in its final stages.

Truman, now enmeshed in the Korean War, waved away Dingell's suggestion. "At the proper time we will take the starch out of them," he wrote back. "I don't think the time is exactly right to do that."[112]

By the time Dingell wrote, in late 1950, it was already too late. As the media had predicted, national health insurance never made it out of committee in either chamber. In February 1950, little-known Senator Joseph McCarthy (R-WI), stood up before a women's group way out in Wheeling, West Virginia, and made national headlines by announcing, "I have in my hand 205 cases of individuals who would appear to be either card-carrying members of or certainly loyal to the communist party who nevertheless are still helping to shape our foreign policy." The chance for liberal reforms—already slim—vanished in the uproar.[113]

As the November 1950 midterm elections approached, Democrats began to run for their political lives. First-term Senate Majority Leader Scott Lucas (D-IL) wrote a letter to Chicago physicians that, as *Newsweek* put it, must have amazed the White House. "The opposition is using my position as Majority Leader ... as the basis for charging that I support ... health insurance.... The incontestable fact is that all the ... proposals for health insurance programs introduced during my leadership in the Senate are bottled up in committee, have not been brought out ... and will not be." Even the Democratic leadership was abandoning the program.[114] The backpedaling did not save Senator Lucas.

Joe McCarthy traveled the state calling him soft on Communism and helped boost Republican Everett Dirksen into the Senate. The Democrats, already divided between their northern and southern wings, now lost fifty-nine seats in the House and five in the Senate—a defeat that finally and fully buried Truman's long-shot domestic agenda.

## Oscar Ewing and the Move to Medicare

When Truman first took office, he had resisted the idea of a Cabinet Agency devoted to health. "Nearly every fellow ... feels that his specialty should be represented with a member of the cabinet," grumped Truman to Senator Sheridan Downey (D-CA), who was pushing for a "health care ministry." "I would have a regular legislature if I listened to them all."[115]

By the summer of 1949, Truman had changed his mind and signed a reorganization plan upgrading Oscar Ewing's Federal Security Administration into the Cabinet as the Department of Health, Education and Security. The change would automatically take effect unless the House or Senate blocked it. The Senate leaped. Senator John McClellan (D-AR) declared that the "prestige and power of a cabinet agency" would "greatly augment efforts of high government officials to force acceptance of [socialized medicine]." The AMA warned against giving Ewing a "higher platform" from which to campaign against the American way. Ewing thought he had been turned into the demon of socialized medicine—"the Man Doctors Hate," as *The Saturday Evening Post* put it. Senators lined up to renounce the reorganization plan during two days of debate and then buried it 60–32. The House also rejected it, for good measure. It was the closest the administration ever came to a floor debate on national health insurance.[116]

After the long string of defeats, Ewing proposed a tactical retreat. At a cocktail party in the fall of 1951, newspaper publisher William Randolph Heart Jr. planted the idea. Hearst said he was all for Truman's health plan, but the sheer scope left him uneasy. "Isn't there some small segment of the problem that you could pick out?" Shortly afterward, the head of New York Blue Cross, Louis Pink, told Ewing that there was no good actuarial data for people over sixty-five years old. This would made them difficult for Blue Cross to insure.

Ewing put the two conversations together: what about starting down the path to national health insurance with people over 65? He took the idea to the Big Three health advisors—Arthur Altmeyer, Wilbur Cohen, and Isidore Falk. When they approved the idea after only three or four days, Ewing knew that they had already hit upon the same strategy themselves.

Now came the hard part—persuading President Truman to retreat. "He didn't like the idea because he didn't like to give up," recalled Ewing. Ewing argued—over several conversations—"that we could not get the national health insurance program through that Congress, or any other Congress for some time, and that we ought to try for something less rather than lose everything." Truman—cussed Missourian that he was—wanted to continue fighting for the whole plan. But Truman generally paid careful attention to his subordinates. As Ewing later recalled, he agreed to "follow my recommendations if I really thought it was the wise thing to do."[117]

A month later, in April 1952, Senators James Murray and Hubert Humphrey and Representatives John Dingell and Emmanuel Celler (D-NY) introduced the new health care bill extending hospital insurance for people over sixty-five years old. The bill attracted little notice, and the president did not even write a message—he did not want to hear the AMA crow over his having backed down. Health reformers—Harry Truman among them—pushed for the reduced health insurance plan across the Eisenhower years. Thirteen years later, in July 1965, Truman's revision would pass into law as Medicare.

YOU ALONE, PRESIDENT TRUMAN

President Lyndon Johnson signed Medicare into law at the Harry S. Truman library in Independence, Missouri. A jubilant Harry Truman—still spry at eighty-one—told LBJ that "no single honor ever paid him had touched him more deeply." In his public remarks, Truman added, "You have done me a great honor in coming here today. You have made me a very, very happy man."[118]

President Johnson explained what they were all doing in Independence: "It was really Harry Truman of Missouri who planted the seeds of compassion and duty which have today flowered into care for the sick, and serenity for the fearful.... Many men can make many proposals. Many men can draft many laws." And then he got to the heart of Truman's legacy: "But few ... have the courage to stake reputation, and position, and the effort of a lifetime upon a cause when there are so few that share it."

Johnson reached back and quoted Truman's very first health message—from November 14, 1945—then turned to Truman and said,

"Well, today, Mr. President ... we are taking such action—20 years later." LBJ then recalled the original congressional sponsors. Hubert Humphrey was now vice president and stood beaming behind the presidents. John Dingell had died in office in 1955; his son John Dingell Jr. immediately stepped in to represent the district (and, as of this writing, is still there, after more than fifty years in Congress). Emmanuel Celler was now the powerful chair of the judiciary committee. Johnson paused to remember Senators Murray and Wagner and Representative John Dingell, all dead.

The ceremony ended with a rare moment in presidential history. One liberal president turned, looked at another, and prepared to sign Medicare with these words: "Perhaps you alone, President Truman—perhaps you alone can fully know just how grateful I am for this day."

Two clashing visions emerged from the Truman administration. First, obviously, was Harry's own fervent belief that all Americans deserved a right to health care. His plans, designed during the Roosevelt administration, would use the Social Security system to guarantee that—as LBJ would put it—America would "never ignore or ... spurn those who suffer untended in a land that is bursting with abundance." That was simply a prettier way to phrase Truman's own description of his days as county judge: "I built a hospital to take care of these people."

Putting national health insurance into play pushed opponents to develop their alternative. During the Truman years, conservatives refined the idea of a private insurance system with some provision for the poor who could not afford or find it. Even the AMA acquiesced. In the next decade, the employment-based private system would take off and grow. Read the Truman documents—such as Oscar Ewing's *The Nation's Health: A Ten Year Program*—and it is hard to avoid an unexpected conclusion: the private insurance system would come to meet many—not all, but many—of the goals that Truman had in mind.

The next generation would wrestle with and refine these contending visions: a Social Security–based right to health care versus a private health insurance with something from the government for the poor. That frame would dominate the health care discussion until Richard Nixon rethought the possibilities. Americans spent more than a quarter-century debating health insurance in Harry Truman's terms.

Of course, Truman would snort at the idea that private markets met his ideals—he was a genuine New Deal egalitarian. Health care should never be delivered as a species of alms. Look across all Truman's speeches and writings, and what jumps out is the intensity of his faith in national health insurance. From the special health message in the first year to the proposal for people over sixty-five in the last, Truman believed. He began and ended his fantastic 1948 campaign promising national health insurance. Here was the presidency as passion, the president as a man with a great gut feeling about what is right. Only one other Democrat, Lyndon Johnson, had such a powerful internal compass or felt health care so passionately.

Still, there is the nagging question: why did Harry not fight harder—why did he not get "back on that train"? He did not come out swinging again until after he had announced that he would not run for reelection in 1952. Why?

In the first round, Truman knew that he was "something of a dub" at public speaking. How could he stand up to the example of the smooth, elegant giant that preceded him? Later there always seemed to be a crisis: nationwide strikes, Cold War flashpoints (such as the Berlin airlift), communist witch hunts, and the Korean War. Finally, health care was always a very long shot in a Fair Deal full of defeated programs.

But then, Harry was used to long shots and, by his own admission, he especially cared about health. We have suggested another explanation. Harry Truman was inventing the modern presidency as he went along. The office had moved to the center of American politics, and it took time to fully work out the implications and possibilities. How to organize the office? What about the pressures for national unity (after a hot war, and during the cold one)? Just how partisan should a president be? How should the bully pulpit work now that the president led not just the country, but the free world? Truman was the first man to fully confront the questions.

There was no notion, in the 1940s, of a permanent campaign. We'll watch as different presidents continued to invent the modern presidency. Still, FDR and Harry Truman had the central insight: Roosevelt understood that nothing would get through Congress unless he himself went public; and Harry, when he finally found his voice, had an inkling about how: get back on the train. The next Democrat in the Oval Office, John Kennedy, finally put Roosevelt's and Truman's intuition into action. Kennedy took to the road—amid an unprecedented media blitz (featuring a new medium, television)—in his effort to win the health care plan bequeathed him by the Truman administration.

Even after that, there would be no permanent blueprint. Each president would have to work out what issues mattered most (amid the cacophony of competing concerns), how much political capital to spend, and just how to explain it to the people.

There is also something more subtle buried in Truman's vision. Like many true Progressives, he believed that changes such as civil rights and national health insurance were inevitable—part of modernity itself. We've seen how Harry dismissed opponents as living in a horse-and-buggy era. The opposition could only delay—it could never stop—a health insurance program. He believed that the things he put on the table would, in a democracy, inevitably win out.

And he was often right. Truman fervently championed a long list of seemingly hopeless reforms. He had no luck with Congress, but he stuck to his guns. Sure enough, many of the long shots he proposed would eventually gather momentum. His call for civil rights proved prophetic; so did his faith that the communist enemies of democracy would someday give up their "delusions." And as for national health insurance—well, the debate goes on, six decades after Harry Truman put the issue before the nation.

# CHAPTER 3

# Dwight D. Eisenhower

*Compassionate Conservative*

Tourists peering through the White House fence could see President Dwight Eisenhower putting on the golf green newly installed on the South Lawn. Ike posed as a bland, amiable, easy-going leader who left Americans alone to enjoy their 1950s prosperity after the uproar of the Great Depression, New Deal, World War, and Harry Truman. The president seemed, wrote one correspondent, "like a man who slipped into the White House by the back door and still hasn't found his way to the presidential desk." Ike did not aim to accomplish much—according to this common perception—and that went double for health care; Republicans offered eight years of calm between Democratic crusades for compulsory health insurance. Truman's autobiography calls losing the fight for national health insurance his life's greatest regret, but Eisenhower's barely mentions the subject at all.[1]

But history has warmed to Eisenhower, and historians now see a significant administration. With a unique style—a calm and meticulous hidden hand—Eisenhower reorganized the presidency, reoriented the Republican party, and wrestled with health care. He fell ill—perhaps more often than any other modern president—and, breaking with precedent, revealed the details: Ike's physicians offered Americans a national seminar on coronary disease. Eisenhower introduced a Republican health care policy that reflected his own personality: a man of liberal and compassionate instincts, unusually solicitous to the people around him, always wrestling with a flinty conservatism bred in his beloved Abilene—the small, dusty, peaceful, church-going town on the Kansas plains. "You mean to tell me," exclaimed a Scotsman when Ike visited Culzean castle late in his life, "that he was the man who was the American president? Why, mon, he acted like a man from the hills." "One of the better compliments paid me in recent years," chuckled Eisenhower when he retold the story. He was the last president born in the nineteenth century, and he always had to balance his nineteenth-century values (rectitude, honor, self-sufficiency, distrust of government, and something close to horror toward debt) with a twentieth-century sensibility (sensitivity, compassion, and a yen for consensus). This chapter tells the story of a president forging his politics and health policies in the clash between two different worlds and times.[2]

## IKE

Dwight Eisenhower's place in history was fixed, writes Stephen Ambrose, "as night fell on the Normandy beaches on June 6, 1944." What else in his life could match the feelings of bucking up paratroopers from the 101st Airborne, their faces already blackened as they prepared to board the planes the night before the invasion? Or the feeling when he forced himself to write (and save) the cable, never sent, announcing the defeat of the allied forces—even as he set the hazardous invasion in motion?[3]

The presidency pursued the military hero as much as the other way around. The Democrats tried to recruit Ike for their ticket in 1948, when President Harry Truman, hopelessly lagging in the polls, threw a stag dinner for the general and quietly offered to run as Ike's vice president. (Truman's *Memoirs* deny the story, claiming that he warned the general away from politics despite the "Eisenhower boom," but later accounts—backed by a recently released Truman diary—confirm the old rumors.) Four years later, an "Eisenhower for President" committee propelled him to victory in the New Hampshire Republican primary while he was still in Europe heading the NATO command.[4]

Stalwart Republicans briefly blocked the way in 1952. After twenty years of Roosevelt and Truman, conservatives itched to seize the White House, repeal the New Deal, and return to an isolationist foreign policy. Senator Robert A. Taft (R-OH)—who had harassed Harry Truman—now carried the conservative banner (supporters dreamed of a Robert Taft–Douglas McArthur ticket), and state party leaders from the South blocked Eisenhower delegates to the Republican Convention. The general outmaneuvered Taft, seated his delegates, snatched the nomination on the first ballot, and swept into the White House (with 55 percent of the popular vote and more than 80 percent of the electoral votes). Republicans narrowly won both House (a ten-seat majority) and Senate (a one-seat majority), though they would hold them for only one congressional term.

President Eisenhower reconciled Republicans to the large, new, active government that the Democrats had built over the past twenty years. "Should any political party attempt to abolish social security and eliminate labor laws and farm programs," wrote Eisenhower to his skeptical brother, "you should not hear of that party again in our history."[5] The New Deal programs were here to stay. But Eisenhower bent them toward his own Abilene values, pulling American government toward private markets, individual entrepreneurs, smaller (and balanced) budgets, and increased authority for state governments.

In health care, the tension between compassion and conservatism yielded private insurance. In 1948, Harry Truman could dismiss it as a failed idea that left most Americans out in the cold; by the end of the Eisenhower years, it had become the American way. The Eisenhower administration policies helped secure the outcome and tried, unsuccessfully, to push it further by offering the insurance industry incentives to market policies to the near-poor and the elderly. Those efforts failed (perhaps because they were too timid), clearing the field—as Eisenhower predicted—for bolder Democratic programs in the 1960s. By the end of the Eisenhower years, the American social welfare pattern had been set. Employers, backed by federal incentives (including tax breaks), offered benefits such as health insurance to most workers and their families; others—the poor, the near-poor, the old, and the sick—would have to struggle for protection under a patchwork of federal and state programs. This "shadow welfare state," as political scientists have dubbed the result, remains in place to the present day.[6]

*Political Values*

In a letter to a childhood friend, Eisenhower summed up his political philosophy of individualism, free enterprise, and fuzzy religiosity: "I believe fanatically in the American form of democracy, a system that recognizes and respects the right of the individual and ascribes to the individual a dignity accruing to him because of his creation in the image of a supreme being, and which rests upon the conviction that only through a system of free enterprise can this type of democracy be preserved."[7]

That left the federal government as a last resort. He had a standard response to questions about the proper role of government: as he put it to the press in 1960, "There are lots of governments, and the thing I object to is putting everything on the Federal Government. I point out to you people all the time, if a city or a county or a State has to raise funds ... they have to go into the market with their bonds. The Federal Government ... can print money. Nobody else can. So, it is always a little caution that you ought to tuck in the back of your minds when you think ... of bringing in new responsibilities and new expenses in the Federal Government."[8]

Almost every discussion about politics elicited Eisenhower's most abiding passion: fiscal discipline. He was ferocious about deficits and incessantly preached against them. Almost nothing in the budget was safe from his cold gaze—least of all defense, which saw steep cuts at both the beginning and end of his administration. In fact, Eisenhower's celebrated farewell address—which warned Americans about a rising "military–industrial complex"—was inspired by runaway military expenditures and the deficits they fostered. In the 1960s, leftists would read the speech as a warning about a power elite undermining democracy as it generated wars for profit; but Eisenhower was more worried about uncontrolled spending.[9]

His commitment to balancing budgets led him to cut spending (the military lost $634 million) in the face of a recession in his final year. "We should strive not only for a balanced budget," he told the press, but "get a small surplus to start paying on this deficit." And then the inevitable Eisenhower take-home message: "Ladies and gentlemen ... It seems to me that this [runaway government spending] ought to have a very significant meaning for all our people, everybody, everybody in this room that is a taxpayer." Democrats pounced on social policy cuts in the face of recession and military cuts despite a growing "missile gap" with the Soviet Union. Ike bristled at the charges (he knew from secret flights that there was no gap), but the charges of inaction would damage Vice President Richard Nixon when he ran for president.[10]

Yet health care was different. Eisenhower often exempted it from his harsh budget constraint. We'll watch health spending tick up while the administration presses the rest of its spending down. Health tapped into that other set of Eisenhower values and sometimes shook his fiscal certainties. Eisenhower's presidency demonstrated the allure—or the inescapable pressure—that would repeatedly drive conservative Republican presidents to except health care from the knife they used to cut domestic programs.

The health care exception reflects a side to Eisenhower that has drawn little attention but that profoundly shaped his management of both issues and his subordinates. Simply put, Eisenhower cared about people. Perhaps this grew out of his understanding of the importance of every soldier to an effective fighting force. Perhaps it reflected his small-town Kansas roots. In any case, it was pure Eisenhower. His empathy came to be embodied in a philosophy of government his aides regularly quoted back to him. In a 1954 memo to the president proposing a health care policy, the first secretary of Health, Education, and Welfare, Oveta Culp Hobby, quoted his instructions to her: "In all things which deal with people be liberal, be human. In all those which deal with the people's money or their economy, or their form of government, be conservative."[11]

Six years later, on January 12, 1961, Eisenhower's third secretary of HEW, Arthur Flemming, wrote in a warm, personal letter of resignation as the administration packed up to leave Washington. "You have provided me with the privilege of observing at first hand your deep concern with human needs.... When you have been called upon to make policy decisions in these areas, you have done so in light of the standard that you established very early in your Administration, namely, that in matters dealing with the people's money, their economy, or their form of government, we should be conservative, but that in all things dealing with people, we should 'be liberal, be human.'"[12]

Eisenhower had a temper that burst and faded, as Greenstein puts it, like a summer thunderstorm. However, his respect for his subordinates (Vice President Richard Nixon was a famous exception)—and their affection for him—runs right through the president's papers. Always the two sides to Ike: the conservative who is deeply skeptical of the federal government and fearful of its deficits and, at the same time, the empathetic leader, concerned about helping people and eager to be liberal, to be human.[13]

## Organization

Eisenhower had a special administrative touch. Fresh from West Point and itching to jump into the war in 1916, he exuberantly oversaw his unit's preparations for the trip to France. "Too much depended on our walking up that gangplank," wrote Ike, "for me to take a chance on any slip anywhere." His superiors were so impressed by his organizational ability that—to Ike's everlasting chagrin—they pulled him off the boat and put him in charge of a new training camp in Gettysburg.[14]

Eisenhower always took administration seriously. To many people, he wrote in his autobiography, "organization seems to summon visions of rigidity ... deadly routine and stodginess in human affairs"—precisely the attitude exuded by Democratic administrations from FDR to JFK and on to Bill Clinton. But Eisenhower firmly rejected "creative chaos." Rather, he insisted, skillful organization is essential to successful enterprises—especially large ones. Good organizations "simplify, clarify, expedite and coordinate." They cannot transform a dunce into a successful leader, but they do offer "a bulwark against chaos, confusion, delay and failure."[15]

Eisenhower brought his organizational style to presidential leadership. He created new positions that are still indispensable: the White House chief of staff, the congressional relations office, and the presidential assistant for national security affairs (now known as the national security advisor).[16] His White House emphasized formal processes, meticulous staff work, the delegation of authority to Cabinet secretaries and a team-based approach to decision-making—a style that almost all Republicans (and no Democrats) would emulate. He expected subordinates to make decisions over their own area; if Ike had to make a decision that belonged to the subordinate, he commented, he'd admonish them the first time and begin looking for a replacement the second. Deference to his subordinates also meant giving them an opportunity to make their case as controversial issues came before him. He treated each opinion with grave respect.[17]

For this style of leadership to work, Eisenhower needed to attract talented people, keep their loyalty, and fashion them into effective teams. Eisenhower's team-building—more fashionable now than it was in the 1950s and 1960s, when FDR's freewheeling was the stuff of legend—led him to pay careful attention to his staff and Cabinet. The administration's files are filled with solicitous, self-effacing notes such as this one to sent Secretary of HEW Hobby on Thanksgiving eve in 1953:

> Now I admit that when anyone gets as high ranking as you are, such a person has gotten beyond the place where he or she can be "ordered about." But I would deem it a very great personal favor if you would get out of this place no later than tomorrow morning [Wednesday] and not be back before Monday. My whole purpose in making this request would be defeated if you would lug off with you in a brief case full of papers.... This request is based on purely selfish reasons ... you are absolutely necessary to this Administration, and we want you to get enough ... recreation and rest in your life that you don't become bored, sick or just plain tired of your job.[18]

Was the Eisenhower style effective? Yes, and no. It minimized mistakes and, by many accounts, led to calm, quiet, steady management. By standing behind his process, argue proponents, Ike defused explosive situations (such as Senator Joseph McCarthy's (R-WI) chase after communists in government) and offered shrewd, steady, nonpartisan leadership through a series of crises at the height of the Cold War (in Korea, Indochina, Suez, and elsewhere). On the other hand, the inexorable process was ponderous and dulling; it could sink bold ideas and make the administration appear indecisive. Appearing to stand above the fray worked during some international crises, but it robbed the president of the bully pulpit that might have boosted some of his favorite programs.[19]

We'll watch how Ike's own values (compassion wrestling with conservatism) and his inevitable organizational process shaped his health policy. But, in his case, there was another important element to the presidency—illness and death.

## EISENHOWER'S HEALTH

Eisenhower suffered as much illness in office as any president since Woodrow Wilson had thirty-two years earlier. Ike's first incident, probably an unrecognized heart attack, occurred on April 16, 1953, a year into his first term.[20] Two-and-a-half years later, on September 23, 1955, he suffered a major heart attack. He first felt ill while playing golf—and decided it was just probably the big hamburger with onions he had eaten for lunch. That night, as the pain grew, he called for his physician, Dr. Howard Snyder, a seventy-four-year-old military surgeon. Snyder also diagnosed indigestion and kept the president under observation at his mother-in-law's home in Denver. When the pain continued, a consulting cardiologist came in, performed an electrocardiogram, and discovered a serious heart attack affecting the front and side walls of the heart.[21]

Eisenhower broke with presidential tradition and ordered doctors and staff to "tell the ... whole truth; don't try to conceal anything." Dr. Paul Dudley White, a well-known cardiologist, became the public face of the medical team. In a famous press conference, several days after the event, he described what happened, soothed fears about the president, and insisted that heart-attack victims could live long and productive lives—a significant matter thirteen months before an election. Later analyses conclude that for all the information the doctors revealed—Ike called the "physiological details" "an acute embarrassment"—they hid the severity of the president's condition from the public. Still, White's frequent media appearances became a kind of national health seminar—educating the public about cardiac health.[22]

Ike's own lifestyle might have subverted his doctor's message. He freely dispensed the recipe for his "vegetable soup," which involved boiling a mess of meat and bone marrow for a full day before draining the liquid and letting it sit overnight for a hard layer of fat to form on the stock. Although this could be removed—as Ike mildly put it—"some people ... like their soup very rich and do not remove more than half the fat."[23]

Eisenhower spent thirteen weeks recovering from his heart attack, first in the hospital, then at his Gettysburg farm. The president's popularity soared as he left the hospital sporting jaunty red pajamas with an answer to the inevitable question—*much better thanks*—stitched above the pocket. Five months later, when Dr. Snyder cleared the president to run for a second term, Eisenhower announced his candidacy. His health became a major campaign issue—Democrat Adlai Stevenson suggested that the shadowy Richard Nixon would soon have his finger on the hydrogen bomb. During the campaign, Ike suffered his second major illness—an acute attack of a recurring abdominal condition known as "regional enteritis," or Crohn's disease, which resulted in recurrent blockages of his small intestine, leading to episodes of pain, nausea, and vomiting. He underwent surgery on June 8, 1956—just five months before election day.[24] The president remained in the hospital for twenty-one days. It simply made the president a more sympathetic figure, and he won in a landslide, with more than 58 percent of the popular vote.

A year after winning reelection, in November 1957, Ike was sitting at his desk when, quite suddenly, he could not hold his pen, read a note, or explain to his secretary what was happening to him. "Words—but not the ones I wanted—came to my tongue." The stroke probably resulted from his physicians' failures. Because of complications from the first heart attack, the physicians should have treated Eisenhower with blood thinning or anticoagulant medicine, and they should have treated his high blood pressure more aggressively. Although the stroke was minor, Eisenhower never fully recovered. "From that time onward," he wrote eight years later, "I have frequently experienced difficulty in prompt utterance of the word I seek." He had to speak slowly and carefully, and if other people didn't particularly notice, concluded Eisenhower, "it certainly is [noticeable] to me."[25]

Two weeks after his stroke, Eisenhower tried to prove both to himself and to the public that he was capable of continuing in office by traveling to a NATO conference in Paris. The trip "was a simple logical test," wrote Eisenhower, "to see whether I was physically and mentally capable of serving as President. If I felt the results were less than satisfactory, I would resign."[26]

Even after Eisenhower passed his Paris test, his fragile health forced him to confront the possibility that he might have to cede the presidency. He coolly contemplated his own mortality. On February 5, 1958, Eisenhower wrote an unflinching "Personal and Secret" letter to Vice President Nixon. Citing the several ways in which presidents could become disabled, and the uncertainties in defining presidential incapacity, Eisenhower wrote out an agreement that, he said, he and the vice president had already reached informally: "In any instance in which I could clearly recognize my own inability to discharge the powers and duties of the Presidency I would, of course, so inform you.... With the exception of this one kind of case, you will be the individual explicitly and exclusively responsible for determining whether there is any inability of mine that makes it necessary for you to discharge the powers and duties of the Presidency."[27]

Eisenhower's health remained a major topic. Reporters routinely asked about even his sniffles: "You seem to have a cold, sir," noted Robert Pierpoint of CBS in September 1959. A month later a reporter from the *Baltimore Sun* followed up, "How's your cold?" When the White House announced a long foreign tour at the end of the administration, one reporter fretted that "this would seem to be a very strenuous trip you are undertaking," and another wondered whether, "in light of your doctors' advice," the president might not be wise to break up the trip with a rest stop in "a warm dry climate."[28]

Eisenhower patiently answered the questions, often earnestly and in detail. He carried on the national health seminar that Dr. Dudley White began after the heart attack. Medicine was at the height of its prestige. Ike's heart attack came only a year after the electrifying news (in April 1955) that Dr. Jonas Salk had discovered an effective vaccine against polio (which killed or crippled almost 20,000 Americans—mostly young—each year)—although distribution bottlenecks and uncertainty had Democrats calling for Secretary Hobby's resignation. Eisenhower used his own infirmities to talk about health and fitness and—a particular focus of his—to discuss whether American youth were going soft as the nation faced its tough, fit Cold War adversaries.[29]

But did all this affect health policy? One reporter put the question directly to Eisenhower six months before he left office and got a sharp "no" for an answer: "Now, I have not, in spite of three illnesses, felt that physical defects ... has [sic] been any decisive factor with me and in the way I have conducted my office. At times I may doubt a little bit my mind and intellectual capacity and my good judgment, but I'll tell you one thing: I never doubt my own heart and where it stands with America. And I don't think that the physical has had a great deal to do with whatever good I've been able to accomplish or the mistakes I have made."[30]

What moved Eisenhower far more deeply than his own health problems were those of his family. In September 1959, Mamie's mother died after a long illness. "I felt a deep sense of personal loss," wrote Ike, "while Mamie was inconsolable." The experience moved Eisenhower to see health policy in a new way. The following month, Secretary of HEW Arthur Flemming was in the Oval Office talking about health care for the elderly. The president "shared with me an experience that Mrs. Eisenhower's family had gone through with the illness of her mother," recalled Flemming later. "She had a chronic illness, extended over a period of two years, which required around-the-clock nursing care. He said it had virtually wrecked them financially." At the meeting, Eisenhower instructed Flemming to prepare a comprehensive health care program for the elderly.[31]

Tellingly, the program that came off the HEW drawing board would have more generous provisions for nursing home care—just what Mamie's mother, Mrs. Doud needed—than anything the liberals would introduce in the ensuing decade, including Medicare. This proposal, like the administration entire health program, grew out of the Eisenhower mix: a flinty urge to pare federal projects and stimulate market solutions, big-hearted compassion—especially for the people around him—and an inexorable (one might say ponderous) organizational process.

## A REPUBLICAN HEALTH POLICY: IKE'S FIRST TERM

When Eisenhower started campaigning for president, he could be excused—even complimented, he thought—"for answering 'I don't know' to certain domestic issues." He was fresh from Europe, and new to politics. His guiding principles, however, were clear: he rejected both "radical left and reactionary right." Centralization of power in Washington, he insisted, could lead only to "ruin" and "lost freedoms."

At the same time, we had to "recognize our responsibility" to alleviate the suffering of those in real need by "private and local institutions," if possible, and by government, if necessary.[32]

Running on this middle ground, Eisenhower found it easy to denounce socialized medicine: "I am opposed to a Federally-operated and controlled system of medical care which is what the [Truman] Administration's compulsory health insurance scheme is." Throughout his administration, Eisenhower prefaced comments on health policy by repeating his campaign promise to "use every single attribute and influence of the Presidential office to defeat any move toward socialized medicine."[33]

However—always the other side of Eisenhower—he usually followed jabs at "socialized medicine" with pointed reminders about the limits of American health care: "Our doctors will be among the first to admit," he declared in an October campaign address, "that—at present—too many of our people live too far from adequate medical aid; that too many of our people find the cost of adequate medical care too heavy."[34]

Speaking in Salt Lake City on October 10, 1952, Eisenhower repeated his mixed message: "Legislation which compels you to join in a Federal health insurance plan is wrong. It is also wrong—morally and economically wrong—to ignore the health problems of those who cannot pay the cost of adequate medical care." What to do? "Federal aid to local health plans that helps make medical care available to those who need it is right." The Eisenhower health policy would keep groping for ways to strengthen private health insurance and bolster local efforts to improve access to health care—always with a wary eye on the budget.[35]

The American health care policy choice would never become a yes-or-no question. Thanks in part to the Eisenhower Administration, Americans would choose between national health insurance (perhaps on the Social Security model) and national policies that subsidized private firms (employers, insurers) and state and local governments that provided the insurance.[36]

## The Department of Health, Education, and Welfare

After his election, Eisenhower proposed a Department of Health, Education, and Welfare (HEW). Led by the American Medical Association, conservatives had squashed Truman's effort to create the department, fearing that it would offer another platform in the drive toward national health insurance. Now that the White House (and Congress) was in safe Republican hands, the proposal did not provoke strong opposition, and

Congress quickly acquiesced. In April 1953, less than three months after taking office himself, Eisenhower swore in Oveta Culp Hobby as the first secretary of HEW (and only the second woman to hold a seat in the Cabinet). Hobby, had reorganized the Women's Army Corps during the war and, as the president cheered, developed "a splendid reputation as an administrator" (always administration). The Texas newspaper publisher had also been a "Democrat for Eisenhower."[37]

Eisenhower had allegedly agreed to let the AMA nominate the chief health aide in HEW, the special assistant for medical affairs. However, Hobby rejected the AMA's nominees—one reporter quipped that "none of their really qualified men would work for a government salary"—and Eisenhower ended up selecting Lowell T. Coggleshell, a liberal physician and dean of Biological Sciences at the University of Chicago, over the medical association's objection. This administration was supposed to be allied to organized medicine—rumors had Hobby declaring it "an AMA administration"—but Eisenhower defied organized medicine more than, say, FDR ever had.[38]

Eisenhower's first budgets took a hard line on spending. In his first two years, total federal expenditure dropped 10.7 percent. But Eisenhower remained sensitive to the importance of at least appearing to tend to health care needs. As he finalized his administration's first budget submission, he upbraided Hobby for being too skimpy on her health care request. Writing from his summer vacation in Denver, Colorado, he told her he was disturbed that she was proposing cuts that Congress had "flatly repudiated" the previous year. "These cuts," continued the president "affect items that are known as 'humanitarian' in their purpose. Consequently, we would be forced to stand before the public ... as being indifferent to the health welfare and educational advantages of the less fortunate of our people." He instructed her to restore the cuts, and to seek savings elsewhere in her department.[39]

The Eisenhower administration began with budget-cutting. Cuts were softened by little fiscal gestures toward "humanitarian" health care measures as an important new department gave health care a place at the Cabinet level.

## Pushing Private Insurance

In 1954, the administration moved to firm up the private health insurance system. Eisenhower used his second State of the Union address, delivered in January 1954, to signal the new health agenda.

As usual, he began with the conservative credo: "I am flatly opposed to the socialization of medicine." Then, the moderate middle ground: "The great need for hospital and medical services can best be met by the initiative of private plans. But it is unfortunately a fact that medical costs are rising and already impose severe hardships on many families. The Federal Government can do many helpful things and still carefully avoid the socialization of medicine." Eisenhower rattled through a familiar list of Federal government to-dos: "encourage medical research," "help the states in their health and rehabilitation programs," and broaden the Hospital Survey and Construction Act (or Hill Burton) so that it might construct rehabilitation clinics, nursing homes, and other facilities for the chronically ill.

Finally, Ike turned to the perilous ground of health insurance. Private health insurance, "soundly based on the experience of the people in their various communities" could and should cover most Americans. But what about high-risk groups such as the elderly, which were difficult to insure?[40]

The administration moved to extend private insurance to such groups by proposing a $25 million reinsurance fund. Reinsurance—basically insuring the insurers—would cover losses that private companies incurred by signing up high-risk people. This approach, pressed Eisenhower, would "protect freedom," reject "the socialization of medicine," and still make "the means of achieving good health accessible to all." It would also blunt Democratic efforts to win more ambitious and expensive programs. Memos flying about the administration termed reinsurance "top priority" and "perhaps the most important of the ... proposals in the health field."[41]

The plan went nowhere. Senator James Murray (D-MT) (who was still submitting national health insurance bills with Representative John Dingell [D-MI]) called it "a paltry, puny, picayune proposal." Murray got personal: "Since President Eisenhower has been getting free, socialized care almost all his adult life ... there is no reason why he personally would have developed any real understanding of this particular problem." Conservative Democrats were only a bit more polite. "The fires of enthusiasm ... which have been kindled in favor of this bill would probably melt water, would they not?" The health insurance companies also rejected the legislation. Neither a White House lunch for executives from fifteen large insurance companies nor Ike's speech to the National Association of Insurance Commissioners moved them. The insurers saw a threat: they would have to open their books to federal officials to prove their losses and claim the (paltry) reinsurance payments. And

who knew what kind of federal intrusions might follow from this opening wedge? The Eisenhower program posed a danger to the first principle of the insurance industry: keep all regulations on the state level,
where the commissioners are reliably friendly.[42]

Even the American Medical Association opposed the bill—to the great
chagrin of the administration, which was, after all, trying to head off
larger government programs. A mystified White House chief of staff,
Sherman Adams, called in officials from the AMA four days before the
final vote and tried to win them over. Why "oppose something ... which
firmly and squarely adopts *voluntary* health insurance as our national
health structure?" reads a briefing memo to Adams. "And yet this opposition is *not* based on possible jeopardy to members of the medical profession." The memo advises the chief of staff to emphasize "the philosophy
of the President on this bill and the strength of his views."[43]

The AMA refused to budge. So did Congress. The bill lost by a single
vote in the Senate and got buried in the House. Eisenhower showed his
famous temper. "Just stupid," he said about the AMA, "a little group of
reactionary men dead set against change." The next day, he complained
to reporters, "I am sure that the people who voted against this bill just
don't understand what are the facts of American life. I don't consider
that anyone lost yesterday except the American people." Ike promised
to fight on. His press conference offers an eerie premonition of a press
conference that John F. Kennedy would hold eight years later—blaming
the AMA for defeating Medicare. The disappointed Democrat promised
to keep fighting for precisely the bill that a disappointed Eisenhower
had hoped to make unnecessary.[44]

Ike could feel both the political and moral pressure to do something
about health care—the question was what form it would take. As he put
it to the annual Alfred E. Smith dinner in October 1954, "We know that
the American people will not long be denied access to adequate medical
facilities. And they should not be. The [reinsurance] program for voluntary health insurance is one further step in achieving this objective in the
American way. It is the logical alternative to socialized medicine."[45]

## Hushing the Budget Hawks

That same year, the administration bolstered private health insurance in
a more important way. During World War II, revenue officials decided
not to tax employer health insurance. After the war, as employer health
plans grew, the temporary policy remained in force but grew increasingly

chaotic as the IRS made ad hoc decisions about what qualified for the tax break and what did not. Of course, the foregone revenues began to add up. After all, tax breaks are a form of government spending—and by the mid-1950s, this one had a real and growing impact on the Eisenhower budget.

In the single most important health care act of his presidency, Eisenhower sponsored the Revenue Act of 1954, which formalized and expanded the tax break—health insurance premiums paid by either employers and employees would be tax-free. The administration went before Congress and—cheered on by a dream coalition of labor unions, the AMA, and the American Hospital Association—made its case for bolstering the American way of health care.

Although the effect on federal revenues could not have been lost on the budget-conscious Eisenhower, administration spokesmen became uncharacteristically coy about the costs. During Senate hearings, Senator Russell Long (D-LA) asked how much the tax exemption would cost:

*HEW Undersecretary*

> *Folsom:* We haven't any estimate on that.
>
> *Long:* If that is something you are gong to benefit everyone with, why haven't you gone to the trouble of finding what the expense will be?
>
> *Folsom:* It is very difficult to estimate ...
>
> *Long:* How much do you think it will cost?
>
> *Folsom:* I don't know.
>
> *Long:* Is it going to be a major loss of revenue?
>
> *Folsom:* No, but it will be a benefit to the people who get it.
>
> *Long:* Do you think it will cost as much as $15 million?
>
> *Folsom:* Oh, probably.[46]

Even this fiercely budget-conscious administration illustrates a principle that appears in every chapter of American health care—expanding coverage means hushing the budget hawks. In this case, a bold package was already in place; it was easy to endorse the political status quo (and it would have been suicide to oppose it). This success insinuates new questions: What if the Eisenhower administration had been bolder—and willing to hush its economists—in the plans it designed itself? Would a more ambitious reinsurance scheme—with real money on the table—have tempted the insurance executives?

The Revenue Act sailed easily through Congress and helped set employer health insurance into the foundation of the American health care. A little-noticed revenue decision in 1943 proved to be the butterfly touch that led to an American health insurance regime that the Eisenhower administration—with a most uncharacteristic fiscal nonchalance—now formalized. The health care debates would continue, of course; but by the end of the Eisenhower years they would be argued in a nation where most people had health insurance. Today, the tax break is still in place, and costs the federal budget more than $200 billion a year.[47]

## The Lost Health Year

The administration's 1956 health budget illustrates the Eisenhower governing paradoxes—generosity and caution, reform and retrenchment. Hobby introduced her HEW budget recommendations by reminding the president of his axiom: "In all things which deal with people be liberal, be human. In all those which deal with the people's money or their economy, or their form of government, be conservative." She then proposed, "during the *third calendar year* of the Eisenhower Administration, we ... concentrate on the health problems of the American people." The health year would include another effort to win the reinsurance plan (which could get health coverage, said Hobby, to 60 million high-risk citizens). Because Democrats had criticized the plan for ignoring poor people who could not afford private health insurance, Hobby proposed federal matching grants for state and local expenditures to pay for the medical care of 5.5 million welfare recipients at a cost of $62.5 million in the first year.[48]

The Bureau of the Budget rejected Hobby's proposal. When Hobby appealed, the director wrote Eisenhower, warning that the $62.5 million program for the indigent would rise to $90–110 million annually. Nelson Rockefeller, undersecretary of HEW, proposed scaling back the spending for medical assistance to $20 million in the first year. The BOB again rejected the spending "from a strictly budgetary viewpoint" but put the essential question to the president: "Is the proposed program 'paternalism' or an effort to address critical health problems among the aged, blind, and others on relief?[49]

Eisenhower gave the green light to Secretary Hobby's scaled-back $20 million proposal. "I recognize clearly the dangers outlined in your memo," wrote Ike to his budget director, "but I am quite certain that the pressures to do something of this nature will eventually be irresistible." If there was no stopping federal involvement, "it would be best to try to establish a moderate program in this field while there is in the

Executive Department a clear comprehension of the dangers as well as the anticipated advantages."[50]

In this prophetic passage, Eisenhower saw a rising tide in social welfare policy. There would be "no stopping" some kind of program that addressed poor people's health care—and, if so, better that it be his solid Republican plan than something from the wild spenders. Eisenhower could feel the political pressures—he made the same point during the Alfred Smith dinner—and struggled to divert them into modest Republican channels.

Ever the cautious manager, the president broke from his Christmas golf vacation and shot Oveta Hobby a note to tell her that approving even the limited indigent appropriation "worries me very much." How could the promise be made to cover 5 million indigent people, asked Ike, "while ignoring the other twenty-five million who cannot afford health insurance? We may be, here, opening Pandora's box. I am always uneasy when I start something [if] I cannot at least faintly see the end of the road." Typically, he ended by urging his Cabinet secretary to get some rest during this holiday season, though he expressed doubt that she would, in light of the "breadth and scope and difficulty of your program."[51]

What the nation saw during this holiday early in the Eisenhower years was a genial president playing golf in Augusta, Georgia. The memos flying in and out of his vacation reveal a president engaged in budget detail, respectful of organizational process, and—as always—torn between the suffering of vulnerable people and the insatiable demand for more. He was no ideologue, but recognized instantly that offering services to 5 million would bolster the case for covering 25 million more. And he understood that some form of coverage was—and should have been—on the horizon. The general in him fretted about an exit strategy. But he took the risk, made his choice, and explained it respectfully while expressing self-effacing concern about the burdens his aides de camp were shouldering.

By the end of the process, health advocates had a little victory—$20 million (or about 2 percent of the HEW budget)—while other programs, especially in education, took heavy cuts. But these were small policies—especially after the BOB was done with them. Eisenhower could read the historical moment and understood the unmet needs, but, bound by budget and process, he produced timid programs that generated little support—from the left or right—and quickly died in an indifferent Congress.

The president mentioned reinsurance again in his 1956 State of the Union address, but after two defeats, the White House lost interest in health care issues. It was not until the 1960 election began to heat up that the topic came hurtling back onto the president's agenda.

## THE SECOND TERM: MEDICARE RISING

Eisenhower had a difficult second term. "I made a grave mistake in my calculations as to what a second term would mean," he wrote in his diary in September 1957. He was the first president affected by the Twenty-Second Amendment, which limits a president to two terms, and he thought that would free him from petty politics. He soon learned differently. "I cannot remember a day that has not brought its major or minor crisis," he wrote after his fifth year, complaining that they all took a toll "upon my strength, patience and sense of humor."[52]

The list of crises began in Egypt in the summer and fall of 1956—right in the middle of the presidential election. The English and French hatched a plan to seize the Suez canal under the cover of an Israeli–Egyptian conflict. "The British and French won the battles but nothing else," wrote Eisenhower, who predicted that "an occupying power in a seething Arab world" would soon regret its folly.[53] At the same time—October 1956—Hungarians revolted against Soviet occupation, only to be crushed by Soviet troops and tanks. Eisenhower handled the twin crises in his quiet and effective way. Brandishing economic sanctions and working through the United Nations, he forced England and France to withdraw from Egypt while negotiating with the Soviets to keep the twin conflicts from erupting into calamity. Eisenhower used his presidency, for the most part, to calm international crises, rather than to foment them.

He was less successful back home. In September 1957, Governor Orval Faubus of Arkansas mobilized the National Guard to stop the integration of Central High School in Little Rock. A screaming mob and 250 National Guardsmen turned nine black children away as they tried to enter the school. Black leaders had been pleading for presidential leadership on civil rights—a national address on desegregation, a national conference for southern moderates, federal marshals in southern hot spots—but these were not the Eisenhower way. While Ike was vacationing in Rhode Island, he met privately with Faubus, who then returned home and, when the courts again ordered the kids to school, promptly stirred up another riot. Eisenhower now faced a direct challenge to federal authority; he ordered a thousand paratroopers from the 101st Airborne (the same unit that had jumped behind the lines the night before D-Day) into Little Rock. No one cheered the president. Civil rights advocates condemned him for inaction as the crisis—and civil rights trouble more generally—escalated. White southerners were furious about the troops.[54]

A month later, in October 1957, the Soviets launched Sputnik, the first space satellite. Many Americans panicked. How had the enemy beaten America into space—and just a year after launching tanks into Hungary? Eisenhower, surprised by "the near hysteria," calmly congratulated the Soviets and told the press that the launch only proved that the Russians "have a very powerful thrust in their rocketry," something that "did not raise my apprehensions." "Look," he snapped when Cabinet members pushed for more spending, "I'd like to know what's on the other side of the moon, but I won't pay to find out this year." The offhand, penny-pinching, reaction only fed popular fears. Complaints about Ike's tough cuts on military spending grew into a full-throated cry about "the missile gap."[55] Ike knew the United States had not fallen behind the Soviets because of information gathered by the secret U-2 spy planes—but he could not say so without sparking the diplomatic crisis that would eventually erupt anyway in May 1960 when the Soviets shot one down. The administration denied everything—an errant weather plane, it insisted, assuming that pilot had injected himself with his poison pin—only to have to eat its words when the Soviets paraded the captured airman and displayed the photographs he had been snapping.

With racial crisis at home and fears about declining security abroad, the Democrats won a midterm landslide in 1958—gaining fifty seats in the House and fifteen in the Senate, for majorities that no party had enjoyed since Franklin Roosevelt had been riding high. It was in this context that the Democrats pushed health care back onto the political agenda.

### Democrats Foment Reform

Toward the end of his second term, Harry Truman had reluctantly agreed to roll back his national health insurance proposal and focus it on the elderly (see chapter 2). In the mid-1950s, three groups resurrected the issue. Social welfare specialists, led (again) by Wilbur Cohen and I. S. Falk, hoped to cover the elderly (and, someday, all Americans) through Social Security; the AFL-CIO turned to the issue and began to match the AMA's firepower; and the surging Democrats were soon impressed by the political bang in health reform.

Congressional Democrats began modestly by passing two programs for the elderly just before the 1956 election. First, they extended Social Security to cover medical disabilities for Americans over fifty. The AMA fiercely resisted, fearing that the federal government would be making medical judgments when it qualified individuals for benefits. The legislation passed over AMA protests—we could have been "tarred and feathered as being against cripples," recalled one AMA official—and the program proved so popular that Congress soon dropped the age restriction. Next, Congress grew a small program that funded states to pay the health care costs of elderly welfare beneficiaries. The states directly paid physicians ("medical vendors" in Potomac parlance), but the AMA was so busy fighting disability that it only wrote a mild letter condemning the government foray into doctors' offices.[56]

In 1957, health advocates grew more ambitious and drafted legislation providing hospital coverage to Social Security beneficiaries. Most Democrats were not interested—the three top ranking Democrats on the Ways and Means Committee refused to sponsor the bill before an unenthusiastic Representative Aime Forand (D-RI) agreed to introduce the measure in August.[57] The American Hospital Association (AHA) immediately joined the AFL-CIO to put unexpected muscle behind the measure. Hospital officials were concerned about the growing number of patients who could not pay their bills. The Chairman of the Ways and Means Committee, Wilbur Mills (D-AR), opposed the Forand Bill but, deferring to AHA requests, convened hearings on the health problems of the elderly on June 16, 1958. The debate over what would eventually become Medicare had begun.

The administration showed no interest. Eisenhower spent his Cabinet meetings between 1956 and early 1959 demanding budgetary constraint and fretting over looming deficits. When nervous Republican legislators, facing the 1956 election, urged the White House to blunt the Democratic moves, the administration simply cranked out a press release listing its programs aimed at the elderly and created a Federal Council on Aging (in April 1956) that brought together relevant domestic agencies.[58]

When Wilbur Mills opened his hearings on the Forand bill in June 1958, the White House dispatched Marion B. Folsom, the secretary of HEW, to throw cold water on the idea. The administration had always opposed compulsory federal health insurance, testified Folsom, and it was confident that the private insurance sector could do the job.[59] Besides, the nation could not afford Aime Forand's $853 million budget-buster. The AMA backed up the administration with a national campaign that, perversely, increased the visibility of a proposal that had no chance of passing. The committee simply took the testimony from both sides and sidestepped the issue with the standard political gesture: it requested a study on the health problems of the elderly from HEW. Meanwhile, the president remained fixed on budget control. In January 1959 the administration even proposed cuts in hospital construction and medical training—popular programs it had always supported.[60]

But Eisenhower did green-light one important program during this middle period—a congressional proposal to offer health insurance to federal employees. Strengthening the private insurance system was always welcome in Eisenhower's White House. The president told the Cabinet that "public opinion would uphold action by the Administration to provide decent treatment of Federal employees on a sound basis." The result was the Federal Employees Health Benefits Program—a model program that is, to this day, a template for national health insurance proposals (such as the one proposed in 2008 by Barak Obama).[61]

*Make It Liberal*

Arthur Flemming succeeded Folsom as Eisenhower's third secretary of HEW in the fall of 1958 and quickly realized the perils of just saying "no" to the health care needs of the elderly. Flemming went to Eisenhower and urged him to move the administration out of neutral.[62] Eisenhower replied, in a memo labeled *Personal and Confidential,* "I agree we must not be reactionary or static in our relations to people." He promised to raise the matter at an Executive Cabinet meeting (always the correct organizational process with Ike). But Eisenhower then went on to "make a few observations—or pose some questions.... Is it not possible that, in the past, we have gone too fast—that we need a bit of time to catch our breath? Progress, in the sense of bettering the opportunities for 175 million people, is not necessarily hastened by additional expenditures." Inevitably, Eisenhower fretted over government deficits and his small government bottom line: "[O]ur ratio of expenditures to the GNP is too great.... It is quite clear that we must *not destroy incentive.*"[63]

Eisenhower's conservatism was dominating his compassion in the fall of 1958. In the popular view, Eisenhower was becoming "uneasy, irascible, crotchety and not quite sure of himself—dismissing politicians as 'sons of bitches'" and growing thoroughly disillusioned with politics.[64] None of this seeped into the extensive correspondence with his subordinates, which remained invariably polite and solicitous.

By the end of 1959, a junior senator with his eye on the White House had discovered the health problems of the elderly. "We knew it was a big issue and getting bigger every month," an aide to Senator John F. Kennedy (D-MA) later recalled. "We felt that it could have a very great effect on … the Presidential election in 1960." Democrats blasted Eisenhower for ignoring this and other social problems.[65]

After the 1958 midterm rout, nervous Republican congressional survivors asked the president about a response to the Forand bill. Flemming deflected by promising the report that Ways and Means had requested.[66] The HEW Report, released in April 1959, duly rejected the Forand Bill and then proceeded to turn up the heat on the administration. America's elderly often lived with precarious finances, exacerbated by health care expenses. And private health insurance was little help. Unwittingly echoing the Ewing report that Truman had used as a call to action in 1948, the Flemming Report revealed that only a tiny percentage of the elderly (9 percent of singles, and 14 percent of couples) had any medical expenses paid by health insurance. Heath costs were forcing more of America's aged onto the welfare rolls, raising government expenditures.[67]

Slowly, reluctantly, Eisenhower responded. He made his first public reference to the problem at the American Medical Association's annual meeting in June 1959: "We must work together," said Ike, to ensure that senior citizens "become independent, useful and creative members of our society." Then the familiar Eisenhower mantra: "In health as elsewhere in American life, our summons to greatness calls for a lively partnership of individual effort, with action by voluntary agencies and private enterprise and, where necessary, Government action at appropriate levels." When Democrats called for bold government programs, Eisenhower responded with calls for partnership and leaned especially hard on the qualifications—"where necessary," "appropriate levels"— to federal action.[68]

The following month, Wilbur Mills convened a fresh round of hearings on the Forand Bill and, in a dramatic turn, Secretary Flemming became the first Eisenhower administration figure to admit that voluntary insurance might not be enough to cover America's elderly. But the Eisenhower administration still offered no alternative.[69]

In October, a fascinating exchange between Eisenhower and Flemming almost hit on that elusive policy—one that might have rewritten Eisenhower's political legacy. Robert Burroughs, a longtime Republican booster from New Hampshire, wrote Ike an arresting memo. "Health protection is the biggest need of the aged and its present lack is the greatest threat to their security," wrote this solid Republican. The Forand bill, he continued, was "defective," and the Democratic leadership had not yet endorsed a solution—although that would be coming soon. The AMA, the insurance companies, and the conservative business groups had "no practical alternative to offer and should not be allowed to hold up progress ... in meeting an urgent need." It was the time for the administration to "take the lead in bringing this protection to retired people." He concluded with a play to Ike's soft spot: providing health care coverage under Social Security would end up "saving considerable money from general revenues." Eisenhower liked the sound of that. He underlined the phrase and put a little arrow in the margin: "saving considerable money from general revenues." Here, perhaps, was a solution to a human problem that could make his inner accountant happy.[70]

Four days later, Flemming and Eisenhower met alone to discuss the issue (with Eisenhower's personal assistant, General Goodpaster, taking notes for the record). "I'd like to send something to Congress," said Eisenhower, who then endorsed a health bill for the elderly based on Social Security. "Work out a pretty good-sized deductible—you know, like these automobile policies." Then Eisenhower turned uncharacteristically personal. Flemming later recalled the conversation: "He shared with me an experience that Mrs. Eisenhower's family had gone through with the illness of her mother. She had a chronic illness, extended over a period of two years, which required around-the-clock nursing care. He said it had virtually wrecked them financially."[71]

Flemming got to work and felt especially encouraged when Eisenhower revealed his plans to the press—putting the private conversation on the public record. Naturally, all hell (and the AMA) immediately broke loose. Medical officials contacted Eisenhower's physician, Doc Snyder, and urged him to reason with Eisenhower. A week later, the president called Flemming back to the Oval Office. "Arthur, I'm sorry," said the president, "but I'm going to have to change signals on you." The president then offered an unlikely explanation. "They have called my attention to the fact that in October of '52, in an address in San Francisco, when I was campaigning ... I said I would not use the Social Security System for this purpose. As you know, one of my principles is that when I make a commitment during a campaign, I'm going to live up to it."[72]

Eisenhower's explanation—he forgot about his campaign commitment—is hard to swallow, for he reminded listeners about it at every turn. What is more likely is that as soon as he went public he heard the opposition roar—conservatives in his administration, Republicans in Congress, his own doctor, the AMA, conservative businessmen.

Still, Eisenhower only backpedaled halfway. "I still want to get something up on the Hill on this issue," he continued. "Work out a federal-state program that will be financed out of general revenues." And then he concluded with a comment that delighted the secretary of HEW: "Make it liberal."[73]

Ike's first instinct—beat the Democrats to a Social Security–based health care program for the elderly—turns the standard historical narrative right on its head. The conventional wisdom sees a president stubbornly resisting the issue as the Democrats forged ahead and Vice President Nixon, nervous about the looming election, pleaded for a plan that might match Kennedy's. In reality, Eisenhower seized the issue two months before Senator Kennedy did and, even after being forced to back off, continued to reach: "Make it liberal." Had Eisenhower stuck to his guns, a lot of things might have turned out differently—his reputation for weak domestic innovation, the history of Medicare, and perhaps even the 1960 election. Instead, the "hidden hand" president let his policies develop through a long, tortured policy process that—finally, almost painfully—produced a policy far too late to shape the national debate.

## Black, White, and Einstein: The Republicans' Medicare

Health care became one of the hottest domestic issues on the Eisenhower agenda during the first nine months of 1960. The new chief of staff, General Jerry Parsons, reported spending thirty-five to forty hours on it in one week in March. The issue divided the administration into rival camps. Secretary Flemming and Vice President Nixon pushed for action. "For the Administration to ignore the problem," warned Nixon at one meeting, "would only serve to help compulsory health insurance get its foot in the door."[74] Others resisted. Bryce Harlow, a high-ranking aide running the Congressional Affairs Office, argued that "if any plan is put through, it will open to door to all sorts of legislation." Why single out the elderly for insurance? "The middle aged and children will follow."

And one "liberal" option, recalled Arthur Flemming, sent Budget Director Maurice Stans right "up the wall."[75]

President Eisenhower stood in the middle—torn between an urge to be generous and his need to be frugal—offering sympathetic reactions to every side. In a meeting in February 1960 he responded to pleas for action by again describing his own experience with Mamie's mother. "The President seemed predisposed to action," concluded Ike's secretary, Ann Whitman, in her indispensable White House diary.[76] But after talking to Bryce Harlow, Eisenhower returned to his eternal query: "How much can be allocated to the Federal Government to do?"[77]

After six weeks of back-and-forth—and five months after asking Flemming to develop a plan—Ike made a decision. Meeting with Vice President Nixon and Gerry Persons on March 18, he went through Flemming's proposal, weighing each feature against the proper "duty of the government," accepting some provisions and discarding others. Fearing that Secretary Flemming might be unhappy with the result, the president asked Nixon to contact him and "stave off" a direct appeal to Eisenhower.[78]

Three days later, the president flipped. He told Flemming that "he could not go along with what, on Friday morning, he had agreed to." "The legislative hassle on the subject," commented Ann Whitman, "is going full blast." The *Washington Post* ran a cartoon that featured the president coolly giving a thumbs down on the Forand bill while being handed his own health report, courtesy of the taxpayers, from the Walter Reed Hospital. His staff thought the jibe "wicked," but it echoed Senator Murray's charge about Ike enjoying socialized medicine while denying government help to others. A month later the president complained when *Life* magazine accused the opponents of the bill of "being extremely hard hearted."[79]

On March 31, the House Ways and Means Committee rejected the Forand Bill 17–8. That should have ended that, but as the *New York Times* reported on April 10, "the question of medical insurance for persons over 65 has become one of the hottest political issues in the nation." "Believe me," commented an unnamed senator the next day, "the heat is on full blast and we are stewing." According to one report, mail was running 30–1 in favor of the plan. Proponents would fight on.[80]

Still Eisenhower temporized. When Republican legislative leaders trooped over to the White House on April 5 looking for "an alternative for those opposing more radical proposals," the president urged them to remember "the impact on the nation of the *total* cost of the many individual proposals." The president again deferred a decision and, interestingly, warned Fleming that he could "talk about his studies" but should not "even intimate that the President was familiar with the details."[81]

Eisenhower deferred to his process and sought consensus among his people—in this case, the hidden hand was a heavy hand. But he himself was torn. In one meeting, with Republican legislators he confessed his "difficulty in arriving at a decision in this field ... since it was a matter of choosing between the lesser of two evils."[82] At another meeting, he lamented that "the only place where black is black and white is white is in moral matters or possibl[y] in arithmetic"—though, come to think of it, he continued, Einstein had done away with black and white even in arithmetic.[83]

Events began to tilt out of the administration's control. In April, both Senate Majority Leader Lyndon Johnson (D-TX) and Speaker of the House Sam Rayburn (D-TX) changed their minds and decided to throw their support behind the Forand Bill. Wilbur Mills reluctantly agreed to disinter the Forand bill that his Ways and Means Committee had buried the previous month. The *New York Times* explained the action by recycling the same metaphor it had used in early April: "Heat from the home precincts has brought the issue of health insurance for the aged to the boiling point in Congress." On April 29, Eisenhower told his full Cabinet that "in the existing political climate ... it [is] just not possible to refuse to take any action."[84]

Two days later, the Soviets shot down the American U-2 spy plane. The administration denied everything but, after seven humiliating days, admitted that the president knew about the flights he had been denying. Ike's most fervent goal, nuclear disarmament, crashed with the U-2. He later called that lost diplomatic hope the greatest disappointment of his career.[85]

On May 2, as the U-2 crisis escalated, Eisenhower gave Flemming "a reluctant green light." "Finally," exclaimed the normally stoic Ann Whitman. The administration proposed federal grants, to be matched by the states, for a program that would pay lower-income, elderly Americans a stipend with which they could buy private health insurance. Though it did not apply to all senior citizens (the liberal goal), the Eisenhower plan offered far more extensive benefits than any plan on the table (then or later), including six months in the hospital and a year in a nursing home. Eisenhower had frequently referred to the expense of caring for Mamie's mother, and the generous benefits may very well have reflected his personal experience. Ironically, Flemming called his plan the "Medicare Program for the Aged." Only the name would survive.[86]

The administration split the difference between two fervent Eisenhower principles. It put its faith in private markets and state governments despite the high costs. A plan with so many moving parts—a federal government program, state government matching programs, hundreds of private insurance company plans, a multitude of beneficiaries shopping for coverage—would cost more than a direct federal subsidy. Eisenhower defended the more expensive approach: "I am against compulsory medicine and that is exactly what I am against, and I don't care if that does cost the treasury a little bit more money there. But after all, the price of freedom is not always measured just in dollars."[87]

Eisenhower rejected a competing proposal from Budget Director Maurice Stans that would simply expand existing welfare programs that paid for health care to the elderly. But, even at this final hour, the president temporized. He entered a memorandum for the record: "The proposal outlined in Secretary Flemming's memorandum [will] be generally followed," recorded Ann Whitman, "(although individual Congressmen [will] be privately notified that a stepped-up public assistance would be acceptable)."[88]

Antagonists on all sides paused just long enough to denounce the belated Eisenhower proposal. The AMA condemned the plan. So did conservative Senator Barry Goldwater (R-AZ), who sniffed "socialized medicine." The AFL-CIO called it "hopeless on every score," and Walter Reuther of the United Auto Workers dashed off a scathing note to the president: "In all candor, I am compelled to state that the plan presented … after so many delays and postponements may meet the political needs of the Republican Party but it will not meet the health needs of American's aged men and women."[89] But even if the Eisenhower administration's proposal had little direct influence, it signaled to Congress that both parties accepted federal responsibility for the elderly and, more concretely, that either the Flemming plan or (in the sub rosa message) an expanded welfare approach would be acceptable. And that's just where Congress was heading.

Even though Wilbur Mills had agreed to vote again on the Forand Bill, he had no intention of passing it through to the full House. Southern political leaders were fighting bitterly for apartheid and knew that if the feds began paying hospitals they would soon be knocking on southern doors asking questions about segregation. Mills scuttled the Forand Bill (by the same margin, 17–8) and reported, instead, a plan increasing federal payments to the states that could dole out money—as they saw fit—for the health care needs of elderly welfare recipients. This simply expanded the medical vendor program passed back in 1956. The safe bill—even the AMA acquiesced—swept through the house 380–23.

The Senate did it with more drama. John F. Kennedy, the Democratic nominee for president teamed up with Clinton Anderson (D-NM), to sponsor a Senate version of the Forand Bill. If it passed, reasoned liberals, at least some of its features might be negotiated with the House. Senator Robert Kerr (D-OK), a Senate baron running for reelection, introduced his own version of the Mills Bill. He wanted something for his district that would not stir up the doctors. Senator Jacob Javits (R-NY) sponsored the administration bill.

In August, three months before the election, the presidential candidates—Kennedy and Nixon—tilted over health care on the Senate floor. The Kennedy–Anderson bill came up for a vote as Vice President Nixon furiously wheeled and wheedled to bring it down. The bill failed 51–44, with the liberals falling four senators short. The administration's plan to subsidize private health insurance could not even hold the Republicans and got buried 67–28. Then the Senate agreed to the middle ground, Senator Kerr's bill, by a whopping 91–2.

In September, Eisenhower signed the Kerr–Mills bill. With its late, ambivalent entry and a wink to paying for state welfare programs, the White House essentially deferred to the southern Democrats and their modest package. On the campaign trail, Richard Nixon admitted that the program was not enough and promised to push for the more generous, voluntary, plan the administration had proffered. Three years later a Senate committee reported that only twenty-eight states had implemented the program (only four with full benefits), covering less than 1 percent of the elderly.[90] That report itself reflected a renewed health care debate led by a new president with a radically different style.

## EISENHOWER'S HEALTH CARE PRESIDENCY

Americans thought their aging, avuncular president played a lot of golf, ignored domestic issues, and turned grouchy if anybody mentioned health care reform. The archives bury that view beneath stacks of meticulous memos—many of them penned from golf vacations in Augusta, Georgia, or Denver, Colorado. Eisenhower delved into details, fussed over budgets, wrestled with himself—compassion versus conservatism—ordered his people to rest up, and instructed the secretary of HEW to announce that the president knew nothing about details or studies (feeding the popular perception of Ike the golfer).

Some political historians have seen through the pose and celebrated Ike's "hidden hand." Standing above the political fray, always mindful of organization and process, Ike waited for consensus to develop before moving forward; others remain more skeptical of Eisenhower's leadership.[91] The health care experience offers support for both sides. Although the Eisenhower style came with costs and benefits, in the long run, the scale probably tilts positive.

On the downside, the White House became almost a caricature of stifling bureaucratic process, especially in Eisenhower's second term. Split between competing views, Eisenhower never stopped switching and temporizing. And the process always left Ike playing small ball—launching creative ideas, but never in big or bold ways. A modest program (from Secretary Hobby) to cover the poor in the 1956 budget, for example, lost most of its funding by the time Ike had adjudicated the inevitable duel between HEW and Budget.

Worse, the hidden hand did away with one of most presidents' crucial strategies—going public. As FDR had understood, an area as fraught and complicated as health care requires the bully pulpit. None of the early modern presidents used it for health policy. Roosevelt never got around to it, Truman mysteriously ducked it, and Eisenhower's governing style ruled it out.

Finally, the White House process turned the administration inward and made it hard of hearing, especially in Ike's latter years. Deft politicians—Lyndon Johnson, John Kennedy, Richard Nixon—heard the health care rumble long before the torturous Eisenhower process could produce a plan. It is easy to imagine—although the paper record shows no direct sign of it—that Eisenhower himself was compromised by illness. He acknowledges never fully recovering from the stroke that felled him the month after Sputnik. The health care back-and-forth in the last year may reflect Eisenhower's declining health as well as his grinding process.

On the upside, Eisenhower worked assiduously at health care, took risks (repeatedly crossing the American Medical Association, for example), and, in the end, crafted a moderate Republican position that shifted the American health care debate. With some help from the administration, the system evolved in exactly the direction Ike was pointing.

Eisenhower successfully bolstered the private health insurance system for workers and their dependents. The tax exemption for workplace health insurance spurred the rapid growth of private plans—a distinctive American institution that now covers 160 million people. In the 1950s the United States chose its unique social insurance route—one based on employment rather than on citizenship.

Eisenhower's faith in private health insurance also led him to support the Federal Employee Health Benefits Program, which insured millions of government workers and demonstrated that the federal government could run a large, federally financed, privately administered, market-based health insurance program. Fifty years later, it now inspires contemporary advocates of national health insurance, who invoke a program Eisenhower approved for ends Eisenhower always dreaded.

Eisenhower tried to induce private insurers to conquer more difficult terrain—underwriting the poor and the old. Two major legislative proposals—the reinsurance plan in the first term and the Flemming plan in the second—both aimed to use government to leverage the industry into the high risk populations. Both failed, setting the stage for the great health care clashes of the 1960s, but with most workers now covered, the debates would be fundamentally different from the debate of the 1940s.

On a personal level, Eisenhower never found health care an easy issue, for it always threatened his deepest commitments—small government, fiscal prudence, free markets, and private initiative. But he stuck to it and even pondered truly daring moves—he and Secretary of HEW Flemming briefly agreed to plunge impetuously ahead with a catastrophic insurance plan for all the elderly under Social Security. We might be writing quite a different history had they stuck to it. But leaping wildly out of bureaucratic process would not have been Ike. Even for compassionate Republican war heroes, that kind of decisive health care action was a bridge too far.

Where did the momentary impulse to be radical—and the sustained impulse to "make it liberal"—arise from? Eisenhower's interest in health care was as much personal as anything else. From the earliest moments of his campaign to the waning moments of his presidency, he consistently spoke publicly and privately about the failings of the health care system, the punishing cost of illness, and the need to help individuals suffering under the burden of ill health. Particularly in private exchanges with his close aides, Eisenhower displayed a personal compassion that matched his public persona. In the end, he repeatedly curbed his deep urge to economize when health care was at stake.

Although we will never know for sure the origins of this compassion, one important influence seems to have been his and his family's experience with illness. Illness does not respect the boundaries of income, class, education, or party. It is an equal-opportunity affliction, and when presidents feel its effects, the policy consequences are tangible. President Eisenhower talked in a deeply personal way about the ruinous effects of Mamie's mother's illness as he pondered his most dramatic initiatives—and even the modest program that came out generously covered exactly the kinds of costs she and her family had faced. The personal dimension is particularly striking not just for Ike, but for all Republicans, because taking the initiative on health problems raises a great deal more ideological dissonance for them than it does for Democrats.

We can underscore the Eisenhower legacy by returning to the final Senate vote on the Kerr–Mills bill. The two senators who voted nay included Barry Goldwater and Strom Thurmond (at the time, D-SC). Four years later, Goldwater would run as the Republican candidate for president, propounding a simple principle: the federal government has no business in health care. In fact, it had no business in any business. Goldwater would get buried in 1964, but his antitax, anti–federal government vision would revolutionize his party and lead, eventually, to a new Republican era. But the Goldwater perspective never gained traction in health care. No president, no matter how conservative—not Ronald Reagan, not George W. Bush—would subscribe to the view that the government had no business helping Americans get access to health care. The second Eisenhower term vividly demonstrates exactly how and why no president—no matter how distracted or disinterested or focused on deficits—can escape the demands for health care reform. In the end, the Eisenhower approach—mixing social concern, federal money, state decision-making, and reliance on private markets—formed a solid foundation for conservatives pondering the health care system. Every Republican administration would return to it.

Finally, the Eisenhower era illustrates five ingredients for winning large-scale reforms in domestic policy, both through what reformers did and what they failed to do. First, a group of experts rises up with a plan—such as the Forand bill, which no one thought worth sponsoring when it first circulated. Second, the plan stirs a powerful, popular reaction (heat from the grassroots, as the *New York Times* kept putting it). Third—and we move now into what did not happen—a bold administration bursts out of its budget-bound administrative process and chooses a plan that will answer the popular movement. Fourth, a president goes public and uses the bully pulpit to stir up support and intimidate opponents. Fifth, and simultaneously, the president works the administrative intricacies of Capitol Hill, where (especially in the Eisenhower era) barons such as Wilbur Mills can bottle up any bill, and the devil with bold alternatives, powerful presidents, or fire from the grassroots. It is a daunting process that illustrates the checks and balances in the American policy process and underscores the central conundrum of modern presidential health politics, already clear after three administrations: no president can escape the issue and almost none can successfully manage it.

CHAPTER 4

# John F. Kennedy

*The Charismatic with a Stricken Father*

No modern president evokes more brilliant images than John F. Kennedy: coatless in January, the vigorous new president takes the oath of office and proclaims that the torch of the American Revolution "has been passed to a new generation" while the old departing general hunches up, bundled against the chill. A youthful profile, caught through the glow of the Oval Office window, contemplates the burdens of leading the Free World. The children, Caroline and John Jr., tumble about the White House, tugging at the president's trousers. Warships circle the placid seas off Cuba during thirteen perilous days in October 1962. Star-studded receptions, state dinners, concerts, recitals, and touch football games all reflect an elegant and vibrant administration after sixteen dowdy Midwestern years.

For every glittering image, however, there is a dark one: the brazen couplings in the White House swimming pool; the sickly politician in almost constant pain, shot full of dangerous drugs; the family mafia with dubious connections, endlessly pulling strings; the public relations machine (and compliant press) that masked the frailties and projected the image of a man who was larger than life. And finally, inevitably, indelibly, the picture of Jackie Kennedy, her dress splattered with blood, clawing her way out of the back seat of the presidential limousine on November 22, 1963.

Kennedy could have been writing about his own legacy when he concluded his book, *Profiles in Courage,* by musing that heroic Americans always remain "elusive," troubling us with their "complexities, inconsistencies and doubts." Kennedy enjoyed more popular support than any modern president; in the first year, his approval ratings never fell below 72 percent and even now, more than four decades after his death, the public faithfully ranks him atop the presidential charts—in some tallies, as the greatest of all. Historians respond grumpily, voting him dubious distinctions such as "the most overrated public figure in American history" (as one group did in 1988), and routinely tick off his failures—a mixed record abroad, a meager one at home, and that muddle of a personal life.[1] But perhaps those who dismiss Kennedy are measuring him against the wrong metric.

John Kennedy was the classic charismatic—a leader who managed to articulate and embody in himself the aspirations and ideals of a nation. The 1950s' fears—born of Sputnik and the missile gap, of social stalemate and a nation growing soft in the face of a Soviet Sparta—were thrust aside by images of youth, energy, and vigor (pronounced "vigaah" on the touch football fields of Hyannisport, Massachusetts). Here was a navy war hero who had guided his comrades to safety, towing one of them by clasping a life preserver strap between his teeth and swimming against the current. John Kennedy led Americans into the messy, hopeful era of civil rights tumult at home and postcolonial upheaval across Asia and Africa. By promising to fight for human rights "at home and around the world," by insisting "that here on earth, God's work must truly be our own," Kennedy called—or seemed to call—a new generation to idealism and public service. Four months after the inauguration, young freedom riders began boarding buses with dangerous dreams of racial equality while more Harvard graduates signed up with the Peace Corps than with corporations.[2]

Kennedy's charismatic style perfectly suited a powerful new medium. His first televised press conference, broadcast live just days after his inauguration, drew an estimated prime-time audience of 65 million viewers. American politics would never be the same. Eventually, Kennedy tested the power of his televised personal style by trying to focus it on individual pieces of legislation—starting with Medicare. Reporters understood immediately that they were witnessing something new.[3]

At the same time—like most charismatic leaders—Kennedy disparaged organization and systems. He did not care about details, did not bother with a chief of staff, and actively discouraged routine and expertise among his close staff. Perhaps that limited what he might have accomplished. Ultimately, Kennedy's legacy lies in his ability to inspire and set the agenda for one of the greatest bursts of progressive legislation in American history. Medicare stands at the heart of this story: it provoked JFK's first all-out campaign for a piece of legislation, and because of him, it would go first when his successor lined up the Kennedy bills after the 1964 landslide. But the charismatic leader himself would never witness the legislative success he made possible.

President Kennedy's health care strategies are well documented in legislative histories. But there is a story behind the usual story: an inexperienced, image-conscious, chronically ill president who badly needed a policy success seized upon a high-risk, long-shot issue. This chapter tells the story of how Kennedy, grieving for his dying father, took enormous risks to advance a health agenda and, in the process, helped redefine the modern presidency.[4]

## I DON'T CARE IF IT'S HORSE PISS: ALL THE PRESIDENT'S MALADIES

John Kennedy radiated youth and vigor while hiding sickness, medical mistreatment, and pain.[5] When he was two, he contracted scarlet fever—an often fatal disease before the discovery of antibiotics—and spent two months in the hospital. After that, he seemed to catch everything—bronchitis, pneumonia, measles, German measles, whooping cough, chicken pox, diphtheria. In 1930, when he was thirteen, an undiagnosed illness caused weight loss and fainting spells, followed by appendicitis. The following year, Jack suffered recurrent episodes of flulike illness with diffuse aches and fatigue.[6]

By his junior year of high school, physicians had focused on Jack's abdomen as the source of his health problems. He went to the Mayo Clinic for a miserable month of testing in June 1934: "I've had eighteen enemas in three days," he wrote a high school friend. "[T]hey give me enemas till it comes out like drinking water." His physicians finally decided he had spastic colitis (which causes diarrhea and abdominal pain), or, perhaps, peptic ulcer disease. Later, they concluded that he had inflammation of the duodenum (the beginning of the small intestine) and the colon (the large intestine). Somewhere along the line, Jack began taking extracts of the adrenal and parathyroid glands, cutting his skin and inserting a pellet that dissolved there, its contents seeping into the bloodstream. The glandular extracts—untested and unproven agents long since abandoned—exuded powerful hormones that had terrible long-term side effects and that may very well have contributed to the development of the Addison's disease (a potentially life-threatening adrenal insufficiency) and osteoporosis (a softening of the bones) that plagued Kennedy's adult years. The adrenal extracts shut down his adrenal glands, causing them to atrophy until they could no longer produce their essential steroid hormones naturally. Later, after he stopped the extracts, he would become desperately ill from adrenal failure (Addison's disease); he remained dependent on adrenal replacement drugs for the rest of his life.

We still don't know the exact source of all Jack's intestinal problems, but there is speculation that, like Eisenhower, he may have suffered from Crohn's disease, which causes diffuse intestinal inflammation and dysfunction. The long bouts with illness quite dramatically illustrate the limits of prewar medicine. His doctors probably did him as much harm as good.[7]

Even as a child, Jack displayed enormous courage and tolerance for pain. He was surrounded by a robust, very competitive family led by a father who always pressed him hard. He and his family were almost ruthless in hiding disabilities. Jack went to Harvard and gamely joined the football and swim teams. By the February of his sophomore year, he was back at the Mayo Clinic, and the following month he spent two weeks in New England Baptist Hospital for an intestinal infection. A year later, in February 1939, it was back to the Mayo Clinic for more inconclusive tests and unhelpful treatments—Kennedy had been "in rotten shape" for months but resisted going back. The diagnoses changed constantly—ulcers, spastic colitis, ulcerative colitis (an inflammatory condition something like Crohn's colitis). The following year, 1940, Jack was playing tennis when he felt something slip in his back—the start of lifelong back ailments likely caused by osteoporosis. Off he went for a new round of treatments, this time at the Lahey Clinic.[8]

Then came the most unlikely turn—Jack's effort to mask his medical problems, enlist in the military, and fight in World War II. He failed the physical for both the Army and the Navy before his father pulled strings and slipped him into the Navy, where (after more string-pulling) he eventually took command of a PT boat (and as the result of still more political juice) finally saw action in the Pacific. On a pitch-black night in August 1943, a Japanese destroyer rammed his PT 109 and split it, killing two men and leaving eleven in the burning water. Kennedy rounded up his men, got them to cling to the floating hull for the rest of the night, and then organized them into teams for the five-hour swim to a small island; Kennedy himself towed one badly burned comrade, the ship's engineer, by gripping the man's life preserver (known as a "Mae West") strap in his teeth as he swam breaststroke. Right after they made land, he bravely, recklessly swam out again across a channel to the shipping lane, hoping to attract rescue, but got caught in the current and almost drowned a second time. The story, picked up by the press, turned Jack into a hero and gave his longstanding back pain a dashing new cover story—war injury.[9]

The following year, Kennedy had back surgery, followed by a stay in a Florida hospital for severe spastic colitis. The Navy retirement board reviewed Jack's maladies and ruled that the chronic colitis was a "service-related injury"—no doubt, they reported, a consequence of "50 hours in the water." Jack had another chronic condition officially elevated into a second war wound.[10]

While visiting London in 1947, Jack developed full-blown Addison's disease. In London, Dr. Daniel Davis made the diagnosis and reportedly gave Jack a year to live—the standard expectation throughout the early 1940s. But new drug therapies that replaced essential adrenal hormones, introduced in the early 1940s (and vastly improved in the 1950s), helped Kennedy control the effects of his Addison's. JFK had another serious illness to cope with, another round of potent drugs to take, and another impairment to hide.[11]

The Addison's never got out into the public view, although there were always whispers. During the 1960 campaign, the Kennedys leaned hard on their physicians to deny that JFK had "classical Addison's"—a revelation that would have undermined his image of youth and vigor. The Kennedy physicians responded to the Addison's story, comments political scientist Rose McDermott, with "a masterful statement, brilliant in its double talk." Richard Nixon asked his own physician about the rumors and, after hearing the details about Addison's, took the high road: "This is a personal subject and we will not use it in this campaign." Later in the campaign, however, someone—we don't know who—broke into the offices of Kennedy's doctors and rifled through the medical records. JFK's, however, were not kept there, and this office break-in might have slipped unnoticed into history if there had not been another office break-in during another Nixon campaign twelve years later.[12]

The medical troubles continued throughout Kennedy's life. In 1955, he underwent back surgery—now more dangerous because of his Addison's—and immediately contracted a staph infection that very nearly killed him. A priest ministered last rites to him (JFK received them four times as an adult), and Joe Kennedy wept for the loss of his son. The antibiotics saved Jack, but he was left with a gaping wound in his back that remained for three years.[13]

All this illness pushed Kennedy into plenty of medical hands. He relied on fine physicians and shady characters. No one oversaw the entire medical program—rather like the organization of the White House when he became president. The greatest danger lay in the sheer weight of medications—by the 1960s, he was routinely taking some twenty-six different drugs. Kennedy's most notorious practitioner was Dr. Max Jacobson—"Dr. Feelgood," as he was known to his celebrity clients—who began injecting JFK's back with a mix of painkillers and amphetamines (and perhaps steroids) during the 1960 campaign. He continued the secret treatments both in the White House and on international trips. When Robert Kennedy expressed concern about what was in those concoctions, Jack cut him off—"I don't care if it's horse piss. It works." Ted Sorensen, Kennedy's indispensable aide, speechwriter, and ghost author, reports being informed that Dr. Feelgood was treating Jackie. Later, Dr. Jacobson lost his medical license when the New York Board found him guilty of professional misconduct.[14]

One of the great medical questions about Kennedy turns on the effects of his pharmacopoeia. Did all those drugs affect his performance? In an analysis of one of JFK's weakest moments—the Vienna summit of May 1961, where Nikita Khrushchev bullied a passive Kennedy and concluded he was a weakling—Rose McDermott notes that Jacobson flew to the summit on a private charter plane at JFK's request and speculates that Kennedy's notoriously weak performance was tangled up in the side effects of Jacobson's amphetamines.[15]

And it went on. Kennedy's personal physician, Dr. Janet Travell, injected his back with procaine up to five times a day—this on top of Dr Jacobson's concoctions. Another White House physician, Admiral George Burkley, insisted that Travell's injections were seriously harming Kennedy's back and creating an addiction. JFK ignored the concern, craving the short-term relief. Eventually, Dr. Burkley brought in a prominent New York orthopedic surgeon, Dr. Hans Kraus, who was soon in a furious row with Dr. Travell over the treatment—he threatened to go public unless the injections stopped. Kennedy eased Dr. Travell aside but, to keep the peace (and, more important, to keep everyone quiet), continued to identify her as the family physician.[16]

The litany of medical troubles testify to an extraordinary level of determination and raw physical courage. John Kennedy forced his way into the military, pushed himself into combat, and served heroically through constant pain. After that, he chose the taxing political life—always juggling high-profile campaigns, almost constant pain, and furtive treatments. In the White House, Kennedy's chaotic operations thrust him into the center of every decision (JFK, like Roosevelt, did not like to delegate). While Kennedy pushed himself relentlessly, family and handlers carefully managed his physicians, his treatments, his pains, and his image, suppressing any hint of doubt about his fitness for office, and especially for the personalized style of leadership he cultivated.

Not many people, and very few presidents, shared anything like Kennedy's lifelong experience with illness, pain, and the ambiguities of medicine—lifesaving and useless, soothing and tormenting. As with FDR, the record provides no direct evidence of how Kennedy's personal health affected his views of health care issues. His lifetime experience with medical follies may have primed him to confront organized medicine, something he did with gusto. His dependence on health care services may have increased his empathy for those without access to it. But that same dependence created political risks for him and might just as easily have made him leery of a close association with health care issues: a pointed interest might raise questions about what lay behind it.

Kennedy did, however, live through another illness that affected him much as Mrs. Doud's illness affected Ike. On December 19, 1961, Joseph P. Kennedy Sr. had a major stroke that paralyzed half his body and left him in a wheelchair, unable to talk. He had been golfing in Florida when the attack hit. For months prior, his doctors had been prescribing anticoagulants (bloodthinners) to forestall a stroke, but the crusty Kennedy had refused to take them and then fought his family's efforts to call a physician after he was stricken.[17]

Joe Kennedy, the domineering and manipulative patriarch, had played a major role in Kennedy's life. Three months after the stroke, Arthur Schlesinger asked JFK how the Kennedys had all avoided the pathologies of wealth and turned out so well; JFK responded, "It was due to my father.... When he was around, he made the children feel that they were the most important things in the world to him." And no ducking the iron will: "He held up standards for us and he was very tough when we failed to meet those standards. The toughness was important."[18]

Evidence from several sources suggests that Joe's stroke deeply affected Kennedy and his views of access to health care services. Larry

O'Brien, a longtime aide, recalled talking to Kennedy about his own father's prolonged illness, which "devastated our family." "It [also] happened with Jack in his own family, and to his credit he was very sensitive to this. With Jack, it wasn't that 'It cost the Kennedy family a great deal of money to take care of Joseph Kennedy over a number of years.' No, his reaction was, 'My God, it isn't going to financially devastate us, but what do other people do if they have a similar problem?'" O'Brien put the effects flatly: nothing had affected his own views on Medicare more than his father's illness. And the same was true for JFK. "Medicare was highly personalized with me and certainly personalized with the President."[19] In a recent interview with us, Theodore Sorensen confirmed O'Brien's recollection of the deep effect that Joe Kennedy's illness had on Jack.[20]

Kennedy was a man of iron will and of considerable intellect and curiosity, with a strong pragmatic bent and without firm ideological convictions. Naturally, political considerations played a major role in deciding where he would move in domestic policy. But he brought with him, as have so many modern presidents, a personal history and experience with health care that opened the Oval Office door to medical issues in surprising and unanticipated ways.

## LET'S DROP THE DOMESTIC STUFF: KENNEDY IN THE WHITE HOUSE

John Kennedy won the White House by a whisker (a margin of 118,547 out of 68 million votes cast) and with no political coattails at all—the Democrats lost twenty seats in the House and one in the Senate. On paper, Kennedy still enjoyed a solid Democratic majority of 65–35 in the Senate and 263–174 in the House, but the winning margin (21 senators, 99 congressmen) were conservatives from the one-party South who routinely voted with Republicans and had been thwarting liberal legislation since 1938. The conservatives had more than enough votes to maintain their grip on power.

In fact, they often didn't even need to vote. The House Rules Committee, dominated by powerful Howard Smith (D-VA), could keep legislation from going to the floor. The committee was composed of eight Democrats and four Republicans, but two of the Democrats—Chairman Smith and William Colmer (D-MS)—voted with the Republicans for a 6–6 tie that kept liberal measures off the floor. To make room for its agenda, the new administration immediately moved to break the conservative stranglehold by adding three seats to the Rules Committee (and selecting loyalists to fill them). Kennedy was stunned to learn the vote would be a squeaker. "The ball game is over if ... we lost [*sic*] this one," he told O'Brien. Even with the influential Sam Rayburn (D-TX) (then in his seventeenth year as speaker of the house) pushing the measure, it barely scraped through, 217–212. As presidential advisor, Arthur Schlesinger later wrote, "nothing brought the precariousness of the administration's position home more grimly than [this] first ... battle."[21]

Kennedy made his own job harder by ignoring the nitty-gritty of legislative process. "He did not have a large amount of patience with working out the details," recalled his aide, Ralph Dungan. "He was interested in the ideas, not the stuff that flows from the ideas [such as] laws, regulations, systems, etc."[22] He was, adds Arthur Schlesinger, "an alien on the Hill." Larry O'Brien, Kennedy's talented director of legislative affairs, added that Kennedy "had been on the Hill fourteen years, but he had [never] been part of the establishment." He had been a junior partner. He never enjoyed the company of congressional politicians. "I mean, he knew them all, they all knew him, but he wasn't an intimate, really, of any of them." And he was not much good at the game of persuasion, Congress style. "It wasn't his nature to put the arm on you directly, frontally," concludes O'Brien. Although Kennedy's charm was legendary—his friends adored him—he never learned to cultivate the legislators whose support was critical to his programs.[23]

The coolness ran both ways. "All that Mozart string music and ballet dancing down there [in the White House]," groused a representative from rural Tennessee. "He's too elegant for me. I can't talk to him."[24] The sophistication seemed fabulous to northeastern elites, but it was alien to many of the congressional bulls from the South and Midwest. The Democratic party would soon crack up over civil rights, but beneath the policy dispute ran long-dormant cultural differences that leaders such as Richard Nixon and Ronald Reagan would adroitly deploy—foreshadowed in the mutual contempt between the Kennedy and Eisenhower styles.

Haphazard relations with Congress were one facet of a haphazard administration self-consciously patterned on Franklin Roosevelt's creative chaos. The disciplined organizational chart—so beloved by Dwight Eisenhower—seemed cautious and stuffy to the new team; the new thinking put Ike's style down as rigid, cautious, and tradition-bound. Kennedy threw that aside for a freewheeling, unscripted, ad hoc executive style. Rather than assign aides to defined tasks, the Kennedy White House expected generalists to move nimbly from issue to issue, free of red tape or formal policy procedures. Fearful of falling captive to a set of experts, Kennedy convened ad hoc groups. He revived Roosevelt's tactic of giving more than one person the same task—he asked both Clark Clifford (a wily Washington lawyer and former Truman aide) and Richard Neustadt (a Columbia professor) to prepare papers on the presidential transition while instructing them not to talk with one another.[25]

Kennedy famously filled his White House with bright young men. "The most striking thing about the administration," gushed Richard Rovere in the *New Yorker,* "continues to be ... the large scale employment of intellectuals." More than FDR, wrote Rovere—even more than the sophisticated capitals of Europe. Not everyone was so thrilled. "They've got the damnest bunch of boy commandos running around ... you ever saw," grumped Adlai Stevenson. And Sam Rayburn wanted less brainpower and more political savvy: "I wish one of them had been elected to dog catcher or something," he muttered to Lyndon Johnson.[26]

Kennedy bypassed the Cabinet and drew power directly into the White House. He scorned the idea of a president who waited patiently for his subordinates to work slowly through the process—boring old Ike, again—in order "to produce more missiles or build more schools." Rather, he insisted, "this nation needs a Chief Executive who is the vital center of action in our whole scheme of government." For the next fifteen years, each president would up the ante on that aspiration.[27]

Alongside the maladroit organization came Kennedy's great innovation—harnessing television to his charismatic persona. His first televised news conferences got rave reviews. As political scientist Samuel Kernell put it, "almost everyone who expressed an opinion agreed that the new president had done well." In the more effusive words of the *New Yorker's* Washington correspondent, Kennedy was "adroit, lucid, diplomatic and frequently informative." This was new ground in the early 1960s, and as political scientists such as Theodore Lowi would famously comment, from that moment on, the presidency became a personal institution. Still, the logic was as old as the Republic: "The only way to get action out of Congress is by creating a public clamor," explained reporter Richard Rovere, to rattle members "when they go back to their constituencies."[28] For a president who disdained the down-and-dirty work of congressional horse-trading and grinding governmental process, going public was a perfect fit.

For all the promise and excitement about the "new frontier," Kennedy's consuming interest was in international affairs. Gearing up for his first Senate campaign in 1951, he declared that "[f]oreign policy today ... overshadows everything else. Expenditures, taxation, domestic prosperity, the extent of social services—all hinge on the basic issue of war and peace." Once he got into the Senate, "it was a hell of a time to get him to spend time on ... anything else," as his longtime aide Ralph Dungan later recalled. "It was true even when he was in the White House. I mean, if you had looked at his time or his calendar ... you would find at least a third to half his time being spent on international questions[,] partly because they were very, very important but also partly because this was the way his mind went." When it came time to write his inaugural address he told Sorenson, "Let's drop the domestic stuff altogether." The focus on international went beyond personal interests. Kennedy shared one great passion—not a word often used to describe him—with his predecessor. As Richard Neustadt put it, "Nothing ... mattered more to Kennedy than ... get[ting] the nuclear genie back in the bottle."[29]

To be sure, foreign policy crises and issues were plentiful. Three months after Kennedy took office, he gave the green light to the CIA-inspired invasion of Cuba that had been in the works when he took office. It was an international fiasco. An embarrassed Kennedy took responsibility and—recognizing the limits of freelancers in the White House—reorganized his national security staff.[30] Two months later, in June 1961, Kennedy met Khrushchev in Vienna for a summit where Khrushchev harangued Kennedy, blistered the United States, asserted Soviet superiority, promised a Soviet triumph over America, and left with the belief that Kennedy was a weakling, easily pushed around. Sure that Kennedy could be bullied, Khrushchev risked installing nuclear missiles in Cuba, precipitating a confrontation between the United States and the Soviet Union, bringing the world as close to nuclear war as it has ever come. The Cuban missile crisis lasted from October 16–28, 1962, and showed Kennedy at his best. He emerged with a reputation as a tough, clever, and resolute manager of international crises.[31]

His stature as an international leader—and celebrity—reached its peak when, in June 1963, he spoke to millions of Berliners in the shadow of the newly constructed Berlin Wall, and declared, "All free men, wherever they may live, are citizens of Berlin, and, therefore, as a free man, I take pride in the words *Ich bin ein Berliner*."[32] Many observers hold that moment—the speech in Berlin, with the outcome of the perilous Cold War entirely uncertain—as the high-water mark of America's international prestige. Again, understanding Kennedy and his successes means understanding the deep power of charismatic leadership and its capacity to move and inspire. After the event—during which the largest crowds Kennedy had ever seen reacted explosively to him and his speech—a euphoric JFK joked that he would leave an envelope for his White House successor containing a sheet with three words on it: "Go to Germany!"[33]

Kennedy had discovered that despite its perils, foreign affairs could provide presidents with freedom to act, lead, and create a legacy in ways that domestic policy rarely could. "It really is true that foreign affairs is the only important issue for a President to handle, isn't it?" he asked Richard Nixon in a nighttime phone call during the Bay of Pigs crisis. "I mean, who gives a shit if the minimum wage is $1.15 or $1.25, in comparison to something like this?"[34] Foreign policy fit Kennedy's passions and his style.

But, of course, no president can escape domestic policy. That minimum-wage boost was the first fruit of the hard-won victory over the Rules Committee. Kennedy had no choice but to engage in the thorny politics of Pennsylvania Avenue. He was exquisitely aware that his party's fortunes in 1962 and his own reelection in 1964 depended on economic prosperity at home. Besides, the crises were piling up at home even faster than around the globe.

In 1960, during the presidential primaries, civil rights protesters had hit upon a new tactic, sit-ins. Four thousand people had been arrested—including Martin Luther King Jr.—even as Kennedy and Nixon campaigned across the country. By May 1961, the freedom riders boarded their buses and ran into the fierce segregationist violence—one bus was chased by a white posse and firebombed; as the young men and women leaped away from the blaze, they were beaten with sticks and pipes as police stood by. The administration belatedly scrambled to provide protection. The following September, James Meredith, an eleven-year Air Force veteran, won a court order opening the door to the segregated University of Mississippi. That sparked a day of riots (leaving two dead), and again, the administration improvised—Robert Kennedy negotiated wildly with Governor Ross Barnett (who proposed a mock battle in which his own men surrendered before superior federal arms) and eventually dispatched federal marshals. The administration remained trapped between the southern segregationist Democrats it needed if it was going to win any legislation and the civil rights activists and their liberal allies, who stood on the moral high ground.

Through most of the Kennedy years, the civil rights pattern remained the same: protestors pushed, segregationists overreacted, a crisis developed, the national and international press reported each move, and the administration, always a step behind, moved to defuse the crisis while clinging to the Democratic coalition of impenitent segregationists and outraged liberals. The stalemate broke during the Birmingham campaign in May and June 1963. The final straw might have been the photo of a police dog burying its fangs into a young black man's stomach—printed on page one of newspapers around the world. Kennedy told Schlesinger that it made him "sick" to look at it, and a month later, he finally introduced comprehensive civil rights legislation. In one of his most eloquent addresses, Kennedy called racial equality a "moral issue as old as the scriptures and as clear as the American Constitution."[35]

Kennedy gamely pushed the Congress to address a series of other domestic issues that constituted his New Frontier and promoted the aura of activism and progress. He sought to boost federal aid to education and succeeded when Congress passed the legislation just before his assassination. (President Lyndon Johnson signed it into law in December 1963.) Unemployment in the United States was stuck at a relatively high 7.5 percent when Kennedy took office. One of his first domestic initiatives, enacted in May 1961, was a bill to combat unemployment in local areas with persistent unemployment—a forerunner to the War on Poverty.

Still, none of his chief domestic priorities—tax cuts, the Civil Rights Act, aid to education, Medicare—became law during his lifetime. He himself saw a big election victory in 1964 as the key to breaking through. And he knew it would be complicated by his embrace of civil rights. With so much at stake, Kennedy needed a popular issue to take to the voters, an issue that suited his charismatic style of leadership. Time and again throughout his administration, he and his advisors returned to the same solution: Medicare.

## MEDICARE RESURGENT

Kennedy grappled with health care in four different phases during his brief time in office. Along the way, he and his aids launched the kind of unprecedented, all-out, grassroots health care campaign that Roosevelt and Truman had hinted at trying. In the end, the administration fell short by a single senator but powerfully changed the dynamics of the health care debate and made Medicare one of the most potent political issues before the country.

## A Fast Start

Kennedy and his staff were not new to health policy. Back in 1956, already eyeing a run for President, Kennedy had cosponsored an omnibus bill on the problems of the elderly that included some health provisions. He had introduced Social Security amendments to include hospital coverage for the elderly in 1958, had proposed his own universal health care plan for the elderly in early 1960, and had served as a prime sponsor of the liberal Kennedy–Anderson Bill (a modified version of the Forand and King–Anderson bills) during the Senate summer showdown that included the orphaned Eisenhower proposal (which appealed to almost no one) and the southern conservative Kerr–Mills alternative (which offended no one). Kennedy–Anderson lost but gave Kennedy an excellent campaign issue.

His experience on the campaign trail further tickled his political antennae. When Kennedy spoke to a rally in Detroit while campaigning for the nomination in March 1960, his remarks on health care got a rousing response. "Most of us felt that this was the point where Kennedy became really committed," recalled one of the rally's organizers. The Democratic party platform strongly endorsed the Kennedy–Anderson Bill, and a reference to health care coverage became part of Kennedy's standard stump speech. Again Kennedy was struck by the intensity of the support for the issue. His running mate, Lyndon Johnson, listened to tapes of their rallies and noticed how medical care for the elderly repeatedly got the biggest applause.[36]

Kennedy enjoyed terrific staff work on the health care issue. He had already tapped Wilbur Cohen, the former Social Security official now turned University of Michigan professor. Cohen had drafted a health bill for Kennedy (in 1958) as well as the Senate version of Kerr–Mills. Immediately after the election, in November 1960, Kennedy asked Cohen to run the transition task force on health and Social Security issues; in January, Cohen delivered a report to the president-elect at the Carlyle Hotel in New York: "The only sound and practical way of meeting the health needs of most older people is through the contributory Social Security system." The team built on the core elements of Kennedy–Anderson and its predecessors, the Forand Bill and the King–Anderson bill. Kennedy responded by asking his transition team to put even more emphasis on the elderly—especially their health insurance and Social Security benefits. A trio of old hands, Wilbur Cohen, Robert Ball (a widely respected specialist on Social Security), and Nelson Cruikshank (a longtime health advocate from the AFL-CIO), repackaged Kennedy–Anderson for early action in Congress.[37]

Their proposal evoked a skeptical response from the Bureau of the Budget. The new director, David Bell, correctly pointed out that this "liberalized version of the Forand bill," focused mainly on hospital costs and offered the elderly nothing for physicians' services or preventive care—despite costs he estimated at $2.4 billion a year. That would require an immediate 0.5 percent increase in the Social Security Tax, with a jump to 0.8 percent after five years. The BOB suggested that the bill cover a wider variety of services while saving money by focusing only on catastrophic—that is, very expensive—illness. The BOB opinion pointed to real problems in the plan and constituted the only careful analysis of the bill in the Kennedy Library archives. However, it had no apparent effect. In Kennedy's State of the Union address, delivered on January 31, 1961, he put it directly: "Measures to provide health care for the aged under Social Security, and to increase the supply of both facilities and personnel, must be undertaken this year."[38]

Nine days later, the president sent Congress a health message proposing the revised Medicare bill that his team had worked up: coverage for 90 days of hospital care, 180 days of nursing home care, 240 home visits by nurses, and a bundle of services and construction programs. The president estimated the cost at $1.5 billion—almost 40 percent lower than the BOB figure.[39]

To all appearances, the Kennedy administration came to Washington primed to launch Medicare in its first days—when presidential capital is invariably at its height. Then, suddenly, the administration pulled up short and abandoned health care for the elderly. The question is why.

### A Cold Shower

Thanks to Franklin Roosevelt, the first one hundred days of every ambitious administration are both charmed and fretful; dreams of bold reform confront the unlikely prospect of matching the New Deal's awesome record. The burden lay especially heavy on the Kennedy administration, which traded so heavily on youth, vigor, and the promise to "get the country moving again."

The administration, keen to sustain the momentum from its rousing inaugural, quickly ran into congressional reality. Kennedy staffers were told, recalled Theodore Sorensen, that with such a narrow victory, they "should forget about any domestic legislation."[40] The scope of the challenge became clear in the effort to remake the Rules Committee. On January 24, just four days into the administration, Kennedy met with congressional leaders, who told him they did not have the votes to carry the change. "If you want a cold shower, you've had it," thought Larry O'Brien, who added that the news threw him into "a state of semi-shock." Losing its first vote would be devastating for the administration. After the meeting, Kennedy asked Rayburn to postpone the vote for a week, then made a balanced budget pledge to lure wavering moderates.[41] The day after Kennedy's State of the Union address, Rayburn delivered the hairbreadth five-vote victory on the rules change.

The administration jumped into "a quick-learning process," Larry O'Brien recalled, about "how congressional relations are supposed to function."[42] He and Kennedy realized they would need at least one feature of Ike's staid procedures—a congressional relations office. The shocked reaction illustrates how Kennedy and his team had not yet developed essential instincts about dealing with the legislature. "When I was a Congressman," commented Kennedy, "I never realized how important Congress was. But now I do."[43]

O'Brien organized weekly meetings between the president and legislative leaders, but there was no talking away the difficulty that the administration faced in Congress, despite the support of Sam Rayburn in the House and Majority Leader Mike Mansfield (D-MT) in the Senate. Medicare loomed as a liability that would bog down the administration and wreck its reputation for effectiveness. Even before the inauguration, Senator Joseph Clark (D-PA) did the legislative math for the White House team: Medicare was three votes short of getting out of the Senate Finance Committee, where chairman Harry Byrd (D-VA) and powerful Senator Robert Kerr (D-OK) were both firm nays. On the House side, Wilbur Mills (D-AR) was also opposed and had the votes to block it in Ways and Means. Moreover, Kennedy needed Mills on other issues. Ways and Means controlled all tax and spending bills, and the administration wanted to expand Social Security in order to pump up an economy just recovering from recession. Inevitably, the AMA piled on in February with a vigorous lobbying campaign against Medicare.

O'Brien saw another problem. Just months before the administration took office, "Congress had made an effort to attend to this problem ... [with] Kerr-Mills." This new program was just going into place, continued O'Brien, and "the very people that you're going to have to convert to Medicare ... have their names on a program and pride in authorship." Selling Medicare meant telling congressional leaders: "You failed." They had an obvious comeback: "You've got to give it more time to prove itself."[44]

The memos prepared by Sorensen and O'Brien for the president's weekly meetings with legislative leaders meetings provide a kind of fever curve of White House interest in Medicare. On March 14 it was number six (after Social Security improvements, water pollution control, customs legislation, and federal aid to education) on the list of presidential priorities—not high, but still on the first string. On March 27, it was down to number eleven.[45] By April, the word in Washington was that Kennedy had ditched Medicare. At an April 21 press conference—as Kennedy dodged questions on the Bay of Pigs fiasco—reporters pushed him about whether Medicare would move this year. His answer hardly inspired confidence: "I don't know. If we had a vote in the House it would depend, of course, on the action of the Ways and Means Committee, so that I'm not—I haven't any information yet as to whether we will get a vote in the House."[46]

Follow-up question: had the administration "reconciled itself to no vote on medical care this year?" Kennedy offered a slender hope. "I would not make that assumption.... It is possible that somebody might offer the bill in the Senate as an amendment to another bill. I don't know that yet, but it is very possible that you could get a vote in the Senate this year. The House is a different problem. You can't get a vote unless the Ways and Means Committee acts."[47]

Meanwhile, the Bay of Pigs dominated the news in April, and the difficult Vienna summit lay just ahead, in May. By July, Medicare had fallen out of sight—number twenty-four—on the weekly list of legislative priorities.[48]

Always interested in box scores, Washington began toting up the Kennedy administration's batting average with the Congress in the fall of 1961. A September 19, 1961, article in *Congressional Quarterly* painted a relatively rosy picture. Of twenty-five administration proposals, the *Quarterly* reported, twenty-one had passed. A reporter for the *St. Louis Post Dispatch* repeated the White House slant on the record: "On the President's desk" the story read, "lies a detailed chart showing that in its first session the Seventy-Third Congress approved for President Roosevelt 11 major bills, all dealing with domestic economy."

Eisenhower, the story continued, succeeded in enacting 14 in his first congressional session. Kennedy had already pushed through 33. According to the White House spin, Kennedy had beaten Roosevelt and Eisenhower. They would keep that box score high throughout the administration. A new generation was in control. The country was on the march. But the administration's risky signature programs—including Medicare—were not yet part of the parade.[49]

## GOING FOR BROKE

Congress remained unyielding on Medicare and many other Kennedy administration priorities. But Kennedy was riding high in public opinion; pollster and advisor Louis Harris reported that no president has ever remained "as consistently high as this [in the polls] over so many months."[50] With a long list of other reforms queued up, who needed the Medicare headache?

Kennedy did, and Lou Harris had explained why in a June 1961 memo to the president. Already looking forward to the 1962 congressional election, Harris argued that the administration had not fully defined itself or framed "the major lines of battle." The president needed "some major and specific score-throughs" that were fast, dramatic and easily understood. Harris suggested education in 1961 and Medicare in 1962 and sketched a bold strategy for Medicare: "Make a frontal assault on the AMA as an obstructive lobby, holding back progress[,] and make no bones about it." The attack would include "grass roots conventions of older people" and a new kind of televised political spectacle: "Take the case directly to the people through three separate television shows ... [including] a fighting, paid political broadcast warning the Republicans of the consequence of their opposition to this legislation in the 1962 elections"[51] And of course, a good outcome in the 1962 election would make JFK's reelection in 1964 that much easier.

The grassroots were already springing up. Union organizers and elderly activists had formed the National Council of Senior Citizens, a group dedicated to passing Medicare. Strategists in the White House and at the Democratic National Committee, brainstorming about an election strategy for the 1962 midterms, agreed that Kennedy ought to follow Lou Harris's advice and come out swinging on health care. The next step was to leak the plan to the press. The Associated Press "broke" the story: "President Kennedy is going to stake his political standing on four explosive issues in the next session of the Congress." Medicare was going to be the toughest to win. Reflecting the language of the White House memos, the story went on to observe, "The President has no illusions that putting across any such program is going to be easy. He was reported to be preparing for the toughest kind of battles."[52]

What would the administration take on first? Sorenson sent Kennedy a memo putting Medicare at the top of the list. But the same stubborn question still confronted the White House: how to shake the program free from Wilbur Mills and his obdurate Ways and Means Committee? The administration broke into two camps.[53]

The political team pushed for a break with the timidity and caution of past campaigns. Go to the people, stir up an irresistible popular movement that would push reluctant conservative legislators. Proponents imagined rallies across the United States culminating in the administration's great charismatic weapon, President Kennedy addressing a rally at Madison Square Garden on national television in late spring, 1962. For the first time, a president would take the fight over a health care bill directly to the public. Proponents of the strategy gleefully circulated memos leaked from the Republican National Committee that showed "how fearful they are of what we are doing"; as one labor official put it, the enemy's trepidation only "reinforces our need to have the President at the Madison Square Garden Rally to further strengthen our hand."[54]

Others vehemently opposed the idea. Wilbur Cohen believed this was no time to abandon the inside game he himself played so deftly. The only way to get Medicare through Ways and Means, he argued, was by stroking Wilbur Mills, earning his trust and offering him round-the-clock technical support. Making his life uncomfortable would only set the cause back. "By gosh," added Larry O'Brien, "[some of these people] became persuaded that ... this grass roots figurative March on Washington ... [would] just sort of roll over ... Wilbur Mills." Below the substantive arguments lay the inevitable fight for turf. Wilbur Cohen resented others—Ivan Nestingen (Cohen's liberal boss at HEW), Kenneth O'Donnell (an important White House aide), Dick Maguire (a White House liaison to the Democratic National Committee)—crowding onto his issues. "Quite frankly, I considered all these other people as being interlopers." After all, he complained, this was "a process for which I was being held responsible." Larry O'Brien thought that "these well-motivated people ... had taken on ... a task that was beyond them." None of them were "engaged in congressional relations," and none of them understood that rallies and speeches "were less than a pebble in the ocean as far as the Congress was concerned." Indeed, he argued repeatedly, the effort might very well be counterproductive.[55]

Kennedy sidestepped the argument by simply embracing both strategies—the administration would try to corral the old bulls in Congress and fire up the grass roots at the same time.

## The Outside Effort

The administration rolled out its public strategy in Kennedy's 1962 State of the Union address. "In matters of health, no piece of unfinished business is more important or more urgent than the enactment under the social security system of health insurance for the aged." Kennedy pointed to the great gaps left by Eisenhower's failure to extend the market. "Private health insurance helps very few [elderly]—for its cost is high and its coverage limited." The elderly had worked hard their whole lives and were not looking for handouts, which was all that Kerr–Mills offered them. "Public welfare cannot help those too proud to seek relief but hard-pressed to pay their own bills. Nor can their children or grandchildren always sacrifice their own health budgets to meet this constant drain." And finally, the highly charged connection to the most popular program in the country: "Social Security has long helped to meet the hardships of retirement, death, and disability. I now urge that its coverage be extended without further delay to provide health insurance for the elderly."[56]

The inevitable question popped right up when Kennedy met the press later in the week: was this "socialized medicine?" Kennedy's answer embellished the link he had made in the State of the Union address: "Well, that is an old argument … it was the argument that was used against the Social Security Act in the 1930s." JFK was constructing an important political retort, one that Democrats would keep returning to in the years ahead. Social Security became a cudgel against the hard hearts resisting Medicare. The Democrats finally had a response with which to reframe the predictable sobriquet about socialized medicine: *That's the same line they used to oppose Social Security.*[57]

During the spring, the White House began organizing rallies of senior citizens around the country. "The grass roots campaign," wrote Kenneth O'Donnell, Kennedy's longtime special assistant, "[is aimed at] mak[ing] people aware of the importance of this legislation." It was always public information—never about squeezing a vote out of recalcitrant congressmen.[58] Administration officials fanned out to campaign for the measure, capped on May 20 by a presidential speech to a great rally in Madison Square Garden, carried live on all three networks.

The effort seemed dramatic and unprecedented. "Presidents have tried to marshal public opinion before this for a favored and politically potent bill," commented the *New York Times,* "but probably never on such a scale as has Mr. Kennedy for health insurance."[59] Harry Truman had tantalized reporters with talk about "getting on a train" and resuscitating his give-'em-hell campaign style to champion stalled domestic programs like national health insurance; Eisenhower had kept his political hand well hidden. Now President Kennedy merged campaigning, policy, and television for the first time. Supporters hoped for a breakthrough.

Kennedy's May 20 speech began amid war whoops and long, loud applause. He celebrated the idea of citizens getting engaged in government—right back to the patriots gathering in Faneuil Hall, who "la[id] down the groundwork of American independence." He cheered physicians: "this is not a campaign against physicians"; "no one would become a doctor just as a business enterprise." And he wrapped Medicare in the popular mantle of Social Security. Kennedy came back to Social Security eight times, knocking home his great effort to reframe the debate: "All these arguments"—it is socialism, it will sap initiative, it is not business for government—"were made against Social Security at the time of Franklin Roosevelt."

The speech was most affecting when Kennedy turned personal and the hall grew hushed. He talked about visiting his father in a New York hospital—joking wryly (and to his biggest laugh) that the old man was richer than the president and could, thankfully, afford the expensive care he was getting. "I visited twice, yesterday and today, in hospital, where doctors labor for a long time, to visit my father. It isn't easy—it isn't easy. He can pay his bills, but otherwise, I would be. And I am not as well off as he is. But what happens to him and to others when they put their life savings in, in a short time? So I must say that I believe we stand about where—in good company today, in halls such as this, where your predecessors—where Dave Dubinsky himself actually stood, where another former President stood, and fought this issue out of Social Security against the same charges."[60]

The president touched important and moving themes, but the conventional wisdom, laid out by journalist Richard Harris at the time, put the speech down as a disaster: rambling, repetitive, and inarticulate. One labor activist who had been organizing the grassroots campaign told Harris, "instead of steam for the Medicare pistons we got a pail of cold water." Sorenson, on the other hand, thought it had been too hot. "It was a fighting stump speech, loudly delivered and applauded. But the President had forgotten the lesson of the campaign that arousing a partisan crowd in a vast arena and convincing the skeptical TV viewer at home require wholly different kinds of presentation."[61]

In fact, the speech had moving passages and moments—long descriptions of the consequences of illness, for example. But, listening to it today, what is striking is the halting, stumbling, somewhat wooden delivery. Perhaps the problem lay in Kennedy's decision, at the last minute, to put aside his prepared text and speak extemporaneously. Perhaps Kennedy's media skills lulled him and his aides into a false sense of security. Perhaps Kennedy was hurting or dulled by some recently administered drug cocktail (or withdrawal symptoms from the same). Or perhaps they had simply crammed the whirlwind weekend in New York too full of activities—JFK had visited his father twice, made public appearances around the city, and—the night before the big speech—attended a gala birthday party thrown for him, also at Madison Square Garden, where Marilyn Monroe—in a flesh colored, low cut dress—stole the headlines when she huskily sang Happy Birthday. Whatever the explanation, the speech did not live up to the reformers' unlikely aspirations: it did not bury the opposition under a popular uprising or stampede Congress into capitulating.

The AMA launched a devastating public relations counterstrike the next day. Edward Annis, the head of the AMA speakers bureau, delivered a sober, dignified address in the stillness of a now-empty Madison Square Garden—still littered with the debris from the rally of the day before. The stagecraft of the cool doctor—who professed ignorance of the political arts—trumped that of the president.[62]

Still, the popular media did not generally judge the effort a failure. On the contrary, *Time* magazine reported the two speeches and suggested an administration success: "Last week in an all out effort to make the nation aware of its efforts, the administration gave the AMA a few lessons in the art of rough and tumble propaganda." And, with some surprise, the magazine reported the efforts to "equate opponents to the bill with opponents to social security." Almost every account repeated the same point: "The cold fact is," as Newsweek put it, "whatever happens, the Democrats can hardly lose." Perhaps Kennedy would score an unlikely but "resounding" victory; more likely, the bill would fail, and the "Democrats would have the best of all issues for the Congressional elections in the fall."[63]

In a larger context, Madison Square Garden marks an important milestone. President Kennedy had taken the tools of presidential campaigns—banners, signs, speeches, rallies, rhetoric, and television—and turned them to serve a single piece of legislation. It seemed, as the *New York Times* had reported, like an old strategy—the bully pulpit—but taken to a completely new level. Future presidents would repeat the effort. It would become part of the standard presidential effort to pass difficult legislation, whether in health care or in other fields. And future presidents would stand forewarned: it takes exceptional skill, organization, charisma, and luck to leverage the outside strategy into success at the insider politics of Congress.

If Kennedy did not win a breakthrough, he had found an answer to the inevitable charge against his reform. "Socialized medicine" now had an effective rejoinder: "opposes Social Security." Over the next weeks, the president kept hammering the point. At a May 23 press conference, for example, he accused the AMA of opposing Social Security in 1935 and extracted a rebuttal from the AMA that became a front-page story in the *New York Times.*[64] Cheered at having the medical association on the defensive, aides scoured the records, permitting Kennedy to shoot back, in a June 4 letter, that AMA leaders had certainly disparaged the Social Security legislation after its passage. "If your organization did not oppose Social Security *before* its enactment—only *afterwards*—I will be glad to point out this unique distinction in my next press conference," he taunted them.[65] A week later, in a briefing memo, Sorensen had Kennedy loaded up again—lamenting the misinformation by "groups that do not understand or accept the role of Social Security in our American way of life."[66] Kennedy didn't use that last shot—perhaps the point had been made well enough.

The president's publicity campaign did not push Medicare though Congress. But it gave liberal congressmen an argument, a leader, and—following the Louis Harris script—a clear battle line symbolized by the sports arena. When Representative Morris Udall (D-AZ), wrote constituents a newsletter about his support for Medicare, for example, he began it by citing the rally: "The 'Battle of Madison Square Garden' between President Kennedy and the American Medical Association has touched off a great mass of mail pro and con on the question of medical care for the aged."[67]

Still speeches and rallies had to be translated into congressional votes.
That left the hard negotiations of the inside game.

*The Inside Game*

Back in January 1962, just as the administration was launching its public strategy with the State of the Union address, Kennedy dispatched
Wilbur Cohen and Abraham Ribicoff, the secretary of HEW, to negotiate with Wilbur Mills. Congressman Mills, reported Cohen, "indicated
that he could probably not get a favorable vote out of the Ways and
Means Committee at the present time on any health insurance bill." But
things were never simple with Mills. He concocted an elaborate strategy
for the administration: a welfare bill would get priority treatment and
pass through the House early in the session. Then, after the bill passed
through committee in the Senate, Clinton Anderson (D-NM) would
tack a health insurance proposal to the welfare legislation on the Senate
floor. Wilbur Mills would then go to conference and—as Mills elabo-
rated with a wink—"after protracted discussions and some compromises he would accept some health insurance provisions." He'd tell the
folks back home that because he needed to get the welfare amendments
passed for the good of the State of Arkansas he "had to reluctantly
accept the 'watered down' provisions of a health insurance bill" that he
had so long bottled up in his committee. Secretary Ribicoff grew "very
enthusiastic" over the plot—a naive response to the wily legislator. The
Mills scheme became the administration's insider blueprint.[68]

By June it was clear that, as O'Brien had predicted, the grassroots
campaign had not caused so much as a ripple in Ways and Means. With
fifty-eight working days left in the congressional session, the administration was pushing forty-eight bills: an impossible load. Something
had to go, and Sorensen asked Kennedy whether it should be Medicare,
which was "less likely to pass."[69] Kennedy immediately demurred, win
or lose—this was electoral gold—and the administration turned to
Wilbur Mills's strategy for getting some compromised form of health
insurance through Congress.

Wilbur Cohen, Senator Clinton Anderson, and the liberal Jacob Javits
(R-NY) negotiated the health insurance plan that Senator Anderson
would add onto the welfare bill. To win, the Democrats knew they would
need Javits to round up some liberal Republican votes. Wilbur Cohen
drew up lists of potential Republicans Javits might corral: Leverett
Saltonstall (R-MA), Winston Prouty (R-VT), George Aiken (R-VT),

and others. Of course, Javits pushed the bill in a Republican direction. Most importantly, he wanted Medicare to pay the premiums for elderly Americans who already had private insurance—eroding the universal philosophy implicit in Social Security. By July, all the principals—liberal and conservative—were growing disgruntled about the compromises they had made. But they all knew that Senator Kerr was hard at work on the other side, lining up votes to bury the Anderson Amendment.[70]

By July 10, 1962, Medicare took the number-one slot in Kennedy's legislative briefing memo. O'Brien's head count stood 51–49 in favor— a squeaker of a win. And the weekly memo asked the critical question: "How far should we compromise with Javits on an option?" And then a cryptic, unlikely question, its meaning lost in time: "Do we want support from the President of the AMA?"[71]

The next day, Cohen announced that they had reached an agreement with Javits. The compromises would not please the liberals, admitted Cohen. There would be high deductibles, and Medicare would pay the premiums for beneficiaries who had private insurance.[72] Presumably Kennedy had signed off on the deal the previous day.

President Kennedy chafed at the compromises he had agreed to. "You can water the bills down and get them by," he told the press. "Or you can have bills which have no particularly controversy [sic] to them and get them by." But the big, important breakthroughs were harder, and he knew exactly what he needed to win those: "[T]his election in November is an important one, because if we can gain some more seats, we will have a workable majority."[73]

Still, Kennedy plunged into the legislative maneuvers as O'Brien identified openings and scrawled suggestions: "Mr. President. Check Sen. Russell [D-GA] on Medicare—motion to table vote Tuesday—perhaps he could vote table and for passage or vice versa—in any event Mansfield still has hope for him—feels this gives you excellent opportunity to check him. Larry."[74] Kennedy had bet his own political capital on a roll of the dice with an odd political trio—Wilbur Mills, Clinton Anderson, and Jacob Javits. Still, it was an agonizingly close call; a July 17 memo from the legislative team put the count "50–50 at best and …"—a little sign of trouble that the White House was slow to pick up—"… Senator Randolph has a problem."[75]

Senator Jennings Randolph (D-WV) had a problem that offered shrewd Senator Robert Kerr a fatal opening. Randolph had faithfully supported health insurance for the elderly, but now his state had overspent its welfare funds and owed the federal government $19 million.

Senator Kerr generously offered help. He would add his own floor amendment to the welfare bill (the same bill Anderson was amending), forgiving West Virginia's debt for a simple quid pro quo: Randolph's vote against the Medicare add-on.

Ironically, Wilbur Cohen—Medicare's great champion—drafted the language that lost the day. According to Clinton Anderson, "Kerr called Wilbur Cohen to his office and said, 'This man [Senator Randolph] has got to have help. How can it be done?'" Wilbur floundered around for a while and finally said, "Well, this nineteen million dollars has got to be cleaned up some way." Kerr browbeat Cohen into drafting the bill that peeled away Randolph and sunk the Medicare amendment. For a $19 million break to West Virginia, Medicare went down, 52–48. O'Brien's 50–50 count had been right on the mark. Randolph's defection made it 51–49; another senator, who had pledged his vote only if it was needed, also peeled away.[76]

The insider strategy had as many perils as going public. Shrewd old legislators knew every trick. Kerr found the weakest link in the administration's fifty votes and bought it off. And—was it merely an irony, or was it a way to rub it in?—he pushed Wilbur Cohen, Mr. Medicare, into offering the technical assistance that brought down the bill he loved.

Kennedy went straight before the television cameras and denounced this "most serious defeat for every American family." Then he tried to turn the defeat to his electoral advantage by serving up both a hope and a villain: "I hope that we will return in November a Congress that will support a program like Medical Care for the Aged, a program which has been fought by the American Medical Association and successfully defeated. This bill will be introduced in January 1963. I hope it will pass."[77] At his press conference, a few days later, he pushed the attack. "This Administration is for Medicare and two-thirds of the Democrats are for Medicare and seven-eighths of the Republicans are against it. That seems to me to be the issue."[78]

From the very start of the campaign, Louis Harris had called for taking the fight to the enemy and defining "clear battle lines." Defeat permitted Kennedy to do just that (perhaps even more than a heavily compromised victory might have done). But the normally cool and detached president took little comfort from the political calculations. "I was taken aback that he took the defeat as hard as he did," recalled Sorensen, who thought Kennedy "never got over the disappointment of this defeat."[79]

Medicare had become personal for Kennedy. There seemed to be something that gave it extra weight in the flurry of crises and decisions faced by the president. Perhaps the fight with the AMA had stirred his fierce competitive spirit. Perhaps he just didn't like to lose. Or perhaps there was something more deeply personal, something that came into play on December 19, 1961—the day of his father's stroke—and that bubbled out of his rambling, extemporaneous remarks at Madison Square Garden six months later.

### REGROUPING

After the July defeat, all the president's men started pointing fingers. Wilbur Cohen and Larry O'Brien, the insiders, ripped the outside strategy as a waste of time that had only antagonized legislators. Cohen was particularly angry at his putative superior in HEW, Ivan Nestingen, whom he repeatedly attacked in later interviews: "incompetent," "naïve," "simplistic." On the other side, liberals thought Cohen had been so eager to compromise that "he would have given away 99% of the bill"; his negotiations with Javits, they felt, produced an unwieldy proposal with limited benefits that would have disappointed the public and that would have been a nightmare to implement.[80]

Senator Patrick McNamara (D-MI), an important member of Congress, led the charge against the high deductibles. But the liberals were especially critical of the private insurance provisions, which they argued would not only subvert universal values but also be complex and confusing. Even Robert Ball, the commissioner of Social Security and part of Cohen's negotiating team, went to talk Kennedy out of sticking with the elaborate compromise. When he walked into the Oval Office, he was stunned to find Wilbur Cohen—JFK always liked dueling advisors. Ball plunged ahead and told the president the plan would lead to "chaos." "Well then," replied JFK, "let's have a little chaos." But Kennedy was not pleased about being outmaneuvered in Congress, and some observers think Cohen's star dimmed in the administration.

The jockeying continued through the fall of 1962 as the administration considered making another try through Congress. Liberals noted that the Anderson–Javits bill had never undergone a thorough policy vetting (a fair critique, applicable to all the administration's Medicare proposals). One memo from the Democratic National Committee called for a "field manager" in the White House to battle Cohen and his supporters. By December, Cohen had backed off the private insurance option, which he conceded was "complex and confusing."[81]

Other matters crowded in on the administration that already had a full agenda. The Cuban missile crisis dominated October 1962. That same month, Kennedy decided to seek a tax cut in 1963—hoping to stimulate the economy in time for his reelection. In Oval Office conversations, preserved on the scratchy, gap-filled tapes of the era, Kennedy committed to tax reduction and insisted on holding domestic spending below $100 billion.[82] Even so, he carefully reserved a place in the budget for Medicare. "I don't think we can probably get medical care," he commented on October 8, "if we don't cover the non-social-security beneficiaries." That is, Medicare would have to pay for elderly Americans who were not in the Social Security system (and not covered through Social Security taxes) by drawing on general revenues. Just three months after the defeat, Kennedy was still holding aside funds for Medicare as he plotted his 1964 budget.[83] A month later, Sorensen wrote the president, "I assume we will go forward again with the following measures," and put health care for the aged first on the list, along with tax reform, a Department of Urban Affairs, and federal aid to education.[84]

The midterms were modestly successful for the administration. The Democrats gained two seats in the Senate and lost five in the House, essentially ducking the usual backlash (Eisenhower had lost twenty-one House seats in the first midterm after his election, and Truman twenty-nine). Still, the congressional calculus remained—southern Democrats ruled. And it rapidly became clear that getting the tax cuts through the finance committees meant placating Wilbur Mills and Harry Byrd (D-VA), who chaired the Senate Finance Committee. Medicare had to go back onto the back burner.[85]

Nevertheless, Kennedy kept his eye on it. "There seems to be some speculation that we have abandoned health insurance for this year," he wrote Anthony Celebreeze, who had replaced Ribicoff as secretary of HEW. "While it may be that events will not permit legislative action in 1963 I believe we should proceed on the assumption that we are attempting to secure it. The failure then will not be ours."[86] Later Celebreeze recalled that Kennedy was "very firmly committed" to Medicare. "We both thought it would pass. It was just a question of time."[87]

When? There are hints that Kennedy was gearing up to revive the popular issue for his 1964 reelection campaign. After all, health care for the elderly had been dynamite on the campaign trail in the last election. In the fall of 1963, Kennedy went to Arkansas to dedicate a public works project and met with Wilbur Mills. Mills was worried about the fiscal soundness of Social Security if it became responsible for the health care costs of the elderly. Wilbur Mills was always playing political poker; but this is one issue he cared about and would return to frequently. Kennedy immediately assigned a member of the congressional liaison staff, Henry Hall Wilson, to work out a technical solution that Mills found acceptable.[88] Hall and Mills reached agreement on the morning of November 22, 1963. As Kennedy's motorcade wound through the streets of Dallas, Wilson sped over to HEW to meet with Wilbur Cohen and report the breakthrough. The two Kennedy officials were working on the Medicare memo when they heard that the president was dead.[89]

This story, of course, may be too poignant to be true, another intimation of future greatness had Camelot only been given more time. One influential labor lobbyist, Andrew Biemiller, dismissed any deal with Wilbur Mills—after all, the representative was always brokering promises and power, and the last deal was usually negotiable for the next. Still, as we'll see in a moment, Cohen would dutifully produce the Medicare memo as the Johnson administration moved into the White House and got down to business.

### KENNEDY'S HEALTH CARE PRESIDENCY

John F. Kennedy restored dash, charisma and chaos to the White House. He left behind an ambiguous legacy that redefined the American presidency. Kennedy oversaw a willfully disorganized administration marked by little systematic process and even less policy analysis. His health care expert (Wilbur Cohen) and his congressional specialist (Larry O'Brien) fumed when neophytes blithely marched onto their turf and persuaded the president to ignore their own expertise. And although Kennedy's congressional scorecard looks impressive—no modern president between Truman and George W. Bush ranks higher—he never saw any of his major legislation enacted into law. Tax cuts, education, civil rights, and Medicare all remained trapped in the congressional process.

At the same time, Kennedy enjoyed a soaring popularity—then, later, and to this day. No president in the polling era (beginning with Truman) could match numbers with JFK's 1,000 days; even today, despite every sordid revelation, he still rides high in the people's rankings. Kennedy was a charismatic leader who grasped the potential of television to project an unabashed, vigorous, powerful, public-spirited American identity: America would beat the Russians to the moon, secure justice at home, and extend FDR's Social Security to health care. The United States entered the era of the video image, full of high hopes and great aspirations.

Kennedy's treatment of health insurance for the elderly perfectly exemplified his ambiguous, tantalizing, and dramatic presidency. Kennedy forcefully applied the new style to the issue. For the first time in the television age, a president went public with the arguments for reform. He stoked the reform's popularity (reporters called each defeat an electoral bonanza), reframed the arguments, put the AMA on the defensive (their denials that they opposed Social Security became front-page news), and handed his successor a hot program more or less ready for congressional action. John Kennedy's efforts set the stage for Lyndon Johnson's Medicare success. At the same time, Kennedy himself failed to deliver health insurance for the elderly, and his management of the legislation was at times amateurish. His legislative team was beaten in the Senate, and the compromise proposal they were pushing probably didn't deserve the effort they put into it.

Why did Kennedy pick this issue? The answer, as we have seen, is not simple. On the surface, it looks like direct political calculation. Kennedy was elected on the promise to do something about health care coverage for the elderly. Labor and the elderly were agitating and organizing. He and Johnson heard the cheers on the campaign trail in 1960. Louis Harris's polls identified a winning issue for the 1962 and 1964 elections. And, as *Time* and *Newsweek* both pointed out, when he lost Medicare in Congress, he got a powerful issue for the hustings. A far less sophisticated politician than the cool, cerebral JFK would have understood the value of pushing Medicare despite the odds.

But there is a difference between advocating a piece of legislation and going all-out to win it. Kennedy supported Medicare before he became president, but not enough to spend scarce political capital on it in his first months in office. He wanted quick victories, and Medicare would offer none. He was more comfortable with foreign affairs, and international crises demanded his attention. There were other domestic priorities than health care as well; health care issues always look alluring from a distance but up close are tough, technical, and politically prickly—presidents beware.

In the run-up to the 1962 election, Medicare rose up the presidential agenda, another familiar scenario. Presidents rediscover health care as the elections draw near. Nevertheless, as the Kennedy administration fought for Medicare in the winter and spring of 1962, more than politics seems to have been at work. The White House and the Democratic National Committee—over internal protests from many of the political pros—invested enormous resources in a national campaign that had few precedents—certainly none on health care matters. And the president himself became identified with the issue—arguably more so than he needed to be were he simply reaching for the electoral advantage that originally seemed to motivate his advocacy.

The issue grew personal as he decided to commit himself and his office to the May 1962 rally in Madison Square Garden. Perhaps his decision to abandon a drafted speech and substitute his own extemporaneous remarks reflected his newfound fervor—for routine occasions, routine remarks suffice. His commitment seemed to grow as he vigorously confronted the AMA in May and June of 1962 and as he and his staff assigned a high priority to Medicare in their weekly conferences with Democratic legislative leaders during June and July. For this few months, no legislative issue seems to have been more important to the president and his aides than enacting health care for the elderly.

When the legislation went down (to no one's surprise), Kennedy seems to have taken the loss personally, in a way that surprised his most intimate advisors. Whether because of his love of a good fight, anger at organized medicine, identification with other sufferers, or—as O'Brien suggested—experience with his father's illness, Medicare came to transcend politics for John F. Kennedy. To the extent that any domestic issue was ever visceral with JFK, Medicare seems to have become so. In this, Kennedy met one of the necessary (though not sufficient) criteria for winning major health care reform legislation from the Oval Office: caring deeply enough about the issue to engage one of the most difficult, risky, complex, and (usually) unrewarding policy issues of modern times.

The administration led its movement without thinking much about the legislative prize itself. After the exquisite bureaucratic caution of the Eisenhower (and for that matter, Truman) years, the haphazard Kennedy process stands out in freewheeling contrast. Proposals received virtually no technical scrutiny. The Anderson–Javits compromise, essentially negotiated by three men, might have been extremely difficult to implement and administer—as Robert Ball and others later complained—but no one in the administration gave it a second thought as it went to the floor of the Senate for a vote. Let's try a little chaos, said a cavalier president. Of course, it was a different era, before professional economists and policy analysts had organized themselves at the heart of the executive (and the congressional) apparatus. And anything the Senate passed would have had to pass muster in conference with Wilbur Mills, who had one of the sharpest red pencils in the Congress. But by ignoring the details and throwing caution to the winds, Kennedy pushed health reform a lot farther than the Truman or Eisenhower programs had ever got.

The contrast between Eisenhower and Kennedy introduces a heretical theme that will become more vivid in future administrations: the more sophisticated the technical analysis, the dimmer the political prospects for health reform. Put bluntly, careful budgetary and policy analyses subvert the political prospects of covering more people.

Kennedy committed to both an outside and an insider process and succeeded with neither. Even so—despite the policy chaos, despite losing health care in every arena—John Kennedy had that intangible, charismatic quality that few presidents can match: the ability to inspire, the capacity to make Americans engage the better angels of their civic selves. Kennedy—whatever his personal flaws—reframed the health care debate and gave it a brash, unapologetic, populist tone planted firmly in the legacy of FDR and Social Security. His leadership supplied an indispensible element—political momentum—that was critical to Medicare's ultimate success and that remains critical to health care reform.

Just an hour after Kennedy's funeral, Larry O'Brien called Wilbur Cohen and told him to deliver the Medicare memo summarizing the negotiations with Wilbur Mills. Cohen drove to his empty office, where his wife typed up the agreement, and then they delivered it to the White House. There, the stunned aides, milling about, promised to give the document to the new president. On that dark, sad Monday afternoon, Medicare passed into the hands of the greatest inside player to occupy the White House in the twentieth century.[90]

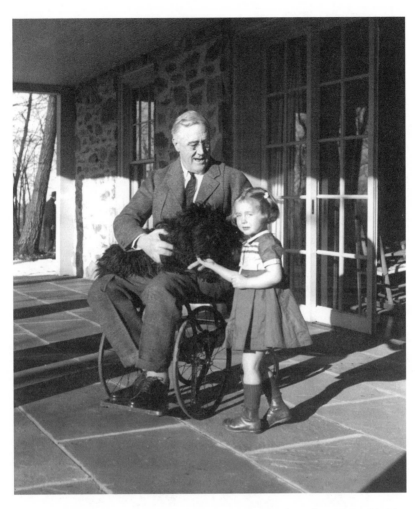

Figure 1. President Roosevelt at Hill Top Cottage in Hyde Park, with Ruthie Bie, the granddaughter of a friend, and his dog, Fala. Roosevelt went to great lengths to hide his disability: this is one of the only photos showing the president in a wheelchair. Photograph by Margaret Suckley; courtesy of the Franklin D. Roosevelt Library Digital Archives.

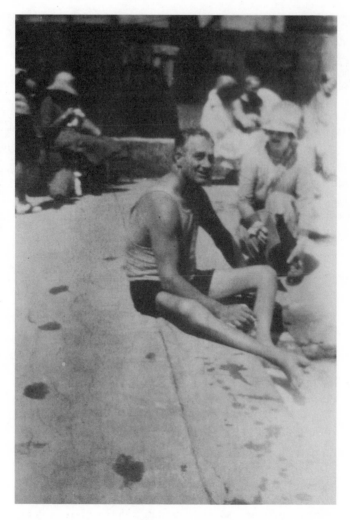

Figure 2. Franklin Roosevelt by the pool at Warm Springs, Georgia, where he developed a rehabilitation program for himself and other polio victims. Compare his muscular upper body to his emaciated legs, the result of polio damage. Photograph courtesy of the Franklin D. Roosevelt Library Digital Archives.

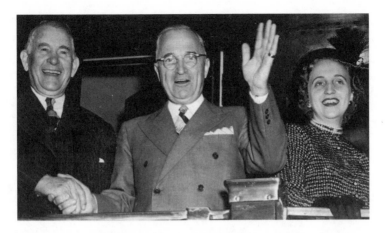

Figure 3. Harry S. Truman flanked by his daughter, Margaret, and vice presidential candidate Alben Barkley during the famous whistle-stop campaign tour that turned the 1948 election campaign. At each stop, Harry would step onto this platform and "give 'em hell." Photograph courtesy of the Harry S. Truman Library.

Figure 4. *The Doctor*, by Sir Luke Fildes, at the Tate Gallery in London. A dedicated physician tends to a sick child while the exhausted mother sits at a table, her head in her hands, and the father hovers in the background. Outside, dawn is breaking. Thanks to the good doctor, the child has made it through the night, and the crisis has passed. The American Medical Association added the caption "Keep the Government Out of this Picture!" and deployed the painting in a fierce campaign against Truman's national health insurance plan. Photo: Tate, London/Art Resource, NY.

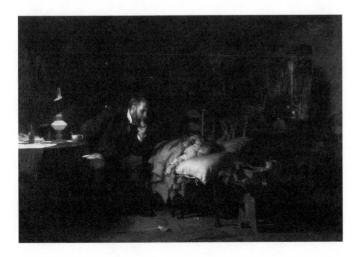

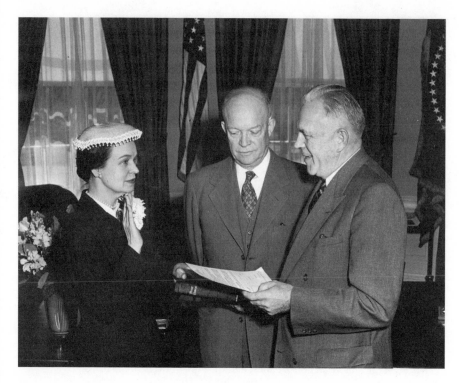

Figure 5. Oveta Culp Hobby is sworn in as the first secretary of Health, Education, and Welfare. Hobby directed the Women's Army Corps (WAC) during World War II and had forged a close relationship with Eisenhower. Photograph courtesy of the Dwight D. Eisenhower Presidential Library.

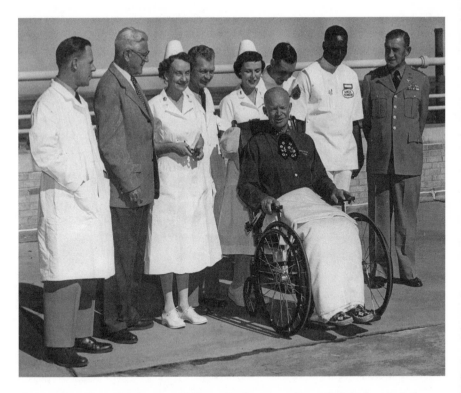

Figure 6. President Eisenhower and his medical team on the roof of the hospital after his 1956 heart attack. Ike's jaunty red pajamas feature five stars (for his military rank) and the answer to the usual question stitched over the pocket: "MUCH BETTER THANKS." Ike was the first president to share the details of an illness with the public. Photograph courtesy of the Dwight D. Eisenhower Presidential Library.

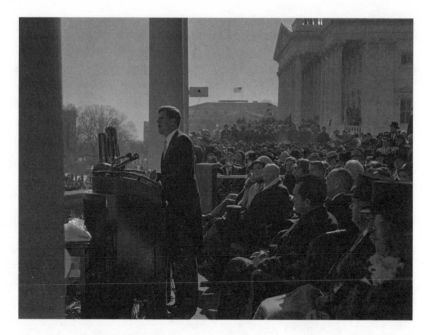

Figure 7. Youth and Age: a vigorous John F. Kennedy delivers his inaugural address without an overcoat while the departing Eisenhower looks on, all bundled up. Photo: © Bettmann/CORBIS.

Figure 8. JFK bends over his disabled father after the elder Kennedy suffered a severe stroke in December 1962. Joseph Kennedy's illness deeply affected JFK. Photograph by Cecil Stoughton; courtesy of the John F. Kennedy Presidential Library.

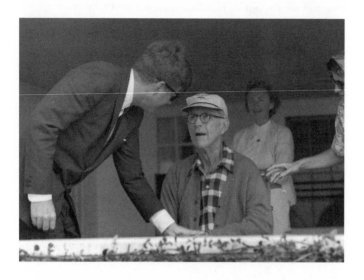

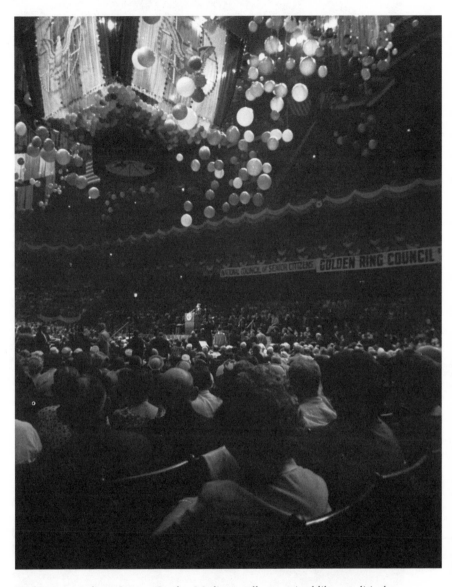

Figure 9. A Madison Square Garden Medicare rally organized like a political convention in May 1962. Kennedy ran an unprecedented public campaign designed to push legislation through Congress. Photograph by Cecil Stoughton; courtesy of the John F. Kennedy Presidential Library.

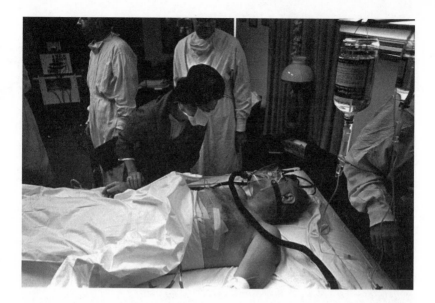

Figure 10. President Lyndon Johnson in the recovery room after gall bladder surgery. Lady Bird leans over him. When rumors circulated that the president had really suffered another heart attack, Johnson tried to squash the falsehood by crudely displaying his scar for reporters. Photograph courtesy of the Lyndon Baines Johnson Library and Museum.

Figure 11. Two titans of Capital Hill: President Johnson meets with Representative Wilbur Mills (D-AR), chairman of the powerful House Ways and Means Committee. Johnson and Mills secretly discussed expanding the administration's Medicare proposal. The wily president feigned surprise when Mills went public with the expansion—and gave all the credit to the congressman. Photograph courtesy of the Lyndon Baines Johnson Library and Museum.

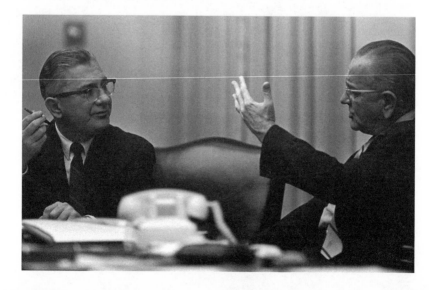

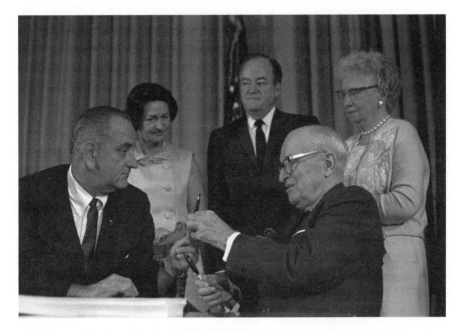

Figure 12. After signing the Medicare bill in Independence, Missouri, LBJ hands the pen to former president Harry Truman, who considered his failure to win national health insurance the biggest disappointment of his life. Behind them are Lady Bird Johnson, Vice President Hubert H. Humphrey, and Bess Truman. Photograph courtesy of the Lyndon Baines Johnson Library and Museum.

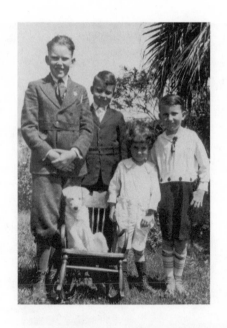

Figure 13. From left to right, Harold, Richard, Arthur, and Donald Nixon. Both Arthur and Harold would die of tuberculosis—traumas that tormented Richard for the rest of his life. Photograph courtesy of the Richard Nixon Library and Birthplace Foundation.

Figure 14. Richard Nixon, his mother, and two brothers: from left to right, Richard, Hannah, Donald, and Harold. Photograph courtesy of the Richard Nixon Library and Birthplace Foundation.

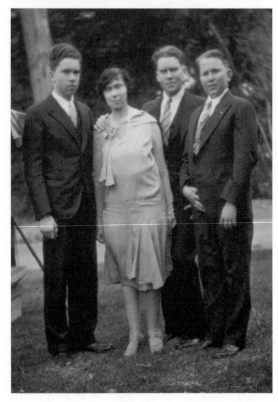

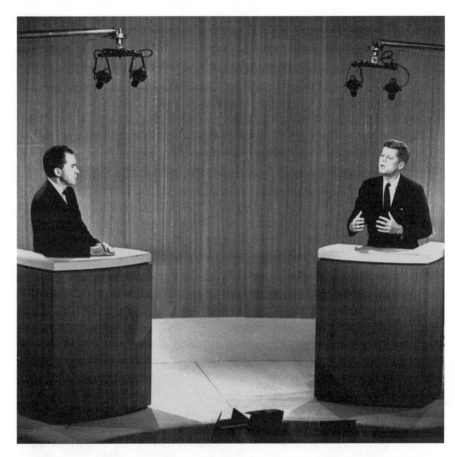

Figure 15. Richard Nixon and John F. Kennedy during the first televised presidential debate. Kennedy had a long list of chronic ailments, but on this night he was the one who looked young and vigorous. Earlier in the day, Nixon had banged his infected knee on a car door, and the pain may have contributed to his pallid, sweaty appearance. Photo: AP/Wide World Photos.

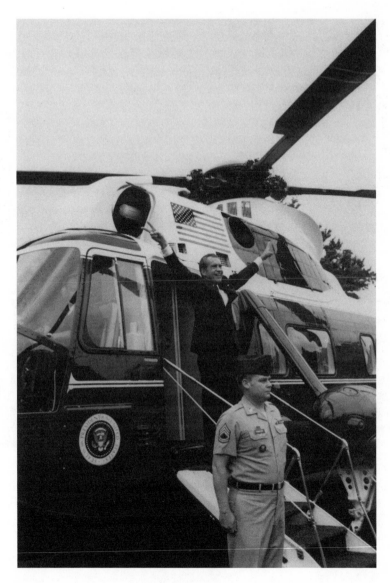

Figure 16. Richard Nixon leaves the White House after resigning the presidency on August 8, 1974. In a rambling, tearful good-bye to his staff, Nixon described his mother as a "saint" for the loving care she had given her dying son and the other tubercular boys whom she boarded and nursed. Courtesy of the Richard Nixon Library and Museum.

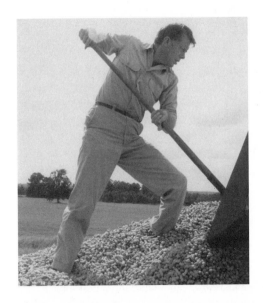

Figure 17. Jimmy Carter shoveling peanuts on his family's peanut farm in Plains, Georgia. Carter grew up on a farm in the pre-industrial South, where hard labor was a part of life. Photograph courtesy of the Jimmy Carter Library.

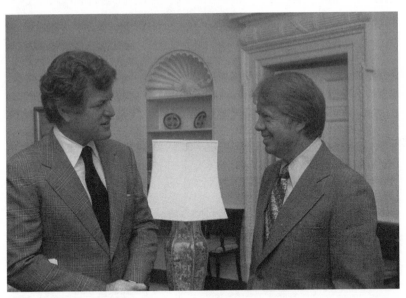

Figure 18. Jimmy Carter and Senator Edward M. Kennedy (D-MA) in the White House. Kennedy pressed Carter to introduce a national health plan, and when Carter balked, Kennedy challenged him for the Democratic presidential nomination. Photograph courtesy of the Jimmy Carter Library.

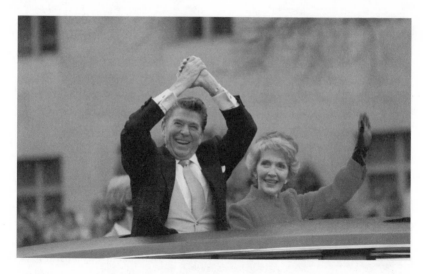

Figure 19. A triumphant Ronald Reagan and his wife, Nancy. Reagan buried the New Deal coalition that had dominated American politics for almost four decades and ushered in a new conservative era. Photograph courtesy of the Ronald Reagan Library.

Figure 20. Moments before the assassination attempt on Ronald Reagan. The bullet deflected off the car door, ploughed into the president's side, ripped through a lung, and lodged an inch from his heart. Reagan's cheerful good humor ("Honey, I forgot to duck") in the face of the trauma made him a hero. Photograph courtesy of the Ronald Reagan Library.

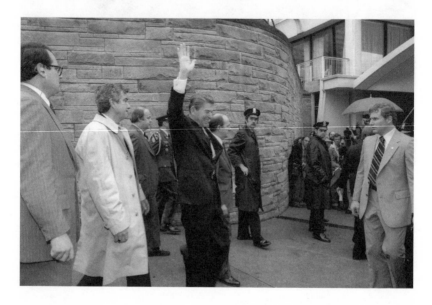

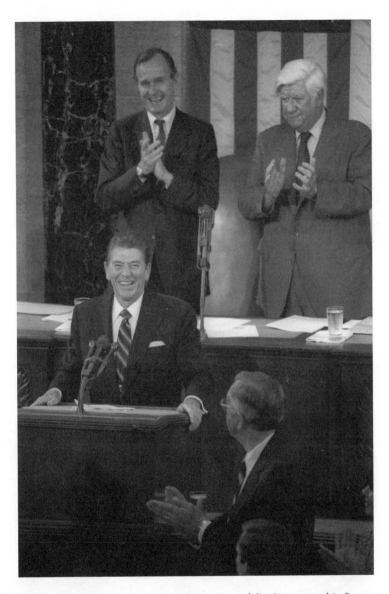

Figure 21. Reagan speaking to a joint session of the Congress—his first public appearance after the attempted assassination. With the press and public lionizing the Gipper, his economic program became virtually unstoppable. Behind him are Vice President George H. W. Bush and Speaker Tip O'Neill (D-MA). Photograph courtesy of the Ronald Reagan Library.

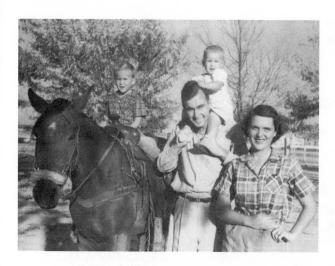

Figure 22. George H. W. Bush with his young family: Barbara, George W. astride the horse, and Robin on her father's shoulders. Robin would soon develop leukemia and die. Photograph courtesy of the George Bush Presidential Library.

Figure 23. President George H. W. Bush with two key domestic policy aides: Richard Darman, director of the Office of Management and Budget, on the far right; and John Sununu, his chief of staff. Photograph courtesy of the George Bush Presidential Library.

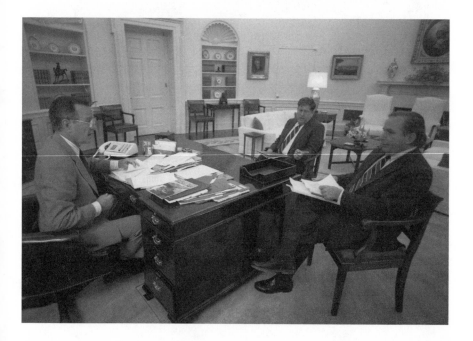

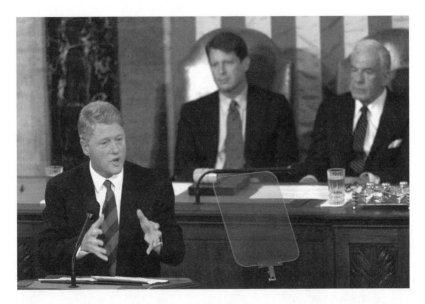

Figure 24. Bill Clinton addressing a joint session of Congress. Behind him are Vice President Al Gore and Speaker Tom Foley (D-WA). Photograph courtesy of the William J. Clinton Presidential Library.

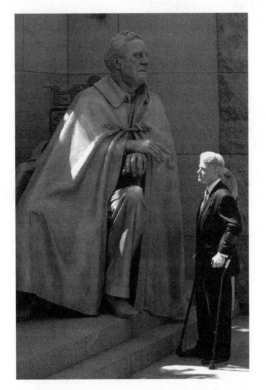

Figure 25. A temporarily injured Bill Clinton contemplates a statue of FDR. Photograph courtesy of the William J. Clinton Presidential Library.

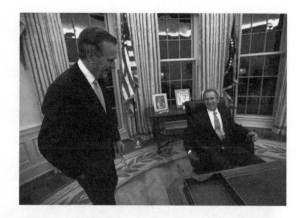

Figure 26. Two presidents, father and son, at home in the oval office. The younger Bush tried to avoid his father's politically fatal indifference to domestic affairs and proved far more receptive to health policy reform. White House Photo.

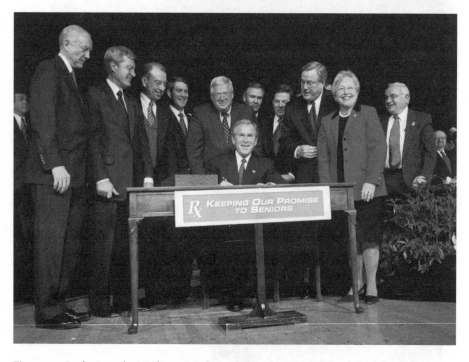

Figure 27. Bush signs the Medicare Modernization Act. Behind him, from left to right, are the key congressional players in the Medicare drama: Senator Orrin Hatch (R-UT), Senator Max Baucus (D-MT), Senator Charles Grassley (R-IA), who chaired the Senate Finance Committee; Senate Majority Leader Bill Frist (R-TN); Speaker of the House, Dennis Hastert (R-IL); Senator John Breaux (D-LA); House Majority Leader Tom Delay (R-TX); Representative Bill Thomas (R-CA), chairman of the House Ways and Means Committee; and Representative Nancy Johnson (R-CT), chairwoman of the Health Subcommittee of House Ways and Means. White House Photo.

# CHAPTER 5

# Lyndon B. Johnson

*The Secret History of Medicare*

If John F. Kennedy swept elegantly into the Oval Office, Lyndon Johnson filled it to bursting. "He'd come on just like a tidal wave," marveled Vice President Hubert Humphrey. "He went through the walls.... He'd take the whole room over. Just like that." "He never, never relaxed," added Speaker of the House Carl Albert (D-OK). Lyndon Johnson vibrated with ambitions, aspirations, insecurities, complicated plots, dirty stories, an astonishing ability to work Congress, an itch to dominate (one might say bully), and a soaring New Deal dream about the Great Society. Health care sat right at the heart of it all.[1]

Johnson took office on that terrible day in November 1963, seized the Kennedy agenda and—invoking the fallen president—began pulling laws out of Congress. He won Kennedy's stalled tax cut in February 1964. He persuaded moderate Republicans to help break an eighty-seven-day filibuster and pass the blockbuster Civil Rights Act of 1964 (in July). He launched the War on Poverty (in August). "You just make this thing work," Johnson said to congressional leaders again and again, "I don't give a damn about the details." The president delegated the details, kept his eye on the principles, and oversaw every jot and turn of the internal politics. On important votes in Congress, he had the highest box score of any modern president.[2]

Medicare and Medicaid were among Johnson's proudest legacies— two sections of the single most important piece of health care legislation in American history. Taken together, the programs weigh in as one of the three largest items on the federal budget after Social Security and (in some years) military spending. LBJ was the most important health care president the United States has ever had.

This chapter retells the Medicare story. Tapes of President Johnson's conversations in the Oval Office and many other archival materials were not available to historians who wrote the definitive histories of Medicare's passage. The information released over the past decade alters both the plot and the lessons about how to manage health reform.

The conventional story emphasized Congress, and particularly Representative Wilbur Mills (D-AR), the shrewd, conservative chair of the powerful House Ways and Means Committee. Through the Kennedy administration, Mills bottled up the Medicare proposal in his committee and refused to let it come to the House floor for a vote. After Kennedy's assassination, Lyndon Johnson picked up the Medicare standard but found Congress and the redoubtable Wilbur Mills just as recalcitrant.

However, continues the traditional story, Johnson won the 1964 election in a massive landslide victory with 61 percent of the vote and carried huge liberal Democratic majorities into the House (295–140) and Senate (68–32). Wilbur Mills accepted the inevitable, changed from a Medicare opponent to its champion, and in a series of brilliant legislative maneuvers, took everyone by surprise and produced the Medicare and Medicaid programs as we now know them. Lyndon Johnson's contribution consisted chiefly of winning the landslide that changed the congressional calculus and loaning Chairman Mills the technical assistance of Wilbur Cohen, who had been drafting health bills through the Eisenhower and Kennedy years for legislators on both sides of the aisle.[3]

Lyndon Johnson himself hewed to this minimalist view in his biography and repeated the now-familiar story: Wilbur Mills took the modest Johnson administration bill (which would have used Social Security to pay some hospital costs for the elderly) and, as the Committee began final action on the legislation, dropped what Johnson called a "bombshell." He suggested merging the administration bill with two alternatives that had been proposed to block it. One proposal, submitted by House Republicans, would pay physician costs (now Medicare Part B) and another, the AMA plan, would cover health care costs for the poor and near-poor (Medicaid). Then, after tripling the size of the bill, Wilbur Mills mildly turned to Wilbur Cohen and asked him to draft the legislation by the next morning.

Opponents, who had been trying to whittle the proposal down, were caught flatfooted; administration officials, who had spent years trying to get a health bill past Mills, were wary. Wilbur Mills's improvisation—if it could be trusted—would add an estimated $400–500 million to the package's annual costs. Cohen returned to the White House and asked President Johnson what do. Johnson was as surprised as everyone else, but he blithely went along and gave the Mills plan the go-ahead. Wilbur Cohen dutifully drafted the bill, and Medicare and Medicaid were born. President Johnson, the cheering bystander, summed up the story: "Chairman Wilbur Mills, so long the villain of the act, was now a hero to the old folks."[4]

Political scientists have drawn the conclusion that understanding Medicare, Medicaid, and, more generally, health care reform, means understanding the subtle operations of Congress itself. The key lies within the institution itself—its intricate rules, processes, folkways, and coalitions. The major outside influence on this infernally complex legislative machine is the nearest election. In a word, Medicare passed because the 1964 landslide turned a "legislative possibility" into a "legislative certainty."[5]

Except that it did not happen that way. We now know—through extensive White House telephone tapes and memos—that LBJ was in on the legislative coup. He cooked up the entire business with Mills—always promising that Wilbur Mills would reap all the credit. Mills later acknowledged as much: "We planned that, yes. Oh, yes."[6] Moreover, as we will see, Johnson played a critical role throughout the process, swooping in to clear the way at various stages, twisting reluctant congressional arms, and suppressing dangerous economic forecasts. LBJ was indispensable, and Medicare was never "certain"—far from it. Wilbur Mills himself began quietly rewriting the story. "Johnson doesn't get the credit he deserves," he later told an interviewer. No other president would "have gotten half of it through."[7]

Our revised history leads to new conclusions about winning health reform. The key lies not just in the congressional process but in the interplay between White House and Congress. For anyone interested in major reforms, the presidency of Lyndon Baines Johnson is nothing less than a primer on how to make it happen—and how even a president with an extraordinary domestic record can lose it all.

## LYNDON JOHNSON'S PASSION

Lyndon Johnson felt the importance of health care in his capacious Texas gut. Many American presidents have dealt with health care issues, but none with LBJ's passion. His own words, often recorded on secret

White House tapes, capture the intensity of his commitment. "Don't ever argue with me ... on health or education," Johnson hectored Vice President Hubert Humphrey. "I don't argue about that any more than I argue about Lady Bird buying flour. You got to have flour and coffee in your house and education and health. I'll spend the goddamn money."[8]

In perhaps Johnson's greatest speech, devoted to the Voting Rights Act of 1965, he looked up at the packed galleries during the joint session of Congress and averred, "I'll let you in on a secret.... I do not want to be the president who built empires or sought grandeur or extended dominion."[9] Here was the rarest of presidential preferences: Johnson actually liked the messy politics of domestic issues.

"There are three big things we are running into," he said in response to an inquiry about the 1964 campaign from well-known journalist Joseph Kraft. "One is peace, one is prosperity, and one is Medicare.... We are really trying to do something for the people. We think the average mother wants peace, she wants her husband to have a job, and they're looking for somethin' to take care of 'em in their old age, and that's what we're trying to do, is to give them a government that appeals to 'em."[10]

Only one president prior to LBJ—Harry Truman—and none since might have ranked a health care program with peace and prosperity as an issue for the American people. The whole area of health care was very near Johnson's core, recalls Joseph Califano, his top assistant for domestic affairs. It was right up there with civil rights.[11] Why did Johnson feel this way? Personal history, deep-seated populism, political ambition, and his own brush with death.

### The Cotulla Populist

"A man's vision reflects his memories," wrote Johnson at the end of his life, and Johnson's early memories turned on hard times in the parched Hill Country of Central Texas. Johnson City, where he moved when his family was five, had no paved roads and no trains until 1917, when Lyndon turned nine. His father, Sam Johnson, was a small-time farmer, cattle and real estate trader, and politician. He served, off and on, as a staunch progressive in the state legislature and Lyndon's favorite childhood memories were political—listening to Sam and his cronies talk politics on the porch at night, running errands for his daddy on the floor of the Texas legislature, and—best of all—the long, happy days of driving from house to house campaigning. But Sam Johnson never quite managed financially, and by the time Lyndon was thirteen, the family had sunk into poverty, surviving with the help of family and friends.[12]

Lyndon's mother, Rebekah, was a cultured woman by the standards of the time and place and had great aspirations for Lyndon. She pushed him hard—and quite against his inclination—to go to college. Johnson struggled to pay his way through San Marcos Teachers College—a "third rate" normal school that had only recently been accredited as a four-year college. In college, Johnson burned at being excluded from the elite group on campus, the Black Stars—dominated by athletes—and retaliated by forming a rival organization, the White Stars, that managed to eclipse (by fair means and foul) much of the elite club's influence; Richard Nixon would have almost the same experience at Whittier college.

Lyndon dropped out after his first year in order to raise tuition money by teaching in a Mexican American grade school in Cotulla, Texas, sixty miles from the Mexican border. Here, Lyndon saw deep, desperate poverty—Mexican workers living at near–slave wages, treated "just worse than you'd treat a dog." Johnson threw himself into teaching. He committed himself, he later told Doris Kearns, to make a difference in the lives of those "poor little kids. I saw hunger in their eyes and pain in their bodies.… I was determined to spark something inside them, to fill their souls with ambition and interest and belief in the future."[13] Here, Lyndon would tell people, in the hard, hot desperate Texas poverty of the twenties, lay the roots of the Great Society. This was one of the deep springs feeding the great aspirations of his presidency. Another was his political ambition.

Roosevelt and the New Deal came along in time to shape Johnson's inchoate populism. By the time he was twenty-six, Johnson was the youngest state director of the New Deal's National Youth Administration. At a gathering of state directors, he met President Franklin Roosevelt, who took an interest in the young Texan. The president "kinda petted me," Johnson later recalled. But nobody knew better than Johnson how to flatter important men, so the petting likely ran both ways.[14] They met again when Roosevelt stopped in Galveston during a fishing trip and Johnson, now a newly minted Congressman, famously plunged into a bold conversation about fishing, warships, and naval power (about which he knew next to nothing). But this was—or would become—a lot more than Texas bullslinging: Johnson fervently admired Roosevelt and positively idolized the New Deal. They would always stand as the golden metric by which he judged himself and his own administration.[15]

Health coverage under Social Security was the lost promise of Roosevelt's New Deal and that made Medicare special to Lyndon Johnson. "[He] looked upon the Social Security Act ... as one of the great legislative triumphs of the ... century," recalled Wilbur Cohen: and that, in turn, "grew out of the very important fact that Mr. Johnson was a ... populist at heart."[16] Johnson's populism, added another White House aide, rested on a bedrock faith that "everybody in society should be given a full and complete chance to make his own way.... Good health was awfully important."[17]

## Health Troubles

Of course, every president has had to cope with his own health issues. Dr. Philip Lee, a physician who served as LBJ's assistant secretary for health, believed that Johnson's own brush with death was another major source of his interest in health care.[18]

By the 1950s, Johnson's lifestyle was a doctor's nightmare. He smoked three packs of cigarettes a day. He enjoyed rich foods—he denounced anything "tossed" (as in salads)—and he ate voraciously. Lyndon had weight problems all his life and took to wearing a heavy girdle—especially in the White House, where the scales tipped past 250 pounds. And, of course, his life was frenzy. "$E = MC^2$ is Albert Einstein's world shaking formula for energy," wrote one journalist, but Washington, D.C., knew a simpler formula. "Energy in its purest form is expressed in the letters $E = LBJ$."[19]

Each time Johnson's career ran into trouble, a health crisis seemed to erupt. The first time he ran for Congress, as a virtual unknown (in a special election held in 1937), he suffered terrible stomach cramps, doubling over, and vomiting. He refused to slow down until, two days before election day, he finally gave in and let the doctors rush him to the hospital, where they found his appendix about to rupture. He learned about his victory in a hospital bed.

During his tough, dirty, long-shot run for the Senate in 1948, Johnson campaigned despite an infected kidney stone that gave him a 104 degree fever and left him vomiting until his stomach was empty. The pain of kidney stones is excruciating—there is none worse. But Johnson barreled through and brushed off the warnings that postponing an operation might prove fatal—to him, losing the election seemed worse. He continued campaigning despite the excruciating pain.[20]

As he prepared to run for the White House in July 1955, Johnson had a health episode that he could not brush off. Under enormous pressure during a tough legislative session, he visited a friend in Virginia where he developed all the classic symptoms of coronary insufficiency—shortage of blood flow to the heart. Johnson's symptoms were absolutely classic—the stuff of medical textbooks. He felt as if his chest had "two hundred pounds on it." Still he refused to call a doctor. It was always politics with Lyndon: if the newspapers got hold of a story about heart trouble, his presidential bid would be over before it began. Senator Clinton Anderson (D-NM)—who would later sponsor the Medicare bill during both Kennedy and Johnson administrations—arrived at the house and immediately recognized the symptoms from his own heart attack. He overruled Senator Johnson and called a physician, who diagnosed the heart attack and told Johnson he was going to go into shock in about ninety minutes—just time to enough to get back to Washington. Johnson sped back to the city lying in the local ambulance (which doubled as a hearse, and was driven by the undertaker).[21]

Lying in the back of the ambulance–hearse, without time to stop and take anything for the pain, the senator finally spoke his great worry: "Doctor," he asked the physician riding up front, "Will I be able to smoke again?" "Well, frankly, Senator, no," responded the physician. Johnson heaved a big sigh: "I'd rather have my pecker cut off."[22]

When Johnson got to the hospital, he wheedled one last cigarette, smoked it, and went into apparent shock. He was grey, motionless, his blood pressure barely detectable. Shock in the aftermath of a major heart attack is ominous. The doctors told Lady Bird the chances of recovery were about even. And, although she meant to keep that from him, Lyndon tricked it right out of her when he turned to her and said, "They're saying my chances are 1 in 10." "Nonsense," she shot back, "they say it's 50–50!" Johnson spent months recovering before returning to the Senate.[23]

Dr. Phil Lee, Johnson's future assistant secretary, thought he saw a major difference between Johnson and Kennedy when it came to health care. Johnson "had excellent medical care throughout his life really, superb medical care." In particular, Dr James Cain, "an outstanding physician" at the Mayo Clinic, treated him after that heart attack and "perhaps made him recognize how important this is." By modern standards, the treatment was primitive—sedation, prolonged bed rest, pain relief. Today, he would have gone straight to the catheterization lab, received clot-busting drugs and perhaps either a procedure to open blocked arteries (a cardiac stent) or cardiac bypass surgery. But these miraculous remedies were nearly a half century away, LBJ got the best available care, and was grateful for it, summed up Phil Lee: "It made him an advocate for health programs in a way that certainly President Kennedy never was."[24]

Dr. Cain would later accompany Vice President Johnson on a tour of Southeast Asia, write a report on Vietnamese health care, and become an informal health advisor when Johnson became President. The Mayo Clinic doctor argued that there were not enough physicians to meet the needs of newly covered Medicare patients and convinced Johnson to convene a commission on the physician workforce.

James Cain, MD, was a presidential first: a physician who had done his patient a great deal of good and saw a government-guaranteed right to health care as something to talk up rather than put down.

## THAT BIG PERSONALITY

And then there was the Johnson personality. Lyndon was big in every way. He stood almost six feet four inches tall, with long arms and large hands. By the time he reached the White House, he was losing his perpetual battle with weight: 230, 240, even 250 pounds—up some 60 pounds from a decade earlier. This enormous man—with a jutting chin, craggy face, and splayed ears—turned his body into an engine of persuasion. The infamous "Johnson treatment" involved towering over the target and touching, clutching, patting, pawing, and talking; no one talked like Lyndon, who deployed stories, jokes, flattery, promises, compromises, threats, or whatever else it took. His old friend, Senator George Smathers (D-FL) said that talking to Johnson was like running into a "great thunderstorm that consumed you as it closed around you."[25]

"His greatest strength," reflected House Majority Leader Carl Albert (D-OK), "was his talent for tenacity. He just never gives up. In that regard, I think he was the most talented man in the world at that time, or any time maybe—any time in our history. I'm sure he was. I think he had a talent for tenacity that no other President has ever had."[26] This force of nature had something more going for him: he was a brilliant politician.

Most people who knew Johnson, whether friends and foes, recalled how he seemed to mesmerize and overwhelm everyone in his path—even

Washington veterans who had long ago become jaded by talent, power, and ambition. Senator Clinton Anderson called Johnson "the smartest politician I ever knew." He added that he figured he'd be saying that "for a long time to come." "Never seen his equal," agreed Bryce Harlow, a conservative Republican aide to Eisenhower.[27]

"I was ... most surprised," commented James Gaither, a White house aide, at "the man's tremendous analytic ability and tremendous knowledge of government." Southern senators generally expected to serve for life, and many grew extremely sophisticated about legislative rules and folkways. Johnson, however, took that knowledge to a new level and combined it with his fierce intelligence. "He asked questions that no one in the room could answer about impact on local government activities and the way the program would be operated, very direct, piercing questions going to the heart of the proposal," remembered Gaither, "and he doesn't move until most all of his questions are answered, and until he has seen all the options and alternatives, and he's convinced it's the right thing to do, and also that he can do it."[28]

Johnson also had an uncanny ability to read people—he backed up his extraordinary intuition with relentless and minute analysis. "He knew all the little things that people did," recalled Vice President Hubert Humphrey. "I used to say he had his own private F.B.I. If you ever knew anybody, if you'd been out on a date, or if you'd had a drink, or if you'd attended a meeting, or you danced with a gal at a nightclub, he knew it! It was just incredible!" This was one of the most famous Johnson traits, and many observers commented on it. "On people and on relations," summed up Wilbur Cohen, "that was something that he knew."[29]

Johnson himself told his biographer, Doris Kearns, "[T]he challenge ... was to learn what it was that mattered to each of these men; understand which issues were critical to whom and why." Without understanding their personal desires and their organizational needs, said Johnson, "nothing is possible." Knowing it "let me shape my legislative program to fit both their needs and mine."[30]

None of this was left to chance. When he was the Senate majority leader in the 1950s, he would rehearse his arguments, anticipate responses, reflect on the appropriate sticks and carrots, plot the meeting—and then make it all look spontaneous, just an accidental encounter in the halls of Congress.

Finally, Johnson's ambition was as oversized as the rest of him. The shock of Kennedy's assassination and the size of the landslide gave him an opportunity. But even the most liberal members of Congress, recalled

Carl Albert, "would have been content with being able to do a few ... [social programs]." Not Johnson. He wanted them all in one term. "He never rested from the time one was passed until you started on another. I'm sure in all the history of Congress there has never been so much Presidential activity in pushing legislation ... as we were able to do in the 89th Congress."[31]

## RUNNING THE MACHINE: JOHNSON'S GOVERNING STYLE

No president in modern times better understood the springs and gears of national government. After his great landslide victory—when he could finally claim a mandate of his own—Johnson gathered his legislative team and gave them a memorable talk, one that every president would do well to ponder. He said, recalled Wilbur Cohen,

> "Now look. I've just been reelected by the overwhelming majority. And I just want to tell you that every day while I'm in office, I'm going to lose votes. I'm going to alienate somebody." And then he took about twenty minutes and traced the history of other Presidents.... And he says, "The President begins to lose power fast once he has been reelected.... It's going to be something.... We've got to get this legislation fast. You've got to get it during my honeymoon."[32]

Johnson knew people would be annoyed, even angry, to be rushed all the time. But he focused on the inevitable clock—his presidential power was always running down, especially for the domestic issues that he cared about most. Democratic leaders and Johnson's legislative team "alternately kind of laughed and commiserated with each other" as Johnson would phone from the White House and prod them to do more. "Well, can't you get another one or two [more bills] yet this afternoon?"[33]

### Working the Congress

Johnson's White House was a perpetual tutorial in managing Congress. There was often a ribald tall tale to illustrate the point—the punch line, if Lady Bird was not present, might be, "he grabbed my balls with one hand and pulled out his pocket knife with the other," or, more pointedly, "the swish, swish, swish, when [Senator] Pat McNamara [D-MI] cut off [Johnson aide, Richard] Goodwin's pecker," by cutting back a White House proposal. But they all went back to the fundamental lesson, which the president famously summarized: "There is but one way for a President to deal with the Congress, and this is continuously, incessantly, and without interruption."[34]

Johnson never left legislation to chance. He consciously built organizational capacity to handle the stream of programs he sent up Pennsylvania Avenue. He kept Kennedy's talented director of legislative affairs, Lawrence O'Brien; then he gave O'Brien his choice of staff from across the administration and pushed his Cabinet to assign their most talented people to congressional relations. He was far more direct about it than Kennedy had been, recalled O'Brien. "Jack Kennedy might not have said to the cabinet, 'Now, I expect you to have the best man [in legislative relations].... Lyndon Johnson thrust himself into this."[35]

He was always ready to intervene, to plunge himself directly into the legislative process. As Medicare ran through the congressional gauntlet, said O'Brien, Johnson "was alert to the ebb and flow from day one until the conclusion. He was totally immersed in it." But he was also careful to leave no footprints and pass off the praise. "We tried like the devil at all times to avoid public comments claiming credit for legislative progress."[36]

"Johnson always acted ... like he was still running the Congress," recalled Wilbur Cohen. "I've been in Johnson's office when he was on the telephone for an hour or two with members of Congress, talking with them, and cajoling them," and giving them the treatment. He understood the members. "The Congressmen looked upon Kennedy as a nice boy, but not a guy who could get what he wanted. I think by and large with Johnson, they looked upon him as a man who was able to outdo them at their same tricks."[37]

Johnson relished the process and missed the congressional melee that he had left behind. The White House tapes capture him prodding Vice President Humphrey about being more aggressive in pushing legislation. "The President can't go see 'em [congressmen]. Hell, I'd love to ... I want to go to the Texas delegation.... That's where I want to be every day.... I don't want to be sitting down here receiving the ambassador from Ghana.... But I can't do it and the Vice President can."[38] On one occasion, the administration lost a roll call at 4:00 A.M. and O'Brien waited until the president was up to tell him. Johnson wanted none of that. "You should have called me right then, because if you're bleeding up there, Larry, I want to bleed with you."[39]

But Johnson could also be brutal to his aides. "Meticulously polite to those in the White House he regards as Kennedy men," scrawled Arthur Schlesinger (the ultimate Kennedy man) in his private journal, "[b]ut when he starts regarding them as Johnson men, their day is over." Johnson demeaned and hazed new assistants to ensure his control. "Whoever he is," Schlesinger quotes Johnson on potential vice presidents, "I want his pecker in my pocket."[40] The quotation is third-hand and may simply reflect the highbrows' view of boorish LBJ—but Johnson certainly talked and acted that way with subordinates. He dragged aides to the bathroom with him, sat on the toilet, and talked business the entire time. He told them how to dress. He completely dominated them, always tailoring the treatment to the psychology of the individual.

Joseph Califano, tells a typical story. In July 1965, Johnson called him to the presidential ranch and invited him into the swimming pool. After a couple of minutes, the men started talking down near the deep end. LBJ, at six feet, four inches, stood; Califano, at five feet ten inches, could not quite touch bottom and had to tread water while Johnson poked him in the shoulder to emphasize each program he wanted action on: transportation, rebuilding American cities, fair housing, racial equality. They were nose to nose, Johnson going poke, poke, poke, and Califano unable to get around the big man, "breathless from treading water" and "electrified by his energy." For this early interview, concludes Califano, Johnson had "instinctively and intentionally pick[ed] a depth of the pool where he could stand and I had to tread."[41]

## Organization

Johnson used his highly personalized congressional manner to run the entire executive branch. Once again, a Democratic president went for a free-form, creative, somewhat chaotic administrative style. Johnson had no chief of staff and, until Califano tried to impose routine, little organized process. He managed by personal relations, and personal relations meant the usual Johnson mix of flattery and intimidation, bluff and bribery. He didn't like formal meetings, and he dominated those that he called.

Like Kennedy, Johnson continued to draw power from the Cabinet Agencies to the White House—and into his own hands. For example, when the president wanted to do something about America's slums, he turned to Califano and O'Brien and told them about an idea he'd heard from United Auto Workers' president, Walter Reuther, to "turn

American cities into gems." He instructed his aides to design the program (later known as Model Cities) and get it through Congress. Califano gathered a team in the White House, going directly to experts in the Commerce Department without a word to its secretary, Luther Hodges.[42] Power flowed away from the Cabinet and toward a small circle around Johnson. "Lyndon Johnson's Cabinet meetings," Califano told us in an interview, "were just tea parties."[43]

Johnson could make this ad hoc, highly personalized governing model work by sheer force of energy, talent, political intelligence, and personal power. And for a time it worked extraordinarily well—there are few parallels in American history for the way LBJ moved Congress. The Model Cities legislation is a good example. It seemed to have no chance in a Congress that was weary of civil rights—and Califano told the president so. The *New York Times* declared it dead in May 1966. But Lyndon pushed and wheedled and bargained and berated and signed the bill in November.

Johnson had his limits, and with time they began to show. After he worked through the Kennedy programs, he began to serve up his own initiatives at the same breakneck speed. Model Cities, for example, went from conception to passage in nine months. A more carefully designed effort might have succeeded where this program soon floundered in the complexities of urban race and class.

Far worse, when Johnson crossed the boundaries of his own experience and ventured onto foreign terrain, the lack of organization and process proved disastrous. Vietnam was the ultimate failure, a great cloud which darkened much of the Johnson legacy. President Johnson could see the trouble coming. "It just worries the hell out of me," he fretted during one telephone call. "I don't think it's worth fighting for." An effective policy process, comments Fred Greenstein, might have permitted Johnson to air such concerns and, just maybe, avoid the blunders that wrecked his administration. In Southeast Asia, the famous Johnson political instincts, his celebrated political gut, was worthless.[44]

For our purposes, however, the war is especially instructive in a different way. Johnson's failures in foreign policy only emphasize his mastery of domestic policy. LBJ was one of the only modern presidents who preferred the messy, complicated, uncertain process of fashioning domestic programs to the freer hand and power of foreign affairs. Where other presidents saw in domestic matters a charivari of clashing interest groups and procedural obstacles, Johnson took heart. In the Congress, he had the home field advantage. In Southeast Asia, he was lost.

## Achilles' Heel

Johnson's policy problems were exacerbated by his personal limitations. For all his extraordinary talent, Lyndon Johnson was profoundly, almost pathologically, insecure. He wanted desperately to run for the presidency but found it hard to commit and permitted himself to be outmaneuvered in 1960, partially because he held back, afraid to plunge into the fray and risk humiliating defeat. Even in 1964, when he was the uncontested Democratic nominee with high approval ratings, he called press secretary, George Reedy, to declare that he was withdrawing from the race. "I don't want this power of the bomb," he said. "I just don't want these decisions I'm required to make." Lady Bird talked him down off the emotional ledge, and the episode slipped into history—but it is a marker (and there were many) of deep emotional distress: Johnson never felt the easy entitlement to the presidential office that Roosevelt, Eisenhower, and Kennedy all felt. The poor boy from Texas did not, in some deep sense, judge himself worthy of leading the Free World.[45]

He was especially sensitive around the easy, sophisticated Kennedys. Johnson was uncertain, bumbling and depressed as vice president and sometimes tried to respond by parroting Kennedy—JFK loved soups, LBJ noticed, and began ordering them at every chance. The sensitivity never completely disappeared. Two years into his own presidency, for example, he was furious and baffled when the media mocked him for being a boor. Johnson had had surgery, in October 1965, to remove his gall bladder and a kidney stone. He was eager to show the nation that there was nothing in the rumors that he had had another heart attack. To reassure the people, he showed the press the big surgical scar down his belly. People laughed at the big man's crudeness—hitting his sore point so painfully that, once again, he considered resigning.[46]

His insecurities and thin skin made him especially vulnerable as protest mounted over the Vietnam War. He withdrew into the cocoon of the White House, cut off friends and allies, and lost touch with the public. His aides puzzled over the way a leader who could effortlessly dominate a small group of men, who appeared vital and charismatic and larger

than life in their company, became wooden, formal, and lifeless in front
of a large crowd or when the cameras were rolling. Johnson's extraordinary skills did not translate onto the airwaves; he could not use the
mass media to touch American hearts and minds.

Still, the problems and limitations of Johnson and his administration—
the agony of civil rights, the quagmire in Southeast Asia, the mass protests, the quickening sense that the Johnson administration had lost
control of events—all lay in the future as LBJ took office and used his
magic to win Kennedy's programs one after another.

## THE GREAT SOCIETY

After President Kennedy's assassination, Johnson reassured a stunned
nation. He managed the task with remarkable skill and uncharacteristic
humility. Although he had resented his exclusion from Kennedy's inner
circle, he now hugged the legacy. He could not emulate Camelot's glamour, but he could hang on to its staff. Johnson essentially maintained
two staffs until his own election a year later—Kennedy holdovers and
his circle of trusted advisors.

More important, Johnson exuberantly seized the Kennedy legislative
program. "I don't know why," said Wilbur Mills, "but he wanted to do
everything Kennedy had espoused in 1960. He had this tremendous loyalty to John Kennedy. Unbelievable. He had to enact everything. Johnson
kept saying, 'I've got to do it because John Kennedy espoused it.'"[47]

Mills thought it a bit perverse: after all, the Kennedys had looked
down on Johnson. But there is not much mystery in why Johnson seized
this cause. He supported Kennedy's domestic policies—they completed
his beloved New Deal—and he understood the power of invoking the
martyred president. As he had scrambled up the political ladder, Johnson
had regularly apprenticed himself—sometimes obsequiously—to powerful mentors; now he latched on to Kennedy's legacy as the key to his
own ambitions. "Everything I had ever learned in the history books
taught me that martyrs have to die for causes," Johnson told Doris
Kearns. "John Kennedy had died. But his 'cause' was not really clear.
That was my job. I had to take the dead man's program and turn it into
a martyr's cause."[48]

Kennedy left behind an impressive, unfulfilled agenda: civil rights,
educational reform, tax cuts, a vaguely defined war on poverty, and
Medicare. Johnson took this legislative list and gave it a distinctive
frame. Speaking at the University of Michigan commencement in

May 1964, he posed a choice between greed and shared purpose that would test the "quality of our American civilization." With a distinct echo of Franklin Roosevelt, Johnson told the graduates, "Your imagination, your initiative, and your indignation will determine whether we build a society where progress is the servant of our needs, or a society where old values and new visions are buried under unbridled growth. For in your time we have the opportunity to move not only toward the rich society and the powerful society, but upward to the Great Society."[49]

John Kennedy's New Frontier found its apotheosis—and most of its domestic victories—in Lyndon Johnson's Great Society. As Johnson seized the Kennedy standards, he was creating a dream combination. The charismatic, now martyred, president had set the national agenda—rallying with the raucous seniors for Medicare, eloquently taking up the moral cause of civil rights. Then the great insider took the Kennedy programs—most of them languishing in Congress—and won every single one. Most were signed within a year. Medicare would be the most difficult, and among the major bills, it took the longest for Johnson to win.

## RENEGOTIATING MEDICARE

Lyndon Johnson tried, almost frantically, to enact Medicare as soon as he took office. Wilbur Mills and his Ways and Means committee stood as the great barrier, and Johnson gave the Congressman the full treatment—he later claimed to have courted Mills more assiduously than he had Lady Bird. Most of their meetings were private and off the record—often dinners at the White House with the two men and their wives—but telephone tapes and oral histories now permit us to reconstruct the negotiations. A great surprise leaps out of the record.

The traditional story—repeated, by Johnson himself, as we noted at the start of the chapter—features the great Wilbur Mills "bombshell." In reality, the bombshell was no surprise to Johnson. He and Mills had been chewing over the details for over a year. Johnson always promised to defer to Mills on the actual package—but then kept egging him on to make it more ambitious. He promised Mills all the credit—at the same time showing that he was perfectly willing to try to work around him.

Johnson's early push got Medicare further than any previous effort. But Wilbur Mills was almost as cagey as Johnson, and in a bit of legislative jujitsu, he took the effort to win the bill and almost used it to scuttle its prospects by draining off the tax revenues. Only Johnson's last-minute savvy staved off the assault. The upshot of all the Byzantine back-and-forth amounted to this: Johnson went into his reelection campaign, asking voters for a mandate on Medicare; at the same time, his deft, quiet inside game had positioned Medicare for passage in the next term.

## Courting Wilbur Mills

Johnson began within weeks of the assassination, with dinners and calls to Mills. What the representative remembered most was the intensity of LBJ's pressure on him to move legislation, especially Medicare. Johnson applied the personal touch; Wilbur Cohen, Larry O'Brien and others ran the technical negotiations. "Live with him," Johnson commanded Wilbur Cohen.[50]

Though Johnson desperately wanted a bill out of Ways and Means, he insisted that he didn't care what was in it. It could be the King–Anderson bill that Kennedy had been pushing. It could be something else. He wanted, he kept repeating, to give Mills authorship, ownership, and credit. Mills responded by floating a series of ideas. In a January 27 memo—a full fifteen months before the drama of the Medicare "bombshell"—the legislative team reported that Mills was already talking about expanding the package. Although they wrote that "Mills has not completely committed himself either to sponsoring or voting for a bill," he seemed to be "heading toward justifying a position for King-Anderson by altering Kerr-Mills to assure broader acceptance of it by the States." Mills would expand the state-run health care plan for poor Americans that he himself had authored back in 1960. The memo to LBJ then describes nothing less than a rough draft of the eventual Medicare package: "The roads he appears to be traveling are: a. Have the Federal Government spend more money [for Kerr–Mills]. b. Install uniform eligibility tests [for Kerr–Mills in the different states]. c. The insertion of physicians' services."[51]

Johnson picked up the thread in previously unreported telephone conversations. On June 9, Johnson phoned Mills and, after talking about an excise tax bill, asked him teasingly how he was doing on the "Mills

Bill." Mills replied that he was concerned about the macroeconomic effects of the increase in Social Security taxes that would be required to expand Social Security and also add on Medicare. "I trust your judgment on that," returned Johnson, deferring to Mills's economic savvy. But Johnson went right ahead talking of the historic significance of the Medicare program and the applause that Mills would rightly win. "The single most important popular thing," LBJ told the Arkansas Democrat, "is the bill you are working with." If Mills reported out a health bill, said Johnson, we would all "applaud you." Over and over, he repeated: "I am not trying to go into details."[52]

Two days later, in a phone call that found Mills just off the House floor, Johnson got into the details anyway. "Find some way to do something about Medicare," he instructed Mills. Mills then expressed the need to cover his and his colleagues' possible flip-flop from fierce opposition to support. "What I've been trying to do," said Mills, "is to get something that we could say was so different from the King bill itself that those of us who have repeatedly said we wouldn't vote for the King bill could vote for it." Johnson shot back quickly and enthusiastically. "That's exactly right. That's what you've got to do to make it acceptable." Mills then floated again the idea of a "three-pronged" bill that included a Social Security cash benefit (then before his own Ways and Means Committee), a hospital benefit (King–Anderson), and an expansion of Kerr–Mills (to cover health care for the poor). Johnson agreed and then upped the ante. "I'd be for all three of those if you could put that fourth one in it." Johnson was pushing for a bigger, more complete Medicare package, presumably the physician coverage that Mills had been discussing with the White House team. That "fourth one," concluded Johnson, has "sex appeal."[53]

Mills had always complained that the administration's Medicare bill lacked any physician benefits. The elderly would be enraged, he thought, when they found out how modest the legislation actually was. Polls taken at the time backed Mills up. Most people expected Medicare to cover physicians' fees. Johnson was right about that fourth one having "sex appeal."[54]

Still, Mills was always wary about reporting a bill out of committee that might lose on the House floor. He and Johnson endlessly counted heads, and Mills invariably fretted about not having the votes. Johnson tried to convince Mills that thirteen Democrats in favor (on a twenty-five-person committee) were enough; that they could probably get fourteen votes in committee; that Mills should forget about the

Republicans: "They're against any proposal I make." His own over-all popularity, purred Johnson, was at an astronomical 79 percent. He needed Mills's help on the "Mills Medicare Bill," and he kept imagining the praise Mills would get. He concluded their June 11 conversation by repeating: "It will be biggest thing you have ever done for your country."[55]

However, Johnson remained wary about Mills's commitment, and within minutes of hanging up with Mills on June 11, he was on the phone with his close friend, Senator Earle Clements, (D-KY), who had served as whip when LBJ was majority leader of the Senate. If Mills backed out and passed a Social Security expansion without Medicare, said Clements, the Senate could then add health care for the elderly to the Social Security package. Mills, in turn, could soften the health legislation in conference and satisfy both LBJ and the physician lobby. Johnson agreed and chuckled: "I always have that [the Senate] to fall back on."[56]

Mills would indeed back out this time. But Johnson had made it very clear that the Congressman had two choices: he could work with the president and earn the credit for Medicare's passage, or he could oppose him and face ceaseless Johnsonian pressure if, as expected, the president was elected to a full term in November 1964. Moreover, Wilbur Mills knew that if and when he moved Medicare, the president would find the funding, help round up the votes, and pass all the credit back to Mills. The ultracautious Representative Mills might have been hesitant to make his dramatic announcement without knowing that Johnson had guaranteed his full support.

## I Always Have the Senate to Fall Back On

The Senate was no slam dunk for Medicare either. In July, the Senate Democratic Caucus had expressed strong support for Johnson's agenda—except Medicare. They split over the health care program. Senator Abraham Ribicoff (D-CT) floated a compromise: let the elderly choose between Medicare coverage and its cash equivalent in increased Social Security benefits. The idea appealed to some Democrats.

Senator George Smathers, an old friend of Johnson's (though they often disagreed on policy) told him to forget about Medicare before the election and just use it in the campaign. "It's a hell of a lot better issue than it is a fact on the books," Smathers told Johnson in August. Echoing Mills, he said the elderly would get angry when they found out how little the administration's program actually gave them.

Besides, he told Johnson, "I don't think you're going to come out with it anyway." He had sat up the previous night drinking whisky with Senator Russell Long (D-LA), an influential member of the Senate Finance Committee, and there was no way Long was going to vote with Johnson.[57]

Blocked by Long and other southern Democrats in the Senate Finance Committee, Johnson decided to introduce Medicare on the Senate floor as an amendment to the Social Security benefit expansion that the House was sending over to the Senate. Senator Ribicoff was working hard for his bill, giving seniors a choice between higher Social Security benefits or Medicare; the Ribicoff plan was a much easier vote, because it was less offensive to organized medicine. Larry O'Brien called Johnson for instructions from the Senate majority leader's office: what should the Democratic leaders do—support the Ribicoff Amendment, or hold firm for King–Anderson? Johnson did not hesitate. They needed to get the more generous King–Anderson bill out of the Senate, or they'd have nothing to compromise with once the Social Security bill went to the conference committee to work out the differences between the Senate and House versions (the House had no Medicare provisions in its bill). "Wilbur Mills will take your pants off unless you have something to trade for," he told O'Brien.[58]

While the Senate debated, the acting director of the Bureau of the Budget, Elmer Staats, weighed in with an economic alarm. "The Bureau of the Budget and the Council of Economic Advisers feel strongly that the tax increases in both ... the Gore Amendment [King–Anderson] or the Ribicoff Amendment ... are too high and would constitute a serious drag on the economy." True to form, the economists opposed the entitlement, in this case because of the large surplus it would have created in the Social Security trust fund. Johnson, in the middle of directing the legislative battle, brushed off the economic quibbles.[59]

He repeatedly talked strategy with Senator Albert Gore (D-TN),who was managing King–Anderson for an ailing Clinton Anderson. On September 2, the day of the Senate vote, he did the head counts with Mike Mansfield (D-MT), the Senate majority leader. When Mansfield reported that he thought he had fifty-one votes but that Carl Hayden (D-AZ) was wobbly, LBJ quickly rang Hayden and pushed party loyalty, election politics, and bragging rights in Arizona. Republican Barry Goldwater, the other senator from Arizona, who was running against Johnson for the White House, was flying back to Washington for the Medicare vote. "Don't you let 'em beat us Carl.... We've got to have these old people."

Johnson then told him that "if we don't need your vote, feel free to go over to the other side." Hayden voted with LBJ.[60]

During the Senate debate, Senate Russell Long proposed that the 5 percent increase in Social Security approved by the House be increased to 7 percent. "Why," returned Senator Gore, "the effect of this amendment would be to kill Medicare forever." The Social Security increase would use up all the tax revenues. "Well, that's the idea," chuckled Senator Smathers. The threat was voted down. Then the Medicare amendment passed the Senate, 49–44. Ten months after LBJ took office, one chamber had finally passed health coverage for the elderly under Social Security.[61]

Johnson seems to have played an essential role in lining up the votes, although we have only found concrete evidence of the call to Senator Hayden. Johnson certainly thought he had made the difference. "I got enough votes to carry it out," he told one well-wisher. "I don't want to leave the impression we twisted arms or forced individuals," he cheerfully added to a legislative aide, "but I'd say we did what we do on a lot of legislation."[62]

For the most part, Johnson passed the credit to his aides. The victory in the Senate paid an extra election year dividend: Goldwater had flown in to vote nay. Bill Moyers, a White House domestic policy specialist, advised Johnson, "I don't think *you* should be kicking Goldwater, but this is a great opportunity for us to beat him to death among these older people if we just play it right."[63]

## Conference Committee Boomerang

The day after the Senate victory, September 3, LBJ practically dictated talking points to the Democratic House leadership team about how to win over Wilbur Mills in Conference Committee. He began by playing to Mills's own sense of importance: "I would try to say to Wilbur that this is a national matter that involves the party.... He's a national fella and he's not just for Arkansas and he's head of the powerful Ways and Means committee and [he] represents everybody." Plus Wilbur could modify the bill any way he wants. "We've given him running room and we'd much prefer to let him modify it." He could compromise us down to Ribicoff. Or, Johnson started to wax ambitious, you could "appeal to him ... for his party and for his country and let's have a *Mills-Anderson-Ribicoff* proposal in the conference." The others did not know it, but this would not be the first time Wilbur Mills heard of that particular combination: *Mills* (that is, Kerr–Mills), *Anderson* (King–Anderson, the administration bill), and *Ribicoff* (a package that included a choice about a Social Security increase) was almost precisely the "three pronged" proposal that Mills himself had floated to Johnson as they talked on the phone back in June. Here, yet again, is a variation of the Wilbur Mills "bombshell" that, in the standard story, would take the delighted Johnson by surprise six months later.[64]

But there was nothing doing. Mills was even reported to be peeved by all the pressure. Which, in turn, set off a rare show of irritation from LBJ: "Well, I wonder, if he's entitled to be peeved, I wonder if I oughtn't to get peeved at him doin' me this way."[65]

Johnson tried a series of fallbacks: push a vote in the House to get the Republicans on the record as opposed; call the House and Senate back into lame duck session after the election and try to push it through then; introduce a measure in the House to instruct the conferees (i.e., Wilbur Mills) to accept the Medicare amendment. But each effort fell short. When Johnson asked Carl Albert for the head count on the motion to have the House instruct Mills, Albert replied that it was 235 against and 200 for. LBJ chuckled ruefully: "Well we've got a hell of a shape, haven't we?"[66]

Frustrated on the House side, LBJ's team turned to the Senate to try to stiffen their resolve in the upcoming conference with the House. O'Brien reported regularly to LBJ on reassurances from various Senate conferees that they would insist on a health care component to the Social Security bill. In the meantime, Johnson conferred privately, and evidently without the knowledge of his own aides, with the Senate members of the Conference Committee. On September 24, he talked to Smathers, asking him to check out reports that the conference committee had deadlocked, and then added: "Don't tell I called or they'll all get jealous." Ten minutes later, Johnson was talking to Russell Long about the prospects for Medicare; Johnson signed off warning Long not to tell anyone that LBJ had called, because "[t]hey'll get jealous."[67]

In the all the back-and-forth in committee, Wilbur Mills almost managed to scuttle the future prospects for Medicare by picking up the strategy Long had used on the Senate floor. Mills himself had tried the same thing in his Ways and Means Committee and came up one vote short: offer a big Social Security increase—usually irresistible in an election year—that would raise the Social Security payroll tax to 10 percent.

This was generally thought to be the upper limit, and if the increase went through, Congress would have used up the federal tax capacity and thus blocked a Social Security–based Medicare plan, regardless of what happened in the election.

On October 2, Mills convened the conference committee and, confident that he had the votes, moved to report the Social Security bill without Medicare. He was shocked to find Senators Long and Smathers—both long-term opponents of Medicare—voting against him and for Medicare. Their votes were decisive, and the committee deadlocked; Congress would report neither Medicare nor Social Security. A dumbfounded Mills stared at Smathers in disbelief for a long moment and then angrily adjourned the Committee. President Johnson's intervention with Long and Smathers seems to have checked the Mills maneuver. Long wanted to be majority whip, and President Johnson's support would be an enormous asset. For his part, when reporters asked Smathers why he switched, he said, simply: "Lyndon told me to."[68]

Although LBJ did not succeed in his first push for Medicare, the effort yielded a major campaign issue. Johnson's intense involvement in the legislative maneuvers had multiple effects: first, if Johnson won in 1965, he would charge back at them full-bore to pass Medicare, and everyone in Congress knew it. Second, he would use every trick—and he knew a lot of them—to drag reluctant Democrats into his column. Third, though they had struggled to a draw, Mills knew that if he chose to move the legislation, Johnson would give him full credit and powerful backing. Finally, Johnson and Mills had essentially sketched the outlines of an ambitious Medicare plan. We have seen its variations in memos (as early as January 1964), in phone conversations (June 1964) and in Johnson's last-ditch, indirect effort to push Mills toward an ambitious, three-pronged, Conference Committee compromise (October 1964). The option was available any time Mills wanted to use it. The election results would, of course, persuade him.

## MEDICARE!

The 1964 landslide made it easy. President Johnson continued to work as a kind of super–majority leader—guiding the legislation, pointing out snares, calling for speed, and clearing an occasional roadblock. But he now tried even harder to keep his fingerprints off the process—and to pass the credit back to Congress.

The election had offered a dramatic choice. A month after being nominated, Barry Goldwater had flown to Washington and cast his very loud "nay" on Medicare. The leaders of the American Medical Association maladroitly organized a "Doctors for Goldwater Committee." On the other side, "Johnson made a great many promises in the campaign," commented journalist Richard Harris, "but none as often or as fervently" as the promise to pass Medicare. The Democratic tsunami, in both presidential and congressional elections, decisively tipped the legislative balance toward the president's agenda. Three Medicare opponents on the Ways and Means Committee went down. No one could miss the implications for Medicare.[69]

## Wheeling and Dealing

The day after the election, Representative Hale Boggs (D-LA), a member of the House leadership, called with his congratulations. Boggs commented on how mean the doctors had been during the campaign and continued:

> *Boggs:* I want you to give me the privilege of being the sponsor of Medicare when Congress meets.
>
> *Johnson:* Those doctors are awful mean.
>
> *Boggs:* Oh, were they mean!
>
> *Johnson:* I want to be sure when we meet in January that we get it through.[70]

A few days later, on November 9, LBJ spoke to Carl Albert and discussed the vacancies on the House Ways and Means Committee left by the defeat of Medicare opponents. Mills no longer had the votes to bury the bill in committee. "We can pass Medicare," reported Albert cheerfully, "we can pass it by discharge petition if we have to, and I think Mills will give. If he doesn't, he's not as smart as I think he is." Throughout the Medicare discussions, the legislators would slip in little requests for their districts. Albert, who represented the then-oil-rich state of Oklahoma, went on to warn LBJ that he might need to rein in the new liberal majority on Ways and Means to prevent it from cutting tax breaks for oil companies.[71]

Russell Long called with his own bit of quid pro quo. The Department of Defense was closing military bases around the country. Long told LBJ that Louisiana's Fort Polk was on the list and asked Johnson to reverse the decision. At first, Johnson stuck up for his secretary of defense: "If it's on the list, ain't nobody can change it." But Long put his IOU on the table. "Mr. President, when I had that vote to kill Medicare, that's not the action I took on you." Johnson replied that he would check whether Polk was really on that list, and get back to Long. A few minutes later, the president left a message for the Louisiana Democrat. Polk would not be closing after all.[72]

Johnson worked fast to get Medicare queued up and ready to go when the new Congress took its seats in January. Three weeks after the election, Anthony Celebreeze sent the president the administration's new proposal, ready for the internal review that preceded formal introduction. The legislation looked very much like the bill Congress had passed the previous summer: a Hospital Trust Fund with its own dedicated payroll tax that would cover up to 180 days in the hospital (along with sixty days of nursing home care and home health visits) for people over sixty-five.[73]

Johnson kept dispatching his staff to smooth out complications. Senator Russell (D-GA), the president's old friend and mentor, was reportedly "on the fence" about Medicare, and Johnson dispatched Cohen to "talk quietly" with the old patrician. James Cain, Johnson's reliable physician, called with a small suggestion that could be quickly cleared up. Jacob Javits (R-NY) came forward yet again and suggested a variation on his own proposal to enhance the role of private insurers. Javits had been trying since the Eisenhower administration, always with the hope that he could round up Republican votes. When Kennedy had found himself holding a weak hand, he had negotiated with Javits; now that Johnson held his royal congressional flush, he instructed Wilbur Cohen to turn Javits down.[74]

When Larry O'Brien thought about leaving the administration, the president gave him the treatment by reminding him what was at stake. He—Larry O'Brien—was going to launch the year "with the most meaningful domestic proposal that had been hanging around for years: Medicare. You'd move with Medicare first: HR1 and S1, the first proposal of the new Congress." The bill numbers signified that Medicare had the prestigious pride of place as the first bills in the congressional hopper. Johnson went on, "[you move] as rapidly and as aggressively as you could." And he promised O'Brien that "by God, he was going to put the wood to the cabinet."[75]

## The Wilbur Mills Story

On January 4, Johnson delivered his State of the Union address. He began as an old colleague and fellow warrior: "On this hill which was my home I am stirred by old friendships." He turned directly to the new members—living, breathing results of his landslide—and told them "twenty-eight years ago, I felt as you do now. You will soon learn that you are among men"—Johnson had come up old-school and did not mention the women in the chamber—"who try each day to do the best they can what they believe is right." Once again, Johnson called for a Great Society that "asks not how much but how good; not only how to create wealth but how to use it; not only how fast are we going but where are we headed."[76]

And then a surprise. Johnson never mentioned his most important program. He discussed health—medical education, community health centers, the importance of health to a great society—but made no mention of Medicare. It was as if that program now belonged to the members themselves. The president would remain very active, moving his most important legislation along. But what the public would see was the Wilbur Mills show. Johnson could sit back and enjoy the master legislator's performance of the script they had prepared (and negotiated, and scrapped over) for more than a year.

Congressman Mills opened his hearings on the administration's bill, and they continued until the legislators had heard the six hundred forty-first witness since hearings began on King–Anderson back in 1961. The AMA, trying to adjust to the new political reality, launched another public relations campaign in which it proposed an alternative bill: a voluntary program that paid physician fees for the elderly, enthusiastically sponsored in Congress by John Byrnes (R-WI). They warned the public that everyone would be sorely disappointed when they went to the doctor's office and discovered that the much-touted administration bill did not do a thing for them. This is precisely what Wilbur Mills believed, and what George Smathers and others had told Johnson. The president kept uncharacteristically silent.

After the hearings, the Ways and Means committee went into closed session, and on March 2, Wilbur Mills pulled the legendary coup. Mills turned to Byrnes and said, "You know John, I like that idea of yours." He then suggested his "three layer cake." The administration bill covered hospital costs. The Byrnes (and AMA) bill would cover physician services for elderly Americans who voluntarily signed up. And a great expansion of Mills's own Kerr–Mills program to cover health care costs for the poor through state-administered programs. These would become Medicare Part A, Medicare Part B, and Medicaid. The package would also include the Social Security benefits increase that had been put aside before the election. Wilbur Mills than turned to Wilbur Cohen, the irrepressible technician, and asked him to draft the language by morning. Cohen asked for a full day, and Mills cut him off—the next morning. "Like everyone else in the room," said Cohen later, "I was stunned by Mill's strategy. It was the most brilliant legislative move I'd seen in thirty years." And so it went down in history. Wilbur Mills received standing ovations when he took Ways and Means back into public sessions, when he went before senior citizens, and when he took the new Medicare to the House floor.[77]

Lyndon Johnson dutifully played his role: expressing delighted surprise, launching into the Texas ol' boy train wreck story (described in the introduction), telling Cohen to go give Mills the go sign that Johnson had privately given more than a year before.

Mills, for his part, frankly acknowledged Johnson's participation. "We planned that, yes. Oh, yes." Johnson had always deferred to Mills on the details, continued Mills. " I'd developed some ideas on it, how we'd proceed" And LBJ pressed him on: "[D]evelop it as you want to develop it."[78]

But Johnson sent all the credit to Mills and went out of his way to minimize his own participation. When the revised pieces of Medicare and Medicaid legislation were ready to be reported to the House floor, LBJ pointedly instructed Cohen that the White House should not issue any statements until they were cleared with Mills, telling Cohen that he wanted Mills to get the credit.[79] Johnson's autobiography, as we noted above, artfully reinforces the legendary Mills story—without ever quite crossing the line into untruth. It is only now, forty years later, that we discover that Johnson coauthored the surprise.

## Dead Cats in the Process

Still, if Johnson ducked the publicity, he restlessly oversaw the process of his legislation. He was acutely aware of each potential snare in the congressional process and kept swooping in to help Medicare negotiate them.

For example, after Mills maneuvered the newly expanded Medicare package through his committee, he gathered with the speaker of the House, John McCormack, and the majority leader, Carl Albert, to call Johnson with the good news. Johnson was already looking to the next potential trap: the rules committee could delay sending the legislation to the house floor. This, in turn, would give opponents a chance to recoup, write letters, and stem the tide. LBJ reminded them to move fast in his pungent Texas way: "For God sakes, don't let dead cats stand on your porch. Mr. Rayburn [Sam Rayburn (D-TX)] former House speaker and Johnson mentor, used to say: 'they stunk and they stunk and they stunk.' When you get one [of your bills] out of your committee, you call that son of a bitch up before they [the opposition] can get their letters written."[80]

Days after this call, Johnson cleared another hurdle for Medicare in the Senate, where he knew that the chairman of the critical Senate Finance Committee, Senator Harry Byrd (D-VA), was a firm opponent. Byrd might try to bottle Medicare in his committee. In a legendary ambush, Johnson invited Byrd to the White House for a meeting with legislative leaders. It was an extremely important and sensitive meeting, LBJ told Byrd, and he was sending a White House car to pick him up. After a closed-door conversation, Johnson ushered the men into an unexpected press conference. With TV cameras rolling, Johnson talked about the successful movement of Medicare through the House Ways and Means committee, introduced the nine Democrats, then turned to Byrd and asked the surprised senator whether there was anything preventing the Senate Finance Committee from quickly holding hearings on Medicare. An uncomfortable Byrd tried to evade a direct answer, saying the bill had not come up before the Senate yet. Johnson pinned him down and squeezed his arm, and not-so-gently pressured him before the rolling cameras. Byrd reluctantly stammered that there would be no delay in acting on the bill.

Afterward, Johnson "had the biggest smile you ever saw on his face.... I guess the only way to describe it was that it was like a fellow who just finished a beautiful steak dinner."[81] Byrd commented ruefully to O'Brien as he walked out to the car: "[I]f I had known what you had in mind, I would have dressed more formally."[82] But he was good to his word and brought Medicare before his committee in the following weeks.

Although the ambush is a familiar story, we can now fit it into the larger pattern. What seemed to be essentially an internal legislative process is now revealed as a far more interactive business—from framing the law to getting it through the complicated congressional process. Success took an extremely deft president constantly operating the legislative machinery—while hiding his hand and deflecting the credit.

## Al Caldy Economics

Johnson did one more crucial thing over the course of the winter and spring of 1965: he managed the economics of Medicare and Medicaid. This was much easier to do in 1965, before the creation of the Congressional Budget Office, which now provides independent economic reviews of all legislation, and a comparable office within the White House, the Office of Management and Budget. But, then as now, the president had to confront arguments that expansions of health coverage were unaffordable. Sometimes Johnson would insist he had fiscal matters under control; at other times, he'd try to keep critics quiet. But he was generally ruthless about clearing financial barriers out of the legislation's path.

Mills expressed concern in a call to Johnson about the costs of adding Part B and Medicaid to the Medicare package in March 1965. Johnson, chewing audibly on his lunch, told him not to worry: "I'll take care of that." First he told Mills that his own fiscal restraint had made the money available. "You see what I've done, Wilbur, ... by withholding and just threatening and ultimatum and being meaner than you or [Senator] Harry Byrd , I am under [budget] this year ... a billion eight hundred million [dollars] under what you [the Congress] appropriated and what I said I'd spend." Having offered up his economic argument, he cuts off the discussion with another Texas ol' boy routine. "You want to put in another 400 or 500 million [to cover Medicare expansion].... What did I say about it? ... I said we had an old judge in Texas one time ... we called him Al Caldy ... old Al Caldy Roberts, and he said, when they talked to him one time that he might've abused the constitution and he said, 'what's the constitution between friends?' And I say 'tell Wilbur that 400 million's not going to separate us friends when it's for health, when it's for sickness, because there's a greater demand ... for this bill than all my other programs put together.' I know that."[83]

Johnson often groused about the budget sharks circling his program. "The fools had to go projecting it [Medicare] down the road five or six years, and when you project it the first year it runs 900 million. Now I don't know whether I would approve 900 million the second year or not. I might approve 450 or 500, but the first thing Senator Dick Russell

(D-GA) comes running in [and] says, 'My God, you've got a one billion dollar [projection] for next year on health. Therefore I'm against any of it now.' "[84]

Cavalier as Johnson may sound here, especially in light of the huge costs the program immediately ran up, his comments signal a theme worth pondering: Johnson, like Kennedy before him, lowballed the numbers and evaded economic projections to smooth the passage of Medicare and the rest of his Great Society Program. The numbers—whether for Truman, Ike, Kennedy, or Johnson—never support the entitlement. An honest economic forecast would have very likely sunk Medicare. Moreover, Francis Bator, a national security aide to Johnson at the time, recently asserted that during 1965, Johnson also suppressed news of the escalation of the Vietnam War, and its attendant costs, so that Congress would not question whether the nation could afford the president's Great Society initiatives.[85]

After Mills had rewritten the bill, Johnson summed up the finances in a long conversation with (really a lecture at) Vice President Humphrey. "I'll go a hundred million or a billion on health or education.... I'll spend the goddamn money." He had given them "the go sign," he said, regardless of the cash required, and he knew that Medicare was finally going to go through Congress "like a dose of salt through a widow woman."[86]

*Medicare Wins*

On April 8, 1965, the House of Representatives met to consider the revised health measure—the first time a Medicare proposal had made it through committee and onto the floor of the House. Mills received a standing ovation, went to the rostrum, and, barely looking at his notes, described what was in the 296 pages of H.R. 1 (by then known, following LBJ's lead, as "the Mills Bill"). When the roll was taken on the crucial vote—whether to send the bill back to committee and substitute the Byrnes bill—Medicare prevailed by just forty-five votes. Only ten Republicans voted with the administration, and sixty-three Democrats defected and voted to bury it back in committee. The Johnson landslide had brought in, by one count, forty-four new Medicare advocates, and the administration needed almost every last one. With the deal done, however, most members got in on the victory; in the final roll call, the House of Representatives voted Medicare up, 313–115.

In the Senate, the sailing seemed smoother. Senator Harry Byrd never seemed to resent the Johnson ambush. On the contrary, he was enough of an old pro himself to recognize another one in action, thought Larry O'Brien, "and probably admired it a little bit." "He is convinced passage is inevitable," reported one legislative aide, and "while he will vote against he will not delay it."[87]

Johnson received a steady stream of reports but only needed to swoop in on a few occasions. The most important dealt, once again, with the matter of costs. In March, Gardner Ackley, chairman of the Council of Economic Advisers, warned the president that the Social Security tax increases Wilbur Mills was using to finance Medicare's Part A were larger than necessary and could constitute a fiscal drag on the economy that might negate the stimulus from LBJ's 1964 tax cut and even push the economy into a recession before the 1966 midterms. Johnson dispatched his economic aides to confer with Mills, who reduced the proposed tax rates.[88]

By mid-April, the economic anxiety about Medicare taxes had spread. Secretary of HEW Celebrezze warned the White House that the newspapers were running articles about Medicare's possible drag on the economy. "He thinks," reported White House special assistant Jack Valenti, "that this is going to be the new attack on the bill." Johnson's first reaction was to apply the muzzle to his economists. He scribbled blunt instructions at the bottom of Valenti's memo: "Please ask Ackley and [Henry] Fowler [Secretary of the Treasury] to ask their friends to pipe down—L." Valenti shot back by scribbling on the same memo: "4/23 Talked to Ackley—bill *is* a drag."[89]

The White House team met quietly and suggested a bundle of technical changes designed to reduce the drag "to a more tolerable figure of $1.6 billion."[90] However, the economic fears framed the administration's strategy in the Senate. With victory assured, many liberals wanted to expand Medicare. They lined up to add benefits such as catastrophic insurance (so that families that ran through the hospital benefits would not be ruined) and outpatient drug payments. Johnson and his team beat back most of these expansions.

In a typical exchange, late in the debate, Senator Robert Byrd (D-WV) touted an amendment to reduce the threshold for Medicare eligibility to the age of sixty. Byrd called Johnson to get support for the proposal. The president—in classic LBJ style—said he hadn't read the amendment and asked Byrd what Cohen and "the boys" felt about it. Johnson knew perfectly well that the boys were busy killing expansions but never let on, and, in a long conversation, never committed. He said only, "All I know is I love you." The Byrd Amendment never saw the light of day.[91]

The traditional Medicare story imagines a rather wide-open liberal shootout in Congress, capped by Wilbur Mills's tripling the size of the program at the last minute. Our revision suggests a very tightly controlled process in which Mills introduced a long-negotiated addition while, on the Senate side, the administration nervously kept its liberal stalwarts in check by reigning in costly amendments that would add benefits such as catastrophic insurance, pharmaceutical benefits, and an increase in eligible age groups. Ironically, health policy liberals would spend the next forty-five years chasing the benefits the Johnson administration defeated during liberalism's high-water mark. Most of the rejected additions would be back: Ronald Reagan sponsored catastrophic insurance (quickly repealed the next year); George W. Bush won pharmaceutical benefits; and as for extending coverage to other groups—stay tuned.

In July 1965, the Senate passed a generous version of Medicare. Later that month, the Conference Committee cut back, by Cohen's reckoning, about $1.2 billion of the $1.5 billion that the Senate had added to the House version. The only administration defeat lay in Mills's insistence that hospital-based specialists—radiologists, pathologists, anesthesiologists, and physiatrists—not be paid with the hospitals under Medicare Part A (which would have made sense, because they were salaried hospital workers); rather, they would be treated as doctors in private practice and permitted to bill Medicare their "customary" fees as any other physicians. This would be far more costly, but Wilbur Mills had promised the AMA that no doctor would be paid under Social Security. Wilbur Mills was the designated hero of the Medicare story, and he got his way. At the end of the month, the House (July 27) and the Senate (July 28) sent President Johnson the Medicare bill that liberals had been fighting for a decade.

Some of the White House staff suggested signing the bill in Independence, Missouri, in honor of eighty-one-year old Harry Truman. Others, including Wilbur Cohen, worried that this might provoke the AMA, which had fought tooth-and-nail with the Truman administration. After all, fretted Cohen, Medicare could not succeed without physicians' cooperation. How about signing at the FDR home in Hyde Park on August 15, the thirtieth anniversary of Social Security? But President Johnson never hesitated.

On July 30, 1965, the victorious White House team, the congressional leadership, and an ecstatic former President Truman met in Independence, Missouri, for an extraordinary signing ceremony. Johnson's remarks—intimate and reflective—ran to the role that presidents play in shaping the course of history. Here was one president speaking to another about what set them apart, about what they believed in, about the risks they had both taken, and about this triumph, which they shared.

## IMPLEMENTING MEDICARE

Johnson could only briefly savor his victory, for his administration now faced another enormous task—it had eleven months to launch the program. The triumphant signing in Independence, Missouri, would be quickly forgotten if 19 million elderly Americans found their health care thrown into chaos when the law went into effect on July 1, 1966. "There were forecasts of disaster," recalled Johnson, "right up to the day Medicare went into effect." "If you miscalculate," he told his HEW secretary, "we're both going to look like the worst kind of damned fools." The administration faced three major challenges: segregation, recalcitrant doctors, and the sheer scope of the task.[92]

### Segregation

Segregation was the great hidden issue lurking in the Medicare debates. Southerners fiercely believed in letting states run social programs—and from Aid to Families with Children (or Welfare, in 1935) to Kerr–Mills (in 1960), they generally managed to keep programs that touched poor and black people under the thumb of state administrators, who understood the importance—as they saw it—of segregation. Social Security was the great exception, and southern Democrats had, at first, managed to keep most southern black people out of the program (by excluding farm and domestic workers). To southern leaders a health program run by the Social Security Administration vibrated with clear danger to segregated health facilities—national regulations and national attitudes would, they knew, quickly follow the money.[93]

Perhaps, as David Barton Smith has argued, the administration was never going to win Medicare until it broke the segregationists and passed the Civil Rights Act (as it finally did in July 1964).[94] But the

Civil Rights Act, in turn, raised the stakes. Title VI of the Act stipulated that "no person in the United States shall, on the grounds of race, color, or national origin, be excluded from participation in, be denied benefits of, or be subject to discrimination under any program receiving federal assistance." To be sure, southerners had inserted plenty of loopholes and qualifiers. But Title VI gave Medicare an explosive issue: what to do about segregated hospitals which "received federal assistance" through the Medicare program.

At first, the administration tried to glide over the matter. "We didn't want it brought up," recalled Robert Ball, who had become a social security commissioner. "[I]t would have been a big barrier to passage in the Senate."[95] But in April, as the Senate debated, Senator Harry Byrd broke the ice and asked the White House point-blank. The White House council, Lee White, wrote Johnson: "Surprisingly enough, this is the first time the question has been raised publicly in all of the deliberations on the Medicare legislation." The justice department straddled the fence. It concluded that Title VI did *not* apply but advised that they could "support a theory that the Title *does* apply" if the president thought it "desirable." Larry O'Brien just wanted it kept "as low key as possible." But Lee White and Bill Moyers both suggested that they should try to fight discrimination, and that—without introducing a separate amendment to Medicare—they should get a reference to Title VI into the legislative record. Johnson apparently agreed. The next day Secretary of HEW Celebrezze wrote Senator Byrd: "The matter has been explored by the Department's legal staff.... I am advised, therefore, that the new hospital insurance program will be subject to the requirements of title VI."[96] The White House overrode a cautious Justice Department legal interpretation and opened a new front in the Medicare campaign. Although the courts might have eventually pushed it, the administration committed itself to a social reform—desegregating hospitals—that made implementing Medicare very difficult in most of the South.

Johnson saw Medicare as more than a passive vehicle of paying hospital bills—he saw it as an instrument of social change. And he understood that by locating enforcement of Title VI deep in an operating agency, he gave the civil rights effort more traction and shielded its officers from legislators seeking to resist social change. Douglas Cater, who had become the chief White House health aide in 1965, reflected the president's view back to Johnson when, he suggested telling a *New York Times* reporter that "you do not agree with the attitude expressed by some bureaucrats that 'Medicare only provides the payments.'" Medicare was about hard-won social change—about making a great society.[97]

When hospitals applied for Medicare certification, they were required to offer proof that they did not segregate. By the fall of 1965, about 1,000 inspectors were heading south to check hospitals for compliance. The administration faced a long list of tricky questions: What exactly counted as integration? Did the hospitals have to achieve racial quotas? Did they have to desegregate by room (an especially explosive issue), or by wards? Did they have to override the expressed preferences of patients (black and white)? And what to do if after threat and bluster, rural hospitals failed to comply? Refusing Medicare funds meant withdrawing care from people who needed it—a blunt instrument that could hurt the people that reformers were trying to help. Still the essential parameters—black doctors and patients could not be barred from hospitals or shuffled into inferior wards or wings on the basis of race—were clear enough.[98]

By May 6, a memo to President Johnson noted that half the hospitals in as many as twelve southern states had still not met the Title VI requirements. Johnson mobilized. He wanted an immediate war council, he scrawled on the memo, with the secretary of HEW (by then John Gardner), attorney general (Nicholas Katzenbach), commissioner of education (Harold Howe), and key aides.[99] With two months to go and the clock ticking, the issue had the president's full attention. He set Vice President Humphrey to calling the mayors of cities where recalcitrant hospitals were located.

On May 23, Farris Bryant, the federal government's Director of Emergency Planning (the equivalent of today's Federal Emergency Management Agency, or FEMA) informed Johnson that compliance would likely be complete by July 1 everywhere except Alabama, Louisiana, Mississippi, and South Carolina. Bryant noted that Governor George Wallace was encouraging noncompliance in Alabama, and recommended waiting before making a final decision about how to manage potentially resistant regions and facilities.[100]

By June, the hard federal line began to develop a momentum of its own. Most southern hospitals were not actively defiant—just dragging their heels in hopes that the administration would cave. When it became clear this would not happen, they backed down rather than risk losing Medicare funds. By July, only 320 hospitals remained out of compliance. By October, the number was down to a dozen.

David Barton Smith offers an example of just how far the federal pressure sometimes went: "Confederate hospital in Louisiana was told ... that they must not only take the 'white' and 'colored' signs off the doors but that they must also label them 'Entrance' and 'Exit' and fix the door handles accordingly. They were also told not just to take the 'colored' and 'white' signs out of the waiting rooms but to label one [the] 'main waiting room' and to cordon off the other [and] put ... in a sign saying 'overflow waiting room—to be used only when the main waiting room is full.'"[101]

Certainly there were compromises and limits. The revolution did not extend, for example, into physicians' offices. But by any standard Medicare's implementation proved an extraordinary engine of social change—in one year, American hospitals underwent a racial transformation that has had few parallels in any sector.

## The Recalcitrant Doctors

Physicians had fought long and hard against Medicare. Now, there was mutinous talk of a boycott. Even brief local resistance—not to mention a general boycott—could be a disaster for the fledgling program. The administration alternately wooed physicians and subjected their leaders to the Johnson treatment.

As the final version of the bill took shape in Congress, the president of the AMA wrote Johnson asking for a meeting. On July 29, the day the Senate voted final approval, Johnson met AMA leaders and gave them the full Lyndon. First, he talked at length about how much "the devotion of our family doctor had meant during my father's final illness." How the doctor came and sat with his daddy all night. How all Americans felt "respect" for and "gratitude" toward their doctors. Even though some might think it corny, he was talking very personally and, at the same time, telling them things they deeply believed. The doctors, who had entered the room in stony silence, began to soften. Then, suddenly, the president leaped to his feet. When the president of the United States of America rises, everyone rises. He stretched and sat down. They sat down. More personal talk about the greatness of doctors. And then, again, the stand up–sit down routine. He was flattering them while letting them know that he was the president, and that no one should forget it. Then an unexpected tack.[102]

The president began speaking about Vietnam. The doctors did not know it, of course, but at that moment the memos were flying back and forth as the Johnson administration wrestled with whether to escalate its war effort. Johnson told the physicians about the people of Vietnam and their medical needs. Could the doctors help? Of course, they responded, perhaps relieved to find an uncontroversial point of agreement. They would organize a program right away. "Get a couple of reporters in here," shouted an apparently grateful President Johnson, who heaped praise on the doctors for agreeing to launch this generous program in Vietnam. The reporters, of course, brushed all that aside and got right to the point. "What about Medicare? Would the doctors support a Medicare program?"

Johnson was indignant. "These men are going to get doctors to go to Viet Nam where they might be killed.... Medicare is the law of the land. Of course they'll support the law of the land." "Tell him," he said, turning to AMA President James Appel, "you tell him." Yes, of course, said Appel meekly. "We are, after all, law abiding citizens."

Johnson had mixed praise, bluster, and intimidation. But beneath it all, he was illustrating the new reality. Medicare was moving beyond Congress—a familiar forum where the doctors could rely on friendly legislators—to the more arcane world of courts and administrative regulations. But Johnson had a final carrot to offer.

He turned to Wilbur Cohen—the physician's archfiend—and dressed him down. Reading the preamble of the Medicare law itself, which promises not to meddle in any way in the practice of medicine, he sternly told Cohen, "Wilbur, I want you to stay here with these gentlemen, and work things out according to my instructions—no matter how long it takes you." After the meeting, reporter Richard Harris heard the doctors buzzing about "how he had talked to Cohen." Today, we'd call it the classic good cop–bad cop routine. But the deeper message of the meeting was unambiguous: they could try the perilous course of resisting the law of the land. Or they could take sensible path of least resistance; after all, here was the government's most important health policy aide at the doctors' disposal.[103]

Negotiations followed, some involving the president himself. Toward the end of August, for example, AMA president Appel shot off a telegram complaining about an administration bill that would create federally sponsored centers to treat heart disease, cancer, and stroke. This federal intrusion into the practice of medicine, said the doctors, was even more dangerous than Medicare. They asked for a delay in the program. Johnson responded that he could help only if they worked with his heart, cancer, and stroke program. He scribbled at the bottom of the telegram: "Tell him for weeks we have been hearing there would be stalling tactics [meaning the boycott]. We will work with them—for them—but they stalled many health items for years and we must act now and coordinate later. I'll spend all fall trying to help—L."[104]

Four days later, Johnson met with the AMA. Again, he showed both resolve and sensitivity. An internal AMA memo described what happened. The president was "critical of any attempt to defer the bill which he said was a traditional ploy in attempts to scuttle legislation, and stated that he would oppose any amendments that would, in effect, 'gut' the bill…. It seemed that our Committee had made no progress with the President. As he left the room, however, he paused at the door and directed [HEW] Secretary Gardner and Wilbur Cohen to remain in the room and try to work out changes in the bill that would satisfy the AMA. We therefore continued the discussion for about an hour."

The result, concluded the doctors, was the introduction of many positive changes. "I think it is fair to say that [we] … succeeded in bringing about at White House level a series of 'improving amendments' which … should allay the fears of the profession."[105] Johnson's mix of drama, firmness, flattery, and accommodation had ushered the medical leadership from opposition to negotiation. Physician leaders, such as Appel, were soon touting their negotiating prowess and crushing the boycotters in the white-coat ranks.

Concessions on heart, cancer, and stroke eased the physicians' opposition to Medicare. That September, a special meeting of the AMA House of Delegates convened to consider a Medicare boycott. The Association of American Physicians and Surgeons condemned AMA leaders for "an indefensible display of collaboration with and complicity in evil." The leadership easily put down the rebellion, both in the House of Delegates and, a month later, at the AMA annual meeting. Douglas Cater wrote Johnson, "This is the result of your patient work with the AMA doctors," and enclosed a UPI story: "The President of the American Medical Association said last night [that] its new policy of negotiating differences with the Federal Government has met with success…. A meeting of top AMA officials with President Johnson led to the adoption … of 30 AMA-backed amendment[s] to the Administration[']s Heart Disease, Cancer and Stroke Program."[106]

By the fall, the fear of a physician boycott had begun to fade. If anything, the administration may have leaned too far the opposite way—conceding too much. It made the rules for paying both doctors and hospitals extremely generous—essentially whatever they charged (plus add-ons) with scarcely any controls or oversight of any sort. The reimbursement regulations led directly to the spike in health care costs that would jolt the program once it went into effect. Still, there had been few precedents for launching a program of this size and scope. Many Johnson aides called it, in retrospect, the domestic equivalent of the D-Day landing in Normandy during World War II. Johnson had managed to win over the physicians, whose cooperation was crucial to Medicare.

## The Scope of the Task

The task was enormous. More than 19 million beneficiaries had to be notified and signed up. The federal government had to set up records, print identification cards, figure out how to pay for services, and manage a host of other details. To make things more complicated, while the hospital services in Part A had been in the works for years and automatically included almost all elderly, the physician services in Part B were a last-minute add-on for which elderly Americans could volunteer. The Social Security Administration had to publicize the new services, explain the choices, answer questions, and track people who signed up. And the government had to set up contingency plans if the rush of new patients overwhelmed the medical system.[107]

Johnson left most of the details to his staff and kept watch for problems and opportunities. He publicized the program to encourage enrollment, suggested that the secretary of HEW present Harry Truman with the first Medicare card, agreed to make March "National Medicare Enrollment Month," and sent Congress a two-month extension request for the voluntary enrollment in Part B (after Wilbur Cohen assured him that it would go through easily). In April, three months from launch, Johnson wrote the secretary of HEW, "I want to be sure that we leave nothing undone to prepare the Federal Government, the states, the providers of hospitals and health services and the American people for the massive job ahead."[108]

By now, the central concern—apart from certifying southern hospitals—was the danger of shortages in hospital facilities. The big issue, Douglas Cater wrote the president, is to "insure adequate hospital services in a Nation already feeling the pinch of inadequate facilities." But the staff was growing confident. He added, "The facts indicate that

*there will not be a sudden, Nation-wide shortage of hospital beds."*
There might, however, be shortages in some communities.[109] Johnson
asked his staff to look into using federal hospitals—belonging to the
Department of Veterans Affairs, the military, and the Public Health
Service—if and where the hospital system fell short.

The week before the launch, as the administration scurried to imag-
ine and cover every contingency, Johnson sent a telegram to his new
allies, the American Medical Association, gathered at a convention.
"ON JULY 1 THE MEDICARE PROGRAM WILL BECOME A REALITY.... PER-
HAPS NEVER—EXCEPT IN MOBILIZING FOR WAR—HAS THIS GOVERNMENT
MADE SUCH EXTENSIVE PREPARATIONS FOR ANY UNDERTAKING.... WE
SHALL CONTINUE TO SEEK YOUR COUNSEL IN THE MONTHS AHEAD—AND
WE SHALL BE AVAILABLE TO EVERY DOCTOR AND EVERY HOSPITAL OFFI-
CER TO DEAL WITH ANY PROBLEM THAT ARISES."[110]

But Medicare launched with ease. There were no bed shortages,
no physician strikes, no lines of crippled or dying elderly Americans
scrabbling at the barred doors of overloaded or segregated hospitals.
Johnson is famous for his acumen with Congress. Medicare showed
that he could be a first-rate administrator as well.

There was, finally, more than a hint that the administration was
scheming to open other health care fronts on the heels of Medicare's
implementation. The administration's list included modernizing hospitals, training health personal (especially nurses), lowering costs,
extending coverage beyond the elderly, and, as domestic advisor Joseph
Califano put it in one memo, a "program of child medical care to start
the country on the road toward a Great Society where no child will be
inhibited in the development of his talents by lack of adequate medical
care."[111] The notes, memos, and minutes reveal the scope of Lyndon
Johnson's health care appetite—and what might have been had the
Vietnam War not increasingly smothered both the president and his
government in its malevolent embrace.


LYNDON BAINES JOHNSON AND AMERICAN HEALTH CARE

The conventional story, authored in part by Lyndon Johnson himself,
explains Medicare's victory as the inevitable result of the 1964 landslide and Wilbur Mills's legislative genius. The full Medicare story,
however, turns on an elaborate interplay between the two ends of
Pennsylvania Avenue—the president and Congress. We put Lyndon
Johnson at the heart of the reform. Indeed, even Wilbur Mills passed

the credit back to the president and suggested that Medicare—in its big, ambitious form—probably would not have passed without him. The new Medicare story offers a revised set of lessons and conclusions that will be reinforced repeatedly in the successes and failures of LBJ's successors.

First, presidents must be deeply committed to large changes such as health care reform. They have enormous discretion in picking the issues that top their agendas. Johnson immediately turned John Kennedy's martyrdom to the Medicare cause. But even with a strong wind at his back, Johnson had to press relentlessly. He spent enormous political capital on Medicare. If a president must pay this high a price at the best of times, the costs during more ordinary political periods will be higher still. Only a president with a deep emotional commitment to improving our health care system would start down such a risky and dangerous path.

Second, speed is essential. Johnson knew this in his bones. Medicare was the first bill he introduced after his landslide victory, and he pressed his staff and congressional allies mercilessly to get it through before "they can get their letters written." As he told his staff, "every day while I'm in office, I'm going to lose votes. I'm going to alienate somebody. We've got to get this legislation fast." Presidents who take the time to think through new reforms can reset the agenda or change the conversation. But, as Johnson explained to his staff, waiting makes reforms a lot harder to win.

Third, presidents would do well to concentrate on the one job that they and they alone can do: creating political momentum. Johnson's 1964 campaign turned the 1964 election into a clear referendum on health coverage for the elderly. Wilbur Mills and his colleagues in both chambers could not miss the message. Nothing boosts difficult reforms like a mandate from the electorate. This, in turn, requires stressing the reform on the hustings.

Fourth, Johnson used his mandate with consummate skill in negotiating some of the most complicated governing machinery in the world. (After all, if the United States operated by the simpler English, Canadian, or even German parliamentary rules, Harry Truman would have passed national health insurance after standing for it and winning election back in 1948.) Lyndon Johnson was better prepared than any other modern president to manage Congress. Legislators not only respected him, they feared him. Any president aspiring to reform health care at the federal level must find his or her unique style for accomplishing what Johnson did with the congressional process. If they themselves do not have the skills, they need a crackerjack legislative liaison team that does. Johnson had both the talent and the team.

Fifth, know when to compromise and when to push. Before the 1964 landslide, when Johnson had a weaker hand, he was ready to give more away to win what he could. After the landslide, he turned around and pushed for more. He no longer needed Republicans and turned Jacob Javits down flat when he tried to reopen negotiations. Again, with the American Medical Association, Johnson drew bright lines around what he would compromise—even in the face of a threatened (and potentially disastrous) boycott. The Medicare experience highlights the subtle negotiating art at which Johnson excelled: know when to give, and when to grab.

Sixth, the most dramatic lesson of the Johnson experience: pass the credit. Johnson saw to it that Mills and his congressional allies received all the public applause. Even in his own autobiography, Johnson artfully retells the train wreck story (never actually writing anything flatly false) as if it were the first time he had heard of the details of the package that, in fact, he had been negotiating with Wilbur Mills for over a year.

Seventh, the heretical generalization that emerged in past administrations is vivid in Lyndon Johnson's experience. Again and again, Johnson muzzled his economists. In a much simpler time, Johnson did this by controlling his staff, flatly telling them not to emphasize the numbers, and underplaying Medicare and Medicaid's long-term economic impact. The net effect was to say: let's do expanded coverage now, and worry about how to afford it later. When the Council of Economic Advisors finally pushed the issue—economic drag—to the surface, Johnson acquiesced and began to squelch additions that reformers are still chasing to this day. It's the same old lesson: expansion never fits the budget. The conclusion runs counter to every contemporary instinct, but it is hard to find an exception. For successful health reform: first expansion, then cost control.

Ultimately, the colorful man we've followed through the chapter was both brilliant and deeply flawed. His own personal and organizational weaknesses led the United States into a foreign policy mess that wrecked his great society and still rocks American politics. He was a difficult and often cruel boss. He was profane, crude, manipulative, and petty. In his rush to legislate, and in his tight control over every policy, he sometimes pushed through maladroit or underdeveloped programs. Still, no twentieth-century president except Franklin Roosevelt managed to win more—and more important—domestic policies. He was a Category 5 governmental hurricane, driven by wellsprings of passion that exploded in every direction, amplified by an unmatched dexterity at manipulating the levers of Washington power. He stands alone as the most effective health care president in American history.

# CHAPTER 6

# Richard Nixon

*A Flower That Bloomed Only in the Dark*

J. K. Rowling might have imagined Richard Nixon: now you see him, now you don't. His dark side roiled just below his granite discipline. Bitterness, anger, and hatred erupted in vindictive fits that consumed him and scathed others. For liberals, he became the closest thing to "he who must not be named."

And yet, and yet—other currents circulated in his cauldron of paranoia, deceit, and opportunism. Secluded in his hideaway office across the street from the White House, the fireplace crackling as the air conditioner hummed, Richard Nixon scribbled on yellow legal pads far into the night, and the stuff of brilliance emerged. Perhaps no other president more fully embodied the stereotype of the wise visionary than this wounded, paranoid man. He hoped grand hopes—for peace and prosperity. He saw things—both in foreign and domestic policy—that others didn't see. He plotted strategies that others could not imagine. And when his inner demons rested, his childhood memories of sickness and suffering pressed him to address the needs of other people.

Richard Nixon was flawed, self-destructive, and alcoholic. Richard Nixon was also one of the most innovative and creative health care presidents. He remade the dialogue on health care policy. Inspired by his own tortured past, he left an important legacy for both liberals and conservatives. To explain why health mattered so much to him is to understand, ultimately, how the personal shapes the political.

## RICHARD NIXON

Biographers cannot resist the urge to psychoanalyze Richard Nixon. Few public figures have revealed more inner thoughts and impulses—in hours of raw recorded conversation. And few, after all is read, heard, and analyzed, remain more inexplicable.

Ironically, this child of devout Quakers—a famously pacifist and tolerant faith—would become known for war and bigotry. He unleashed ferocious bombing of North Vietnam and invasions of Cambodia and Laos. He even mused about going nuclear—a threat that so frightened his secretary of defense, Melvin Laird, that Laird instructed his subordinates to check with him before following orders from the Commander in Chief. In private conversations, Jews were "kikes." Henry Kissinger, his national security alter ego, was his "Jew boy." African Americans were inferior beings on whom government assistance was wasted.[1] But the simple images—warmonger, bigot, paranoid, genius—conceal more than they reveal. Richard Nixon was full of contradictory things; he was constantly darting between light and dark.

*Childhood*

Nixon was born at home on January 9, 1913, in the small California town of Yorba Linda, where his father, Francis, a former handyman and trolley motorman, had a lemon orchard. Yorba Linda recalled the western cow town in a B movie: a few rundown one-story wood structures straddled a muddy main street.[2] The family scraped by in a modest, single-story frame house until Richard was nine, when oil companies pushed the family off the land to exploit the black gold that lay under the lemon trees. The Nixons moved to nearby Whittier, his mother Hannah's hometown, where they opened a general store. Frank Nixon was rough, argumentative, and moody. He would not chat up the customers who kept the family business afloat; the job of running the store fell to Hannah. The family became economically secure, at least until the children started getting sick, but the Nixons were never well off.

Frank was tough on his sons. One day, for example, he discovered that Richard and his older brother, Harold, had disobeyed him and gone swimming in a nearby irrigation canal. Frank rushed over, pulled the boys out of the water, shouted, "You like water? Have some more!" and threw them back in. An aunt finally stopped him, screaming "You'll kill them, Frank! You'll kill them."[3]

Many observers trace Richard's lifelong anger and self pity to this painful father–son relationship. Howard Phillips is typical: "the dominant factor in [Richard Nixon's] psyche was rejection by his father, and his love-hate relationship with his father was mostly hate."[4]

Richard's mother provided the emotional support. Although Hannah practiced an iron self-control—by modern standards, she was distinctly aloof—in Richard's mind she came to symbolize all that was good, kind, and caring. Hannah inspired his dream of becoming an American spiritual leader.

Richard's childhood pictures reveal a handsome, serious, round-faced little boy staring with almost startling directness into the camera. He grew into a thin, quite attractive young man of middle height, with a full head of dark brown hair, prominent nose, and engaging smile. The second-oldest of five, Richard was always different from other children. He was serious and smart, a dreamer and a loner, a bit of a prig and a do-gooder. He was uncomfortable in groups, preferred reading to conversation, and lacked close friends. Richard never managed to win a comfortable place in any circle.

One can imagine how boisterous rural boys treated this slight, awkward, bookish child. There is no mention in most biographies of bullying, but it is hard to imagine that it didn't figure somewhere in Nixon's childhood. Asked how Richard defended himself as a child, his younger brother Donald replied: "Dick used his tongue more than his fists."[5] By junior high school, he was a champion debater. As he grew older, he relied on grit, verbal dexterity, and dogged ambition to capture the rewards that others attained through membership and privilege.

Nixon was accepted by Harvard but chose local Whittier College because he could afford it. He tried out for athletic teams and then warmed the benches (he was a third-stringer on the football team). Rejected by the elite men's club, the Franklins, Nixon founded a competing organization, the Orthogonians; in his senior year, he represented his club in the election for class president and beat the candidate from the group that had spurned him. From Whittier, Richard went to Duke Law School where, like LBJ, he worked his way through school and famously lived for a time in an abandoned shack. He hit the books so hard that classmates tagged him "gloomy Gus."[6]

During World War II, Nixon joined the Navy and served in the pacific. He arranged supply shipments—and the removal of wounded troops. Nixon became a superb poker player and won substantial sums. He always relished bluffing and bold gambles.

For Richard, life was constant struggle. He saw himself as a victim, surrounded by privileged villains for whom everything came easy: intellectuals, liberals, the Ivy Leaguers, the press, political rivals—and, above all, the damn Kennedys.

## Sickness and Death

Illness ravaged the Nixon family and deeply wounded young Richard. Tuberculosis, an ancient scourge that antibiotics finally conquered during Nixon's adulthood (though it is surging again today), first touched Richard when he was ten. An X-ray showed a shadow on his lung that a local physician interpreted as possible tuberculosis. For five years, the doctors forbade him to play sports, although when the problem did not progress, they concluded that the finding was a false alarm—likely a scar from a pneumonia that Nixon had at age four. The X-ray technology of the day made such misdiagnoses common. Richard was exposed to tuberculosis throughout his childhood, so he probably did harbor some TB in his chest; the germs often take up residence and lie dormant for decades.

Two years later, tuberculosis struck for real. Nixon's younger brother, seven-year-old Arthur, grew weak and feverish. He stopped eating.[7] As his health declined, a local physician, Dr. H.P. Wilson, called in a specialist, who performed a spinal tap—a procedure that involves inserting a needle into the spinal column through the spaces between the bones of the lower back and extracting a small amount of the fluid that bathes the spinal cord. This remains the standard approach to diagnosing infections in and around the brain. Doctors examine the fluid under a microscope and use special stains to search for bacteria that might be causing an infection and the kinds of symptoms that afflicted Arthur. Tuberculosis shows up as microscopic red rods when stained with the dye. That's what the doctors saw in Arthur's fluid. Today, antibiotics can fight the disease, but in 1925 there was no treatment. Arthur died after awakening long enough to recite a sad little prayer: "If I should die before I wake, I pray thee Lord my soul to take."[8]

Although Frank Nixon truculently refused an autopsy, the doctors labeled the cause of death tubercular encephalitis, which meant that the tuberculosis bacterium had actually invaded the brain. When Arthur died, Nixon allegedly saw his father cry for the first time. Twelve-year-old Richard was himself being monitored for a tuberculosis infection, and one can only imagine the sense of dread he must have felt. Certainly the event had a profound effect on him. He became even more withdrawn and developed a driving ambition to make up, somehow, for Arthur's loss.[9]

Five years later, when Richard was in his first year at Whittier College, Arthur's death was still on his mind. He wrote an earnest recollection entitled simply, "My Brother, Arthur R. Nixon." It began,

> We have a picture in our home, which money could not buy. It is not a picture for which great art collectors would offer thousands of dollars. There is nothing outstanding about its frame or coloring.... It is probably unnoticed by most of those who come to visit us, for they all have seen pictures of small boys.... However, let us examine the picture more closely. The first thing we notice, perhaps, is that this particular boy has unusually beautiful eyes, black eyes, which seem to sparkle with hidden fire and seem to beckon us to come on some secret journey.

Nixon goes on to recount the birth, happy life, and wasting death of his little brother. He concludes after remembering Arthur's final words:

> And so when I am tired and worried, and am almost ready to quit trying to live as I should, I look up and see the picture of a little boy with sparkling eyes and curly hair; I remember the child-like prayer; I pray that it may prove true for me as it did for my brother Arthur.[10]

In this cloying expression of love and goodness, there is an eerie premonition of the notes that President Nixon would scribble to himself as he obsessed alone in the White House. In these quiet moments, he would exhort himself to be compassionate, courageous, spiritual, moral, and good—to elevate the nation while his presidency collapsed in lawlessness and deceit. "Above all else," he scrawled at 5:00 A.M. on New Year's Day, 1974, "dignity, command, faith, head high, no fear, build a new spirit, act like a President, act like a winner."[11]

Even after Richard's scare and Arthur's death, tuberculosis was not finished with the Nixons. Perhaps their cow was the source of the problem. Frank insisted that the family drink fresh milk—infected cattle can pass tuberculosis to their human masters. Doctors urged Francis to have the cow tested, but he obstinately refused. Richard's older brother, Harold, was the next victim.

His tuberculosis was diagnosed in 1927, two years after Arthur's death. It had probably been festering for a while, since Harold had had chronic colds and coughs for years.[12] A fierce conservative, Frank Nixon refused to have Harold hospitalized at the public veterans hospital in Los Angeles—he dismissed that as "socialized medicine."

Instead, he sent Harold to a series of private sanatoriums in southern California.[13] These places treated TB patients with rest, open air, and isolation—the conventional, if largely ineffective, treatment of the time. When the Nixons ran out of money and went into debt, Hannah moved with Harold to a four-bedroom house in Prescott, Arizona; the hot dry climate, they hoped, would slow the disease. To make ends meet, Hannah took in three boarders who also had tuberculosis and nursed all four boys. Several died.

The adolescent Richard was left with his irascible (today we might say abusive) father while the mother he idealized disappeared to care for strangers suffering from a deadly and contagious illness. Frank drove Richard and his younger brother Don to Prescott for summer visits. In 1929, Hannah became pregnant and moved back to Whittier. Harold's health waxed and waned until he died in 1933, when Nixon was twenty years old. Once again, Richard was powerfully affected. According to his mother, "he sank into a deep, impenetrable silence.... From that time on," she continued, "it seemed that Richard was trying to be *three* sons in one, striving even harder ... to make up to his father and me for our loss."[14]

If the young Nixon commemorated Arthur's death in an over-wrought college composition, the mature Nixon memorialized Harold in public and private speech—sometimes when he was under stress, often when he was thinking about health care policy. The president's thoughts would return, again and again, to his mother, tuberculosis, Prescott, Arizona, and the financial trauma that came with illness. For example, in September 1972, Nixon had an Oval Office conversation with Dr. Charles Hoffman, the newly elected president of the American Medical Association. As Nixon sought Hoffman's support for the administration's health insurance program, the conversation turned to the financial strain of serious illness:

> *Nixon:* We have a little experience with this. And this of course occurred at an age when this disease was not under control. The only known therapy was bed-rest. My older brother was— had tuberculosis. He contracted it when he was seventeen and he died when he was 22. For five years my parents, now they earned enough, but they borrowed, they sold property. They did everything. They put him in hospitals. They took him to Arizona for two years. He stayed in a very expensive hospital and then he finally died. But I know what it did to that family. Because my father and mother were very proud people, they

wouldn't put him in the public health "line." They wanted to
pay it all themselves. But I think the rest of their lives they owed
money.

Hoffman:  My first wife had tuberculosis and she was sent for two years—I
was in medical school and we didn't have any money. We were
absolutely ...

Nixon:  You remember that's what they did then. They put them in
those damn—and you just lay there.

Hoffman:  Just lay there—bed rest, right.

Nixon:  ... It didn't work.[15]

And again, on August 8, 1974, at the most baleful moment of his life,
a weeping Nixon said good-bye to the White House staff just before
boarding the helicopter and flying away in disgrace: "Nobody will ever
write a book, probably, about my mother. Well, I guess all of you would
say this about your mother—my mother was a saint. And I think of her,
two boys dying of tuberculosis, nursing four others in order that she
could take care of my older brother for three years in Arizona, and seeing each of them die, and when they died, it was like one of her own."

Illness would affect Nixon directly at other times during his career.
Shortly after his election to the Senate in 1950, he had back and neck
pain that several physicians attributed to tension. He developed a relationship with a New York internist, Dr. Arnold A. Hutschnecker, who
specialized in psychosomatic medicine and became Nixon's therapist and
confidant for eighteen years. During the presidential election campaign
of 1968, the New York Times ran a story hinting that Hutschnecker had
treated Nixon for a psychiatric illness—the campaign denied the story,
but Nixon broke off the treatment.[16]

In 1960, during his grueling campaign against John Kennedy, Nixon
developed an infection of the knee joint. Such infections cause the knee
to redden, swell, and grow intensely painful; cures generally require
intravenous antibiotics, rest, and elevation of the leg. Despite repeated
treatments, including two weeks in Walter Reed Army hospital, Nixon's
infection waxed and waned through the remainder of the campaign.
When Nixon faced Kennedy in that fateful, nationally televised presidential debate, the vice president was running a fever and had just banged
his inflamed knee against a car door. The pain and fever accounted for
the pallor that emphasized Nixon's supposed five o'clock shadow and
for the beads of sweat that pooled on his upper lip, making him look
nervous and ill-at-ease. In contrast, Kennedy, his face artificially full and
round from the side effects of the steroid supplements he used to treat

his Addison's disease, appeared robust and fit. Perversely, the healthy vice president fell victim to a transient illness that under the glare of television lights enabled the chronically ill Kennedy to seem more hale and vigorous.[17]

Nixon repeatedly testified that his own medical experience, particularly the death of his brothers, shaped his thinking. It pushed Nixon—again, by his own account—to remake the American health care debate.

### Character

The suffering that Nixon experienced on his voyage to the presidency—personal, social, medical—formed his complex character.[18] There were also other personal streams feeding the Nixon presidency, and they almost all ran both light and dark.

First there was Nixon's enormous intelligence, which impressed and humbled many of his aides.[19] Assistants recalled Nixon's steel-trap mind. He seemed to retain every detail from policy documents and briefings—and, at the same time, managed to keep the big picture in mind. Elliot Richardson, who served Nixon as secretary of three Cabinet departments (HEW, Defense, and Justice), would later say, "He is a realist whose realism ... is infused with cynicism.... He takes the long view, and that capacity helps to explain the fact that he is perhaps the leading strategist we have had in the White House since World War II. He constantly thought about how to adapt the policies of the United States so as to accommodate our more long term national interests."[20]

However, his brilliance flourished in isolation. In this, he couldn't have been more different from many of his presidential brethren—FDR, LBJ, and JFK—who refined their thoughts and made their decisions amid the jousting of advisors and experts. As Reeves puts it: "In the mountains [of Camp David] Nixon was forever plotting, planning revolutions, great and small, sometimes to build a better world, more often just coups against his own staff and Cabinet. He saw himself as a man of ideas, and of surprise moves, his real work done alone with his yellow pads, or with [aides] Haldeman and Erlichman, his agents of control and organization, whom he saw as his two arms."[21]

Nixon engineered his most memorable strategic triumph, the opening to China, shuttered away from Washington's foreign policy establishment. Nixon and Kissinger, the Lone Ranger and Tonto (though who played which role remains lost in the fog of dueling egos and memoirs), designed and executed the coup.[22]

Nixon's desire for solitude freed his mind while it hobbled his presidency. His substantial talents were often hidden. This was nowhere more apparent than in the management of his own public image. Few presidents had less personal charisma. As president, his smiles seemed forced, his arms akimbo, Pinocchio-like, as if guided by some inattentive puppeteer.

Through much of his career, Nixon made up for these deficits by being smart, shrewd, and ruthless. The traits powered a meteoric political rise. Between 1946 and 1952, Nixon shot from first-term Congressman to Vice President. The key to this ascent was Nixon's grasp of public hopes and fears, his ability to identify and exploit weakness, and a gift for redefining public debate. In early political races, he pointed fingers, fabricated, and brawled. Furious Democrats dubbed him "Tricky Dick," but his gutter tactics often worked.[23]

In the White House, Nixon constantly pushed aides to win over the public, sell his policies, and manage the press—which he heartily detested. But there was always a Nixon paradox. President Nixon wanted nothing to do with the public relations that had won him the presidency. Despite his success in debate and campaigning, he recoiled from the spotlight. According to John Erlichman, his key domestic advisor, Nixon "abhorred what he called 'hokey' public-relations, and would turn down 90 percent of the P.R. proposals that came to him." At the same time, Erlichman believed that "once among the people, he performed well and seemed to enjoy the interaction.... So Nixon propagandists were dealing with a paradox. They were not unlike florists who were trying to sell a flower that would bloom only in absolute darkness."[24]

Health care is one issue that can only be cultivated in sunlight. Nixon's team crafted innovative health care plans that would fade in part because he either would not or could not design a public relations effort to sell them.

Another paradox: Nixon was a talented public manager whose introversion and paranoia hobbled his management. He came to the presidency well prepared to run the office, having served as vice president for eight years in Eisenhower's tightly organized White House. Like most Republicans, Nixon favored methodical process. He reshaped the Executive Office of the President by creating the Office of Management and Budget (OMB). OMB became a critical tool enabling future presidents to ride herd on a far-flung federal bureaucracy; it offered some control over a budget that adds up to a fifth of the national economy.

Nixon put another lasting managerial imprint on the presidency by creating a Domestic Council modeled on the smooth-running National Security Council. This reform grew out of a brawl during the first year of his presidency. Nixon had hired Daniel Patrick Moynihan, a flamboyant, hard-drinking, Democratic government professor from Harvard, to run domestic policy, and told him to redesign the nation's welfare program. Moynihan ran headlong into a conservative, bespectacled, pipe-smoking economist, Arthur Burns, who constantly fought the Irishman over welfare policy. According to Erlichman,

> The Burns-Moynihan domestic operation contrasted markedly with the smooth and orderly operation of Henry Kissinger's National Security Council. The President began asking Roy Ash [an industrialist who was consulting on White House operations] and the others who were studying the organization of the Executive Office of the President why he couldn't have a domestic policy operation analogous to the NSC and as pain-free.... The Ash group met with the President and the Domestic Council evolved.[25]

Nixon got what he was after. His Domestic Council became a well-oiled machine that churned out a steady stream of domestic proposals.[26]

The Executive Office of the President leaped from 292 people at the beginning of the Nixon administration to 583 by its end. Nixon vastly increased the number of tasks performed directly in the White House, and dispensed with the old pretense that the White House staff was there to assist both the president and the policymakers in his Cabinet. Nixon built a White House that made its own policies. And that, in turn, finally shattered a worn-out shibboleth: the idea of bipartisan policymaking. Functions moved into the White House just as the White House was growing increasingly attuned to politics and elections. Nixon was the first president to say it out loud: "We are in a continuous campaign."[27] Every president has followed in Nixon's footsteps—the White House staff sets policy with its eyes always fixed on the political prize.

Nixon wrestled power into the White House in part because he saw the federal bureaucracy as teeming with enemies who wanted to bring him down. He disliked and mistrusted many of his own Cabinet secretaries and saw them as prone to "going native"—becoming captives of liberals and Democrats populating the vast federal agencies that surrounded his isolated White House team. After all, Democrats had constructed the sprawling federal establishment over the past thirty-five years. "If we don't get rid of these people," Nixon wrote in his memoirs, "they will sit back on their well paid asses and wait for the next election to bring back their old bosses."[28]

However, Nixon's own character kept him from taking full advantage of his redesigned White House operation. He simply could not stand the personal interactions it required. Instead, he walled himself off behind a triumvirate of aides: John Erlichman, a California lawyer and former Nixon advance man who became his domestic policy advisor; Robert Haldeman, a longtime Nixon campaign *apparat* and former advertising executive, who became chief of staff and chief enforcer; and Henry Kissinger, the brilliant, egotistical professor who ran the foreign policy operation.[29]

In August 1969, seven months into the administration, one of Erlichman's aides, Kenneth Cole, wrote Robert Haldeman a memo that spelled out the limited lines running into the Oval Office: "President Nixon only wants to deal with a very limited number of advisors on a regular basis.... It would be very difficult if not impossible for any top level staff member to gain enough Presidential confidence to deal effectively with the President on a regular basis."

The memo went on to recommend that the president interact regularly with only five top officials: Kissinger, Erlichman, Haldeman, Bryce Harlow (Nixon's congressional liaison), and the chair of the Council of Economic Advisers. Within months of his arrival in the Oval Office, Nixon had cut himself off from the outside world.[30]

At Nixon's insistence, this tiny circle kept White House staff and Cabinet members at a distance so that he could spend long periods alone with his yellow pads. The triumvirate Erlichman, Haldeman, and Kissinger was Nixon's hammer. It pounded home Nixon's unhappiness over personnel performance or press leaks. It delivered bad news—even demanding resignations.

When Nixon ventured into public, his White House operation would carefully choreograph him: aides told him where to stand, who to greet, when to greet them, and what to say—he was usually primed with talking points. FDR, Ike, or LBJ would have scorned this kind of direction. When Nixon felt ill at ease in public, he would launch into monologues that minimized any real interaction.

It is hard to imagine a man of Nixon's temperament as a successful legislative president; certainly he was never comfortable in the give-and-take of congressional relations. Like his rival, John Kennedy, Nixon had trouble closing a legislative deal. His frustrated legislative director, William Timmons, once felt compelled to pencil at the bottom of Nixon's talking points for a congressional meeting, "ASK HIM FOR HIS VOTE."[31] However, Nixon understood the importance of congressional politics and, with typical perseverance, pushed himself—at least early in his presidency—to work at it. Erlichman recalled: "The morning after a White House social event, Nixon's desk would be dotted with little scraps of paper—notes he'd made during talks with Congressmen as they came through the receiving line... Nixon would pepper me with questions and complaints he'd picked up the night before. Within a few hours my staff would produce answers to enable the President to telephone those Congressmen that same afternoon with complete follow-up."[32]

Until Watergate and his own paranoid style brought him down, Nixon actually accumulated a workmanlike legislative record by forging alliances between conservative Democrats and Republicans to beat back Democratic initiatives and advance his own agenda—he won a higher percentage of congressional votes than Ronald Reagan, George H. W. Bush, or Bill Clinton.[33] Whatever his other failings, they did not include lack of understanding or application—Nixon knew what he had to do to succeed and, when he was able, applied himself to the process.

Still another paradox of the Nixon presidency—one that figures prominently in the health care story—was his attitude toward and management of domestic affairs. Like so many presidents, Nixon was partial to foreign policy. He found domestic affairs a bramble patch of tangled political interests and unsolvable problems. When he got directly involved in domestic issues, he most often focused on politically charged topics—race relations, crime, the economy—that might make a difference for his own reelection, or for his larger goal—displacing the Democrats and making the Republicans the majority party.[34] As Nixon put it in a note he sent Erlichman after his 1972 reelection: "I want you to concentrate on selling domestic programs and answering attacks on them, rather than developing those programs.... Substance in the case of foreign policy is infinitely more important than substance is in the case of domestic policy."[35]

Early in the Nixon presidency, Haldeman would note that memos on some domestic policy issues came back from the president unread. As a result, Erlichman became a virtual deputy president for domestic policy with—as he put it—"carte blanche in ... many areas."[36] And yet Nixon sometimes plunged into domestic issues. He was too savvy a politician, and too broad a strategic thinker, not to understand the importance of domestic policy for his legacy. Robert Finch, a longtime Nixon friend and his first head of HEW, confided to an aide: "You watch that man.

He's going to surprise people. He wants to be remembered in history, and, as a student of Theodore and Franklin Roosevelt, he knows that presidents who come up with progressive social programs are likely to make a name."[37]

Moynihan had introduced him to the history of Benjamin Disraeli, the Tory Prime Minister who had been a major social reformer in late nineteenth-century Britain. "You know," Moynihan told Nixon, "it is the Tory men with liberal policies who have enlarged democracy." Nixon warmed to the comparison.[38]

Ultimately, Nixon sought to portray himself as a centrist innovator on domestic affairs, and he exhorted the Cabinet (of course, he despised Cabinet meetings) to bring him bold new programs. In January 1970, Nixon wrote Erlichman: "In your discussion with the Domestic Policy Group, you should emphasize one great basic theme. The opposition in Congress is attempting to cement in all of the Great Society programs and simply to increase the amounts of money appropriated for those programs. We are attempting to initiate new approaches with reform. This is a basic difference."[39]

Nixon's domestic initiatives were sufficiently aggressive to send shivers through conservative allies. Presidential speechwriter Pat Buchanan warned the president in January 1971:

> We have a serious political problem developing on the Right.... Originally localized, the infection is spreading and now being broadcast, through the press, to the party structure nationally.... The President [according to conservative critics] is adopting a liberal Democratic domestic program, indistinguishable from what an Ed Muskie or Ed Kennedy would propose—and the President's ability to drag the GOP along behind his proposals makes him a more effective "President Liberal" than any Democrat could possibly be.[40]

Buchanan was prescient. He and his friends on "the Right" would have been even more concerned had they understood the full extent of Nixon's pragmatic affection for government as an instrument for improving lives. "I am a government man," he told an Oval Office meeting of private health care leaders in September 1971. "I have been in government most of my life. I have great respect for people in government."[41]

Nixon was an enigma even to his own conservative allies. Like few other presidents, he was hidden in public view. His actions took the presidency to breakthroughs in international relations, bold proposals for domestic politics, and treachery in the Watergate affair. Behind the contradictory record stood a man who was himself a bundle of contrasts. He was infected, to use Buchanan's metaphor, with a legacy of personal struggle that left him bitter and paranoid. But he also carried, like the TB that likely lay dormant in his lungs, a memory of suffering and deprivation that enabled him—when his demons were in check and the times were aligned—to imagine a better world for all Americans. This tortured man was capable of remarkable things—as his health care presidency would demonstrate.

## THE NIXON PRESIDENCY

The 1968 election campaign echoed the tumult of the era. During the spring primaries, an assassin murdered Martin Luther King Jr.—and the cities erupted into race riots (again). The Vietnam War raged. The United States had deployed more than 500,000 troops, bombed North Vietnam, and inflicted enormous casualties. Peace talks began and quickly stalled. The war dragged on. Nixon ran on the promise that he would end it, echoing Eisenhower's 1952 campaign promise to end the Korean War. In a country racked by urban riots and racial conflict, Nixon promised national unity.

The Democrats were divided—dispirited by the assassination of Robert Kennedy after the California primary and wracked by an antiwar insurgency led by Senator Eugene McCarthy (D-MN). In a tumultuous national convention, the Chicago police attacked raucous antiwar demonstrators. The Democratic establishment muscled aside its rebels and nominated Vice President Hubert Humphrey, who was closely identified with LBJ's Vietnam policies. The once-reliable southern Democrats—outraged by the administration's civil rights policies—bolted for segregationist George Wallace. Nixon seized on the racial tension to battle Wallace for the southern vote—shrewdly setting out to lead a new Republican majority rising out of Dixie.

Nixon watched his big lead (after the blood and chaos of the Democratic Convention) dwindle through the campaign. He managed to squeak by with 43 percent of the popular vote—beating Humphrey by less than 1 percent. Nixon's slim electoral mandate was undermined further when the Democrats maintained control of Congress with margins of 57–43 in the Senate and 245–189 in the House. Nixon became the first newly elected president since Zachary Taylor in 1848 to face a Congress entirely controlled by the opposing party. He took office with an approval rating of 63 percent and was quickly tested by troubles both at home and abroad. Twenty-five years of steady economic growth was coming to an end, inflation began rising, and the Vietnam War ground on.

## Triumph and Folly

Efforts to negotiate an end to the war continued to founder, and a major antiwar march on Washington in October 1969 demonstrated that Nixon now owned the Vietnam War. In response, on November 3, 1969, he appealed to "the great 'silent majority'"—a hugely successful political metaphor invoked to claim the support of a stalwart, patriotic mainstream for his controversial escalations.[42] A precipitous pullout, said the president, would be irresponsible and dishonorable. On April 30, 1970, Nixon steeled himself by watching the movie *Patton* and then announced a "limited" invasion of Cambodia to put pressure on North Vietnamese supply lines. A burst of new protests on college campuses followed. On May 4, National Guardsmen shot and killed four students at Ohio's Kent State University (including two women who were walking to class). The protests grew and spread.

Recognizing the need to calm the fury, Nixon began the "Vietnamization" of the war—he reduced the number of U.S. troops from 550,000 in 1969 to 60,000 in 1972. U.S. casualties fell from over 300 per week to under 10. The maneuvers neutralized the war as a 1972 election issue. In early 1973, the United States concluded a peace deal with the North Vietnamese. Nixon had delivered on his promise to end the war, though it had taken four years and tens of thousands of lives.

Bold thrusts marked the rest of Nixon's foreign policy. In July 1971, Henry Kissinger secretly flew to China and began the negotiations that resulted in Nixon's triumphant visit to Beijing in February 1972, where he met Mao Tse Tung, the Chinese communist leader. The new relationship with China changed the dynamic in international affairs, allowing the United States to play China off against the USSR. The Soviet Union's anxiety over the U.S.–China relationship helped facilitate Nixon's détente with the USSR. Nixon went to Moscow in May 1972, met with Soviet Leader Leonid Brezhnev, and negotiated a nuclear arms limitation and an anti–ballistic missile treaty.

Nixon returned triumphantly from the Soviet Union on June 1, 1972. The 1972 presidential primaries were ending, and Nixon was well positioned for the fall campaign. But winning was not enough for Nixon. He had to crush his opponents—he was certain that they felt the same way about him. On June 17, a team of burglars working for Nixon's reelection campaign broke into the Democratic Party headquarters at Washington's Watergate Hotel. They were there to replace a failed bug that was recording the Democrats' conversations. A security guard caught them. Six days later, on June 23, 1972, the Oval Office taping system recorded a conversation between Nixon and Haldeman in which the president suggested that they enlist the FBI and the CIA in an effort to portray the break-in as a national security matter. As soon as those words left his mouth, Nixon's presidency was doomed. We don't know whether the president knew about the break-in beforehand, but the White House tapes revealed him coldly obstructing justice and covering up the crime. When courts forced the tape's release two years later, the June 23 conversation became the "smoking gun" that forced Nixon to resign.

A steady stream of Watergate revelations crippled Nixon's second term. In the spring of 1973, Haldeman and Erlichman faced indictment for their roles in covering up the burglary. On April 29, Nixon summoned them to Camp David where he asked for their resignations. Erlichman recalls visiting the president's cabin: "Nixon, in a checked sports coat, came in the room from his bedroom. Neither of us sat. His eyes were red-rimmed and he looked small and drawn.... He told me he had hoped and prayed he might die during the night. 'It is like cutting off my arm,' he began, and could not continue. He began crying uncontrollably."[43]

Other resignations and indictments followed, as well as dramatic congressional hearings and impeachment proceedings. Between April 30, 1973, when he publicly announced the resignations of his two primary aides and November 30, 1973, the president spent only thirty days in Washington—and ten of those were at Walter Reed Hospital, where he was treated for pneumonia.

Dark rumors began to circulate—about drinking and drug abuse in the White House. When the British Prime Minister's office called the White House to consult on the Arab–Israeli (Yom Kippur) War on October 11, 1973, Henry Kissinger took the call and told a subordinate to put off the conversation, saying, "When I talked to the president, he was loaded." In December, Nixon acted crazily at a small dinner party—leaping wildly from subject to subject. Senator Barry Goldwater (R-AZ) was stunned by the behavior and the next day bluntly asked presidential aide Bryce Harlow, "Is the president off his rocker?" "No," replied the aide, "he was drunk." Goldwater continued to worry that "all might not be well mentally in the White House."[44]

Al Haig, Nixon's new chief of staff, took over more and more daily responsibilities, becoming a virtual deputy president. At one point,

Nixon looked at the former general and muttered, "You fellows in your business ... you have a way of handling problems like this. Somebody leaves a pistol in the drawer. I don't have a pistol." Haig began worrying about suicide.[45]

But even as the scandal metastasized and Nixon's drinking got out of hand, he managed the Israeli–Arab war, his most dangerous international crisis. Nixon rallied to make the crucial decision to resupply Israel as its arms stores dwindled, and with the help of Haig and Kissinger negotiated an end to the war—averting a showdown with the Soviet Union, which was poised to aid the faltering Arab states.

### Domestic Policy

The ignominy of Watergate should not eclipse the many achievements of this six-year presidency. Two themes dominated Nixon's tenure in domestic affairs: first, a bold and sometimes cynical political effort to woo southern and blue-collar voters into the Republican fold; and second, a Disraeli-like effort to address real problems with government policies.

In service of the first goal, he crafted the Republican Party's southern strategy. His 1968 election campaign emphasized "law and order"— designed to appeal to anxious white voters. After watching one of his advertisements, Nixon exulted that the ad "hits it right on the nose. Its all about law and order and those damn Negro–Puerto Rican groups out there." Nixon's vice presidential choice, Spiro Agnew, had made national news by suggesting that law enforcement officers shoot looters after Martin Luther King Jr.'s assassination; Agnew confronted liberal orthodoxy by arguing that "misguided compassion" led to urban chaos.[46] In office, Nixon nominated two conservative southern jurists— both with checkered histories on racial rulings—to the Supreme Court, scoring points with segregationist voters in the South while enraging northern liberals, who blocked both appointments. Nixon opposed busing students to reduce racial segregation in schools. His hard line on Vietnam reflected, in part, his calculation that blue-collar voters (in fact, the Democrats' right wing) would defect to the Republicans if he faced down student protesters and took a tough line ("peace with honor") against North Vietnamese communists.

At the same time, Nixon and his staff worked conscientiously with Congress to respond to national problems. This reflected in no small measure the effective functioning of both OMB and his new Domestic

Council. The late 1960s witnessed the emergence of the environmental movement. The first U.S. celebration of Earth Day took place on April 22, 1970. Nixon responded to public pressure—supporting some environmental initiatives, moderating others, and opposing still others. On July 9, 1970, Nixon proposed the creation of the Environmental Protection Agency and the National Oceanic and Atmospheric Administration—one to regulate pollution and the other to research environmental degradation. The latter agency would ultimately become a thorn in George W. Bush's side when its scientists supported the existence of global climate change. In December 1970, Nixon signed the Clean Air Act, which aimed to reduce automobile emissions by 90 percent over six years. At the same time, he "impounded"—withheld—funds appropriated under the Clean Water Act when he judged expenditures too high.

The Nixon administration aggressively (if unsuccessfully) sought to reform the nation's welfare program along lines laid out by Daniel Patrick Moynihan. Nixon signed a $25 billion tax cut in 1972 that included the first investment tax credit. He imposed national wage and price controls in 1971 to control inflation (a radical intervention for a Republican president). He presided over the expansion of Social Security in 1972 to include disability benefits and the indexing of Social Security payments to inflation. He broke with the Bretton Woods agreement and let the market set the price of the dollar—opening a volatile new era in currency trading. And he won general revenue sharing, which—though opposed by many Democrats—served the Republican agenda of shifting political control from Washington to the state governments.

Nixon even managed a mixed record on race relations. Though he criticized busing and desegregation, he quietly pushed integration on the ground. He supported two important civil rights acts (the Voting Rights Act of 1970 and the Equal Employment Opportunity Enforcement Act of 1972). Despite his personal bigotry and political stunts, Nixon understood that race relations had to improve for the sake of domestic stability. During his tenure, the percentage of black students attending all-black schools in the South fell from 68 percent to 8 percent. Seeing an opportunity to create disarray in Democratic ranks, in 1969 the Nixon administration introduced its "Philadelphia Plan," which imposed Affirmative Action on the fiercely segregated Philadelphia construction unions. This pitted labor unions against civil rights leaders. Nixon then beat back union efforts to gain a congressional ban on the Philadelphia plan, which eventually spread to fifty-five cities. The Nixon administration also introduced "set-asides" for minority businesses in federal contracts.[47]

Bitter and isolated as he was, Nixon was able to make extraordinary progress in foreign affairs and amass a creditable record in domestic policy. We are left to wonder what he could have accomplished if his personal demons had not consumed him and his administration. Hints emerge in his management of health care policy.

## THE HEALTH CARE PRESIDENCY: FIRST TERM

More than any other Republican, and more than most Democrats, Nixon was a health care innovator—he devised breakthrough strategies and new legislation. He did not wake up each morning thinking about health policy, but his childhood traumas gave the issue special meaning to him. He left a richer health policy legacy than almost any other president.

The Nixon administration addressed health in two phases. During the first term, 1969–72, it showed methodical Republican policy development in all its ponderous splendor. During the second, 1973–74, as Watergate ripped through the White House, a desperate administration took big gambles. The result was a dramatic departure from previous Republican policy, and a proposal that inspires Democrats to this day. In both phases, Nixon showed himself a capable public manager, delegating detailed policy work while staying on top of the big picture.

### A Republican Plan

Nixon was the first president to inherit Medicare. Through his career, he had toed the Republican line and opposed compulsory federal health insurance. Now, his administration was responsible for running the program Republicans had long fought—a program whose growing expense shocked even its supporters. Would Nixon move to dismantle or drastically roll back this Democratic violation of bedrock Republican principle?

A second major question loomed. Liberal Democrats had always seen Medicare as the opening battle in a war for national health insurance. "Medicare was the first step … and the next step [was] coming," recalls Edward Kennedy's chief health policy aide, Stan Jones.[48] History, they thought, was on their side. Ted Kennedy (D-MA)—whose brother had died running for the presidency in 1968—was just one of the Democrats circling for a run at the Oval Office in 1972. In 1969, Kennedy introduced his ambitious cradle-to-grave national health insurance proposal. How would the administration respond?

Nixon's political career offered some clues. Even as a second-term representative making his name as a Red-baiter, Nixon had joined liberal Representative Jacob Javits (R-NY) to sponsor a health plan for low-income elderly Americans.[49] In contrast to other Republican health plans, the Nixon–Javits plan carefully avoided a means test.

A decade later, Vice President Nixon was running hard for president. Nixon feared that the Eisenhower administration's cautious health proposal was too little too late. Once again, he teamed up with Jacob Javits, now a senator, to cosponsor a more progressive measure. On the floor of the chamber, Vice President Richard Nixon and Senator John F. Kennedy fought the first skirmish of their election by dueling over their health care plans. Until the last hour, Nixon furiously worked the chamber—seeking votes for his own proposal and peeling votes away from Kennedy's. Neither won. The Democrats proposal evolved into Medicare, passed under Lyndon Johnson, and now fell into the Nixon administration's hands.

Nixon tipped his hand as soon as he appointed the gracious, mild-mannered California Republican, Robert Finch, as secretary of HEW. If you wanted to run Democratic health programs out of town, Finch was not the gunslinger to hire. In fact, Finch immediately turned around and tried to hire Dr. John Knowles—a patrician, New England liberal who was head of the Massachusetts General Hospital—as his assistant secretary for health. The AMA firmly opposed Knowles, and the nomination died.[50]

Nixon and his advisors clearly had no intention of taking on Medicare, which had already joined Social Security as the third rail of American politics (touch it and die). But how would the administration respond to Democratic plans for national health insurance? The story of Nixon's first year is one of fits and starts. In effect, the Nixon administration was searching for an ambitious Republican alternative to the Democrats' signature issue.

*First Efforts*

On March 12, 1969, Nixon shot an impatient memo to his top domestic aides:

> In about five weeks we will have completed 100 days since the Inauguration. I would like to have this week a summary of the legislative proposals we have already sent to the Congress, and a hard analysis of what other

legislative proposals will have been sent to the Congress for action before the
100 day period expires. I think we are going to have to put some deadlines
on the departments with regard to those legislative proposals that we think
have some substantive political meaning. From what I have been able to see
to date, most of our directives have been responded to in an unsatisfactory
way.... There is very little prospect for action.[51]

A strange attitude for a Republican. In vivid contrast to Eisenhower,
Nixon would not ignore FDR's—or LBJ's—one hundred days.

Secretary of HEW Finch had already expressed alarm that so many
Americans did not have access to adequate health services even as
Medicare and Medicaid put new demands on an overloaded system.[52]
By July 10, 1969, President Nixon himself released an HEW health
report declaring that the problem is "much greater than I had realized.
We face a massive crisis in health care costs."[53]

Secretary Finch soon ran into trouble. The HEW Civil Rights Division
was pushing school desegregation, against the president's express
wishes. Nixon (or, rather, his hammers) fired the division's chief, Leon
Panetta. Panetta would become a prominent Democratic representative
(from California), Bill Clinton's chief of staff, and Barak Obama's CIA
director. As Finch fell from favor, Erlichman took charge of domestic issues. Erlichman was a Christian Scientist and, according to the
rumors, did not care for health reform. The issue slipped quietly onto
the back burner.[54]

In his first State of the Union address, delivered January 22, 1970,
the president promised a dozen major pieces of domestic legislation. He
emphasized reforms in welfare, revenue-sharing, and economic opportunity for all Americans, and then noted: "I could give similar examples
of the need for reform in our programs for health, education, housing,
transportation, as well as other critical areas which directly affect the
well-being of millions of Americans."

Health care remained on the administration agenda, but down in
the fine print. Perhaps it did not drop completely out of sight, thanks
to the president's own view, shared with his speechwriters in February
1970, that "a key domestic issue [in the 1972 campaign] will be health
care."[55] That month, Erlichman formed an Initial White House Study
Group on Health.

The health policy team soon rolled out a big idea. Because the
administration's leaders (including Nixon, Finch, and Erlichman) were
from California, they were familiar with the Kaiser Permanente Health
Plan—one of the original prepaid group practices. A group of health

policy advocates had been promoting this type of plan as a more effi-cient way to provide health care. The idea caught the imagination of Nixon administration officials, who coined the term Health Mainte-nance Organization (HMO) as a catchy way to sell the concept. The idea met multiple administration needs: it promised cost-reduction and efficiency that would contain Medicare and Medicaid costs and pro-vided a dramatic new approach to delivering health care—the kind of bold thrust that appealed to the reclusive gambler in the Oval Office.

Nixon was interested enough to invite Edgar Kaiser to come brief him on the concept. He told his aides in February 1971, "This [the HMO idea] is a private enterprise one. The reason he can do it—I had Edgar Kaiser in here to talk about it and I went into it in some depth—the rea-son he can do it is all the incentives are towards less medical care." In March 1970, the administration proposed that Medicare and Medicaid patients be permitted to enroll in health maintenance organizations—the first time the federal government championed HMOs.[56]

The administration had plucked a new idea from a group of special-ists who had repackaged Kaiser Permanente as a model for injecting market competition into health care. Nixon and his health advisors came to see the idea of HMOs competing for enrollees as a solution to every health care problem—costs, access, coordination, and preventive care. With fits and starts and controversy, both Republicans and Democrats would eventually embrace this Nixon administration concept. HMOs would become a fixture in the health policy firmament—inspiring the Clinton Health Plan in 1993–94, the managed care revolution of the mid-1990s, and George W. Bush's Medicare Modernization Act of 2003.

## The Health Care Disraeli

In the second half of 1970, two forces gave health another push. First, Nixon replaced Robert Finch with Elliot Richardson. The son of a prominent Boston surgeon and veteran of the Army Medical Corps during World War II, Richardson was a tall, trim, articulate Boston Brahmin and Harvard graduate. Although he embodied all the traits that Nixon despised, he was a deft manager, had a sense for health issues, and earned Nixon's confidence—at least as much as anyone from outside the president's inner circle.

Second, the White House began looking ahead to the 1972 presidential campaign. In July 1970, an extraordinary memo from the Domestic

Council to Secretary Richardson launched a new health policy initiative:

> It would ... be helpful to the President if you gave some thought to what our position on health might be in 1972. This involves both *what* we can say and *when* we can promise delivery. For instance, we might want to be able to say that we have initiated a program that provides adequate medical care for all Americans (for all poor Americans) or (all disabled Americans) or (all America's children) or that we are going to provide such care by 197?. On the other hand, we might want to say that we have protected all, or some part, of American society from the catastrophic cost of serious illness.
>
> Naturally, budget indications are important, but they should not in any way act as an absolute restraint in developing these choices.[57]

The memo is remarkable for its brisk, nonideological tone—all kinds of alternatives are on the table. Richardson responded. Paper began flying through HEW, the Domestic Council, and OMB (headed by George Shultz, a pragmatic manager and former economics professor at the University of Chicago). Using the new domestic policy apparatus, Republican policy management reached new heights of thoroughness, rigor, and, critics might say, ponderousness. The result was the first fully developed Republican national health insurance proposal.

In December 1970, Nixon met with the Domestic Council's Subcommittee on Health, darting back and forth between his light and dark sides. The president had received a briefing paper on health care issues the evening before, which (contrary to Haldeman's claim that Nixon didn't read domestic reports), he had extensively annotated with observations and questions in the margins. However, Nixon opened the meeting by complaining that there were "more leaks out of this Administration than public statements out of most." Then—flipping persona—he called for a program that showed that the administration was serious about health care. "[The] country," he told his advisors, "doesn't think we have a program. [We have] good people preparing papers—but [we] must make the country know we care."

Like a good chief executive, he tried to motivate his staff, praised their work, deferred to their judgment about details, emphasized that he wanted the program sold, and promised to include it in the forthcoming State of the Union address: "[You are the] best group of experts, done good work, know [the] president's biases, [my] concern [is about] deterioration of [the health care] distribution system, keep quality high...."

[You should take] a long-range view.... [I] will support anything that the group recommends—I don't know enough. [I will] hit highlights in the State of the Union address—[we should follow up with a health] message 1–2 weeks after SOTU [State of the Union]—The PR should be big.... We should get out the big guns."[58]

The president suggested that Vice President Spiro Agnew become the administration's point person on the health plan. Nixon also floated the idea of holding regional meetings on health care "like foreign policy," that the vice president would chair. Then Nixon flipped persona again, and the meeting ended on a entirely different note. A conservative economist, Martin Feldstein, interrupted to argue against any insurance plan that would include first-dollar coverage—people would demand too much health care if they didn't have to pay something. Nixon shot back: "60–70% [of patients] are hypochondriacs.... I want to see 2 or 3 psychiatrists comment [on the plan]—some experts on psychosomatic illnesses."[59] Perhaps Nixon's personal experience with Dr. Hutschnecker was nagging at him? In any case, the dark cynic reappeared to close the meeting.

Over the next month, health care memos flowed into the Oval Office, and the president diligently checked off options and suggested alternatives. He met repeatedly with domestic policy advisors. In January 1971 James Cavanaugh, a health policy expert, joined the domestic council staff. Cavanaugh remembered how Nixon plunged into health care: "He would say that [he wasn't interested in the details] but then he tracked the details. He was not an absent President. He had always read whatever we sent him."[60] In contrast, Vice President Agnew couldn't grasp the complex issues involved in health policy development, and he dropped out after a few meetings.

The program that emerged reflected Nixon's opinions on the health care issue as he repeatedly expressed them. His comments at a Cabinet meeting on February 16, 1971—three days before public release of the plan—are typical:

I can sum up my own attitude in a nutshell—I have very strong convictions and they are reflected in this program. Very strong convictions—In a period of reform—you don't reform for the sake of reforming. The important thing to remember is that if you look over the course of history of nations—the history of reforms is that where reforms have really done good in a nation is where they have been highly sophisticated zeroing in on what was wrong but made very careful—very careful not to destroy more than they constructed. And where revolutions or reforms go beyond that—They set a country back rather than going forward—I think there's a great deal wrong with the

American medical care system, but ... anyone important who is seriously ill in the foreign country and come and—is looking for the best medical care in world—He does not go to those countries that have socialized medicine although some of them have very good doctors. They come to the United States.... Our free medical system with all of its faults, does at the highest levels produce the finest medical care in the world. What we have tried to do here is develop a program that will correct what is wrong with the healthcare system without destroying what is right.

Nixon's thoughts about health care always ran on three lines: First, he would be the American Disraeli and solve a problem that his family knew all too well. Second, this would help his own reelection. Third, he had to stop Kennedy's plan, which would be a disaster. As he later put his criticism: "When I go to the doctor, I ... want to make sure that he is a good doctor. It is the quality of health care that is important here. I think ... that ... as long as we can retain some degree of volunteerism, some degree of private initiative within the whole healthcare system ... that means that the quality of our healthcare will be higher than if we simply throw up our hands and say, well, we'll have one monolithic system in which all the doctors are in it and we lay down all the rules"[61]

You could disagree with Nixon, but you couldn't argue he didn't have a well-formed viewpoint. The nation, thought Nixon, needed targeted, well-crafted reforms—not a new Medicare for the entire nation. Some poor and working-class Americans did not have insurance, and the government should help them get it. Full stop.

The administration's program, released on February 19, 1971, broke new ground in two ways. First, the Family Health Insurance Plan would provide health insurance to all poor and unemployed Americans with an income up to $5,000. The very poor would get free coverage. Those with higher incomes would share premium expenses. Second, the plan would, for the first time, require private employers to provide health insurance to their employees. Federal authority would reach into the private health insurance market in an unprecedented way; although the required benefits were limited, administration officials were proposing a "comprehensive" plan—a genuine alternative to the Democrats. Among the many reforms sprinkled through the bill (more community health centers, more money for the war on cancer, more physicians), the administration promoted a nationwide network of HMOs.

Nixon extended a Republican line of reasoning that had begun under Eisenhower: The United States should continue to rely on private health insurance, but the system had failings that government could remedy.

Some observers viewed all this as preelection politics—an attempt to usurp the Democrats' issues—and that it certainly was.[62] But it was also more. Nixon took pride in his health plan. In January, a month before the plan was released, he met with the all-important Ways and Means Committee leaders Wilbur Mills (D-AR) and John Byrnes (R-WI). Mills agreed to hold health insurance hearings in April after the committee had waded through welfare reform and tax issues.

The *New York Times* called the plan a credible alternative to the Kennedy program. Nixon commented a few days later to Erlichman and George Shultz: "Well this is a hell of a good program—with surprisingly good reception.... It deals with the problems and is still fiscally conservative."

The conversation continued:

*Erlichman:* Elliot [Richardson] is testifying before Kennedy's health subcommittee today....

*Nixon:* Oh boy.

*Erlichman:* Well, he's been looking forward to it with great relish.

*Nixon:* Well, he'll know the subject.

*Erlichman:* He's highly enthusiastic about this program.

*Nixon:* Well, he'll know the subject. Some of them will not know the subject.

*Shultz:* Elliot, from the bit I saw on his *Face the Nation* performance—I saw yesterday—he seemed to be doing extremely well.

*Nixon:* I didn't see any of that. But he'll do it. He'll handle the congress.[63]

Meanwhile, the health insurance issue seemed popular. A Harris poll released on April 26, 1971, showed that 80 percent of Americans were concerned about the costs of care and that 38 percent feared that their insurance might not cover them adequately in case of illness. By then, virtually all the major interest groups—the American Hospital Association, the American Medical Association, the insurance industry—had introduced their own comprehensive health insurance proposals. By July 22 proposals clogged the congressional hopper.[64] The stakeholders were braced for action. On June 8, Nixon commented to aides in the Oval Office:

> Here we come to health. If the media can make the environment an issue, then they sure as hell will make health an issue—with the help of Teddy Kennedy. That's why health—regardless of where it is in the present poll—will probably go up. It will go up because health costs are up and the doctors are giving people bad medicine or they're not giving people enough or it's costing too much or whatever the case may be and so forth and so on.... So what we're playing in the health game is really a defensive maneuver. In addition, of course[,] to trying to deal with the real problem ... effectively.[65]

Always the same three rationales, jumbled together: winning the next election, blocking Kennedy (and other Democratic proposals), and solving a problem that struck those painful childhood memories about "not giving people enough medicine."

Of course, getting large changes through Congress is always difficult. Republicans on Ways and Means asked for a delay to remedy what they perceived as flaw in the Nixon proposal: the economic pain it would inflict on small employers. The administration agreed that John Byrnes should introduce an amendment that would exempt businesses with fewer than ten employees—a standard provision in all future legislative proposals.

There was the other great challenge: managing Wilbur Mills, whose true views were always elusive. Mills fancied himself a potential Democratic nominee for president. LBJ had assiduously courted Mills: now it was Nixon's turn, and with rare magnanimity, Nixon echoed LBJ about spreading the political credit to get the job done:

> *Erlichman:* I think Mills as of now is favorably inclined to your approach. He is in favor of the president's approach right now. He's trying to figure out a way to outdo you because he'd hate to give you credit for the thing—but his position is favorable to what we've advanced and he's having a hard time coming up with anything to change....
>
> *Nixon:* John—why don't you make an agreement with Mills—he takes credit one week and I take credit the next week. [Laughter] Seriously, seriously ... I am not concerned about his getting credit ... anyone can get credit ... but anybody who's in their right mind knows that Wilbur Mills is not going to be the nominee of the Democratic party for president, ... he might be the vice president, or he might even make the speaker, which is more likely.... My point is we're arguing about whether we

> should get credit or Mills should get credit, and I don't think it
> makes all that much difference. The point is it's done![66]

Neither Wilbur Mills nor the Congress would be moved so easily. The finance committees were still trying to swallow the huge, unexpected Medicare and Medicaid expenditures. Senate Finance Chair Russell Long (D-LA) remained dubious of any proposal that would increase federal spending—even the very modest $3 billion a year that the administration projected for its proposal. And the wily Louisiana Democrat was touting his own plan: catastrophic insurance that had the government picking up the costs after individuals (or their insurers) had spent $2,000.

Despite the president's interest, the White House did not lobby the issue. The idea of deploying the vice president had fizzled, and the president rarely spoke out publicly or twisted arms privately on health matters. National health insurance made little progress for the remainder of the 1971 session.

### A Do-Nothing Congress

In the winter of 1972—his reelection year—Nixon reintroduced his national insurance and HMO proposals. Elliot Richardson reported (or perhaps imagined) progress.[67]

By now, however, Nixon was consumed with his dramatic visits to China and Russia in February and May 1972. His interest in domestic issues receded and—the old problem—he was not available to sell the plan: on May 30, Cavanaugh wrote Kenneth Cole, who had become the lead White House domestic advisor on health:

> The best method of selling the program is having our people out traveling across the country doing substantive events, remarks before associations, and getting the right message across on T.V. news spots.... Most of the White House Press Corps now believe that the President is firmly behind and interested in the cancer program.... It takes a series of events to bring this credibility about. It just can't be done by issuing a Presidential Statement or "just spending another $100 million to get attention" ... Most of our visible White House spokesmen stay away from the health program when commenting on the domestic program. The selling of the health program has been left exclusively to Richardson [and others] at HEW who ... have not been able to capture very much public attention.[68]

Nixon did hold occasional meetings with interest groups to drum up support for his health plan. As always, he seemed as intent on beating the Kennedy plan as on winning his own. He told the president of the AMA in September 1972 during an Oval Office meeting,

> The proposal on the Democratic platform—the Kennedy proposal—We have a lot of reasons why we would hope to whip it ... —just talking politically which you can't do. And one of the reasons is that this kind of philosophy must be put down. Put down really good right now. You know that program costs 60 billion dollars. 60 billion dollars! ... Where the devil are you gonna get the—Where are you gonna get the hospitals? Where are you gonna get the medicine? Right now you're overloaded. You haven't got enough doctors. You haven't got enough nurses. You haven't got enough hospitals with Medicare. Nobody thought of that before they put it all together.... We all fight for the establishment. We don't want to change the way things are. We don't want to do things in a different way because it may endanger our way of doing things.... I don't mean ... some screwball scheme like this 60-billion-dollar one—But on the other hand, you must not just stand on the status quo.... We must not just stand there.[69]

By the fall of 1972, Nixon was in the thick of his reelection campaign. Like Harry Truman in 1948, he seized on congressional inaction on health care. "They didn't pass the health bill," he told Erlichman in October. "Now's the time to fight Congress—this Congress didn't pass the health bill."[70] At the end of the campaign, Nixon began to blast the Democrats for proposing too much and passing nothing. On November 3, Nixon told a national radio audience:

> No American family should be denied access to adequate medical care because of inability to pay. The most important health proposal not acted on by the 92nd Congress was my program for helping people pay for care.... One of the clearest choices in the 1972 Presidential election is the choice between the comprehensive health insurance plan, which is a private plan that I have just described, and our opponents' plan for a medical system which is paid for by the taxpayers and controlled by the Federal Government.[71]

Nixon headed into the election with a strong hand. He faced a weak opponent in Senator George McGovern (D-SD). He had neutralized the Vietnam War. He had scored coups with both China and the USSR. Domestically, he could claim achievements in tax policy, revenue sharing, and the environment. And his southern strategy was breaking almost a century of Democratic domination.

In health care, he had pioneered two concepts that would have a tremendous impact: using HMOs to improve efficiency and mandating employer insurance to spread coverage. Most future health reformers—Democrats and Republicans—would pursue variations of Nixon's plan. His gut feelings on the issue (childhood memories, beating Kennedy, winning reelection, winning praise, solving a problem) all led him to be bold.

At the same time, his efforts to actually win the national health insurance that his administration concocted were desultory at best. Like Truman, he had not devoted much political capital to the fight. Some read Nixon's diffidence as evidence that he didn't really care. According to this view, he proposed national health insurance purely as a defense against Democratic proposals in general, and Kennedy's in particular.

Of course, beating Kennedy always mattered. However, as his private conversations and well-marked memos testify, Nixon cared a great deal about health care and devoted considerable attention to it. He failed for some obvious reasons: the AMA opposed his HMO concept. A fractious Democratic Congress, divided among many approaches to health reform, could agree on one thing: it did not want to give credit to a Republican president. Moderates and conservatives were wary of increased health spending when Medicare had unleashed health care costs—and had made cost growth more politically fraught by feeding on visible tax dollars (rather than hidden private insurance premiums). Finally, there was that last, personal matter: Richard Nixon never liked selling his programs—either to the Congress or to the American people.

Although polls showed—as they always show—that the public cared about health care coverage, actually moving a comprehensive program through Congress was invariably a long shot. It required the mobilization of public opinion to push legislators and confront hostile interest groups. Like Harry Truman before him, Richard Nixon had floated a groundbreaking health care plan that would inspire future reformers. And, like Truman, Nixon failed to go out and sell his plan. Presidential leadership could not assure political success, but the lack of presidential leadership once again assured failure.

## THE COMPREHENSIVE HEALTH INSURANCE PLAN: 1973–1974

On November 7, 1972, Richard Nixon won his smashing victory—carrying forty-nine states and over 61 percent of the popular vote. Only one candidate in American history had won a larger percentage of the electoral college (FDR in 1936). Nixon's coattails were short. The Democrats picked up two Senate seats, for a margin of 56–42; Republicans gained twelve House seats, but Democrats led, 239–192. Still, the president had much to be proud of.

Pride, however, was not much in evidence at the White House. Nixon watched the results alone in the Lincoln Suite. The next day he met his staff. "We need new blood, fresh ideas," announced the president; he turned the meeting over to Haldeman, who brusquely demanded everyone's resignation. Later in the day, Haldeman fired the entire Cabinet.[72]

Nixon retreated to Camp David for several weeks, where he made plans for his newly acquired political capital. "Goals for the 2nd term," penned Nixon on one of his yellow-lined pads: *Substance, Political, Personal.*" Under *Substance,* he wrote out a long and ambitious list: "Russia—SALT; China—Exchanges; Mideast—Settlement ... Crime; Education; Health; Land Use; Race.... " Under *Personal:* "Restore respect for office; New idealism—respect for flag, country; Compassion—understanding."[73]

## Why Does It Have to Be So Aggressive?

In the Cabinet shuffle that followed the mass resignations, Elliot Richardson moved to the Defense Department, and Casper (Cap) Weinberger, who had been director of the Office of Management and Budget, replaced Richardson at HEW. Weinberger's reputation for merciless budget cutting had earned him the moniker "Cap the Knife." Washington observers assumed that Weinberger's brief was to impose discipline on HEW's subversive Democratic holdovers. But things were never quite what they appeared in the Nixon presidency. Cap the Knife would bring comprehensive health insurance closer to reality than any of his predecessors.

The fortress around the president opened for the new secretary of HEW, who enjoyed unprecedented access to Nixon. The two men met regularly along with health advisor James Cavanaugh. Nixon instructed Weinberger to produce a national health insurance program that could pass the Congress. The president gave general directions: a "public-private" plan that assured universal insurance that augmented private sector coverage and used government to fill gaps. The president was interested in his legacy, surmises Cavanaugh, "and [he] had identified health as an area where he wanted to leave a mark."[74]

Nixon had motives beyond his legacy. For one thing, Robert Teeter, the Republican pollster, joined some of the meetings and reported polls measuring the power of the health care issue. As Watergate emerged,

Nixon seemed desperate to divert attention and recapture American hearts. Health was one of the straws at which he would clutch.

Shortly after Weinberger arrived at HEW, the supposedly fearsome new secretary surprised his health aides by asking for a top-to-bottom review of national health insurance. Stuart Altman, a young economist who had emerged as a key health policy advisor in the Richardson regime, recalls the unexpected marching orders: "[Weinberger said] I don't want any options off the table ... he said it was the most important piece of legislation ... our previous plan had not gotten any traction and he wanted a plan that people would take seriously."[75]

By April 30, 1973, Erlichman and Haldeman were gone and Cap Weinberger's influence grew. As the tight circle around him crumbled and the White House fell into disarray, the president began to rely on Cabinet departments. In May 1973, Kenneth Cole, who had replaced Erlichman as the head of domestic affairs, wrote Alexander Haig, who had replaced Haldeman as the White House chief of staff: "The President has expressed a strong desire to work more closely with members of his Cabinet, and to insure that the Cabinet plays a more active role in the formulation of policy than it has in the past. As we well know, the President's first step to expand his own channels of communication with the entire Cabinet, and to shift more responsibility ... back to the Cabinet, away from a highly centralized White House staff, was to terminate the Counselor system"[76]

The president was making a virtue of necessity. For Weinberger the result was that for the first time in the Nixon presidency a Cabinet secretary had almost total control over the direction of health care activities. He became head of the Domestic Council's Committee on Health. He had the ear of the increasingly desperate chief executive. Altman recalls: "He [Weinberger] wasn't frozen out. He had the ability to go talk to the President.... He got his way.... The White House staff did not dominate him.... There was not an independent force [in the White House by that time].... Weinberger was in control much more than [Eliot] Richardson [had been]."[77]

On December 7, 1973, Weinberger sent the president a memo: "A revised [national health insurance] proposal is now ready.... Recent developments on Capitol Hill seem to make it advisable for us to reach agreement on an Administration proposal and announce it by the end of the year."[78]

It was difficult to cut health spending, continued Weinberger, when Americans had no health care safety net. The best way to cut waste in

HEW was to provide basic coverage to everyone. He also noted the action on Capitol Hill: Ted Kennedy and Wilbur Mills were negotiating a joint proposal, and Senator Russell Long was pushing his perennial bill covering catastrophic health costs.

> The absence of a proposal for NHI has temporarily placed the Administration in a very negative posture in the health area.... We have been working diligently ... to construct a proposal which would correct these deficiencies while maintaining the basic structure of the Administration's original plan.... I urge that it be one of your major domestic initiatives and that you make this known within the Administration. I further recommend that the plan be ... part of your State of the Union Message.[79]

The Comprehensive Health Insurance Plan (CHIP) was a more ambitious version of the first term plan. It required that all employers provide comprehensive coverage to all their employees. This time, the administration limited employee cost-sharing and mandated generous benefits. A government program (federal and state) would cover Americans who could not obtain private coverage; there were no income limits on eligibility for this coverage. Although this plan was more expansive than its predecessor, the total cost in additional federal on-budget expenses remained less than $5 billion.

CHIP would become the essential blueprint for national health insurance. For the next thirty-five years, Democratic proposals would offer variations—increasingly less ambitious variations—of the proposal that emerged in the final months of the Nixon administration.

At the time, the first resistance sprang up from within the administration. On December 13, 1973, a week after Weinberger's memo, Nixon dropped in on a meeting of the Domestic Council to quell dissent. As they waited for the president, several Cabinet secretaries groused about the plan. Why was national health insurance so important? Why did it have to be "so comprehensive" and "so aggressive?" When Nixon stepped into the room, he sternly explained his position. As usual, his talking points mixed defense (stop Kennedy) and offense (this was a solid program):

> I know that there are some of you who question why we need to have any proposal at all. Let me give you some of my reasons.... First, there is the threat of a Kennedy type plan.... There is no question that at some point in time, there will be a serious move to push legislation through the Congress and we must have a proposal to counter it. You simply can't fight something with nothing.... I do want to emphasize, however, that I feel this is an important program and we need to develop a sound program. I want you to know that I place a very high priority on this effort.[80]

Nixon told them that he wanted a final plan by the end of the month and left. The grumbling stopped. Nixon may have been a crippled president, but he could still bring his Cabinet to heel. Stuart Altman left the meeting feeling that he and his colleagues in HEW now had free reign: "I never had so much power," he jokes.[81] At the same time, however, Nixon—the sometimes savvy policy manager—also instructed Weinberger to try to accommodate the administration skeptics.[82]

The administration planned to formally introduce the plan after Congress returned in January 1974. However, empowered by the meeting, Weinberger immediately began leaking key elements to the press. The White House was pleased with the reaction. On December 14, Cavanaugh wrote Weinberger, congratulating him on the "good play" he was getting for his health plan. Dan Rather of CBS News referred to a Weinberger press briefing on health insurance and announced that health care "is building as a 1974 congressional campaign issue."[83]

In late January, Weinberger sent Nixon a final decision memo. It was a classic, well-designed presidential options paper in which Weinberger presented his plan, the objections to it, and his response to those objections. The memo revealed that economists in the administration and business interests outside it still had strong objections. The Council of Economic Advisors (CEA) wanted the president to abandon the idea of employer mandates and substitute a tax credit that would push people to purchase private insurance—an AMA proposal that has become popular once again among today's Republicans. The Department of Commerce piled on, recommending that employers be required to cover only hospital care.

Weinberger pushed back: "To follow the CEA approach would, in effect, mean the abandonment of an Administration national health insurance proposal. The Commerce recommendation would result in a less comprehensive plan than we previously submitted. Either proposal would jeopardize the Administration's having a serious contender among the bills now introduced in the Congress."[84]

Under the president's direction and political protection, a strong secretary of HEW had produced an aggressive health plan. It had been vetted within the administration. Opponents had had their say. It was now up to the president.

On January 30, 1974, Richard Nixon stood in the well of the House of Representatives, looking past the nation's leaders—representatives, senators, Cabinet secretaries, supreme court judges, generals—and out at the American people. This should have been a moment of triumph.

The Vietnam War was over. The administration had deftly managed the Yom Kippur War. Relations with the Soviet Union and China had not been better in thirty years. Nixon began his State of the Union address:

> Tonight, for the first time in 12 years, a President of the United States can report to the Congress on the State of a Union at peace with all nations of the world. Because of this ... I have been able to deal primarily with the problems of peace ... rather than with the problems of war.

Nixon could now try to hear gentler voices, the side of his tangled character that yearned to embody his mother's compassion. Halfway through the address, Nixon announced the plan that Weinberger had developed:

> The time is at hand—this year—to bring comprehensive, high-quality health care within the reach of every American. I shall propose a sweeping new program that will assure comprehensive health insurance protection to millions of Americans who cannot now obtain it or afford it, with vastly improved protection against catastrophic illness. This will be a plan that maintains the high standards of quality in America's health system. It will not require additional taxes.

Of course, Nixon's health plans always came with a shot at their rivals. The president gave Kennedy equal time:

> Other plans have been put forward that would cost $80 or $100 billion, and that would put our whole health care system under the heavy hand of the Federal Government. This is the wrong approach.... The right way is one that builds on the strengths of our present system, not one that destroys those strengths.... Most of all, let us keep this as the guiding principle of our health programs: Government has a great role to play—but we must always make sure that our doctors will be working for their patients and not for the Federal Government.[85]

This time, Nixon was willing to throw himself into public advocacy. Appearing on February 5 before the annual meeting of the American Hospital Association, Nixon gave the kind of talk he had failed to give in his first term. His handwritten notes reveal the familiar two-step— propose and attack: "1974—a year which could be historic in progress toward better medical care—It must be right ... people want it—danger is target wrong kind of program."[86]

In the talk itself, he called comprehensive health insurance "an idea whose time has come." He described his CHIP proposal, blasted the Democrats' comprehensive programs, boasted of the administration's own accomplishments, decried the gaps in the nation's current system of insurance coverage, and then returned to his personal health care touchstone:

> Forty-five years ago my oldest brother contracted tuberculosis. In those days we did not have the new methods of treatment which handled tuberculosis very effectively and very quickly, and for five years my oldest brother was bed-ridden. My mother took care of him, took him to Arizona for three of those five years. It was, of course, a very great burden on the family from the standpoint of separation. It was, from a financial standpoint, a disaster. As a matter of fact, we recovered from it. We were able to go on and seek our education and the rest, but that example could be repeated today in millions of American homes ... not with regard to tuberculosis. We can be thankful ... that the advances in medical science would not require five years of bed rest as a possible, not cure, but possible way to arrest the disease. But there are other diseases.... You know, everybody in politics has some particular program that he believes in very deeply because of his own personal experience. I have related a personal experience, one from my own family, which indicates why I believe we have got to move in this area so that other families of modest means will not be drawn, basically, to bankruptcy because of the inability to handle medical problems of a catastrophic type.... There is no [domestic] area in which I think people are more concerned and in which a greater contribution can be made than in the field of health.[87]

Again and again, Nixon returned to his lost brothers. Beneath all the partisan cunning and policy calculation lay a wounded man's childhood trauma. The personal touchstone focused Nixon's personal urge for "compassion—understanding" (as he had written at Camp David after the election) on ensuring that all Americans got the health care they needed.

On February 6, the administration sent its CHIP program to Congress, where it was introduced by Representative Wilbur Mills and Senator Robert Packwood (R-OR). Of course, this was no triumphant moment. His closest aides had resigned and faced indictment. His own hold on his office was shaky. He was isolated, traveling between Key Biscayne, Camp David, and San Clemente. He rarely appeared in public. The pathetic details soon leaked out. The president wandered about the White House at night, drinking heavily and babbling to the portraits. He would appear at the Oval Office around noon—eyes already glazed from liquor. Secretary of the Treasury William Simon thought he looked like a "windup doll." Nixon's son-in-law, Edward Cox, told Senator Robert Griffin (R-MI) that he feared Nixon would "go bananas" and kill himself. Al Haig quietly moved to keep prescription drugs out of the president's hands.[88]

In this bleak hour, President Nixon turned back to health care. In retrospect, the president's born-again interest seems even more poignant because of the events unfolding on Capitol Hill. The congressional barons were in motion, and their ponderous minuet created an opening for health insurance. A powerful president might have been able to seize the chance; even this wounded president came close.

## The Power Brokers and the Stripper

Nearly two years earlier, in the run-up to the 1972 presidential campaign, two aides to Senator Edward Kennedy, Stan Jones and Lee Goldman, had had a wild idea. Wilbur Mills's interest in becoming president—or at least, moving beyond Ways and Means Chair—might create an opportunity for national health insurance. Mills would be looking for issues that could draw national attention. Maybe Kennedy (the ultimate health care liberal) and Mills (the conservative scourge of liberal health plans) could craft a joint proposal. Mills might even see this as a shot at running as Kennedy's vice president. When the staffers approached Kennedy, the ruddy-faced senator looked incredulous. Then, slowly, a mischievous grin. He gave the go-ahead to test the waters with Mills.[89]

Rather than approach Mills directly, Jones and Goldman took a more devious route. Mills and Kennedy were scheduled to testify together before the Democratic Party Platform Committee in June 1972. Jones asked Wilbur Cohen, who was cochairing the Committee, whether he would suggest that Mills and Kennedy work together. Cohen, the irrepressible health care warhorse—we've seen him work legislation under Roosevelt, Truman, Kennedy, and Johnson, had developed a close relationship with Wilbur Mills and was tickled by the suggestion. A day later, Mills shocked his health aide, Bill Fullerton, by telling him to find out whether Senator Kennedy was serious about reaching common ground.[90]

Over the next several months, Kennedy, Mills, and their assistants met secretly in Mills's hideaway off the House floor. Kennedy and Mills spent most of the time talking politics, but in the last few minutes of each session, they got down to business: they answered a series of questions posed by their aides and then raised additional issues to be staffed out for the next meeting. Eventually, they reached an agreement that then went to House lawyers, who, stunned by the strange alliance, drew up the legislation.[91]

As part of the compromise, Kennedy abandoned key tenets of his own approach. He agreed to finance insurance through Social Security taxes rather than general revenues—essentially copying Medicare. Kennedy made a larger concession in order to limit program costs: patients would pay coinsurance and deductibles . Today such copayments are standard, but at the time liberals—and especially labor—fiercely resisted them as financial barriers to health care.

With the proposal in hand, Kennedy turned to his political base. He met with a group of labor union titans, including Leonard Woodcock, president of the United Auto Workers (UAW), and Andrew Biemiller, second in command at the AFL-CIO (and a key architect of Medicare). They sat around Senator Kennedy's comfortable, wood-paneled suite packed with stirring reminders of the legendary family: photographs of Jack and Bobby, of the patriarch, Joe Sr., and the matriarch, Rose. And—intimations of a new Camelot—there were also pictures of Teddy's three young children hanging alongside their exuberant drawings.

The meeting did not go well. The union heads fiercely opposed copayments: this, they argued, violated bedrock principle. Kennedy responded by describing the positions of the important members on the House and Senate finance committees; there was no chance of a better deal. The union leaders did not budge. Kennedy stuck to his guns. For a liberal presidential hopeful, this was a brave break with his key (and at the time, still-powerful) supporters.

On April 3, 1974, Kennedy and Mills took their surprise proposal public. In the world of Washington health care policy, this was a major event. There were now two unlikely health plans on the table—the administration's CHIP bill (which leaned toward moderate Democrats) and Kennedy–Mills (which, although it broke with liberal orthodoxy, represented the liberal alternative to CHIP).

A short time later, two key aides Stan Jones (from Kennedy's office) and Stuart Altman (from HEW) found themselves on a health care panel in the mountains outside Santa Fe. Jones, a tall, lanky, relaxed man with a broad, comfortable smile, a ready laugh, and a flat Midwestern accent, would later become a minister. Altman was a short, fast-talking Jewish economics professor from Brooklyn with a New York twang, a quick mind, and a caustic wit. The unlikely pair had much in common: political shrewdness, a commitment to universal coverage, and a bold new health insurance proposal they were responsible for marketing. They were both working for savvy political pragmatists—Weinberger and Kennedy. In the New Mexico mountains, they dreamed up a bold plan: combine CHIP and Kennedy–Mills.

Back in Washington, the principals—Kennedy, Mills, and Weinberger—all signed on. The aides began meeting secretly in the basement pub of a Capitol Hill church to work out a compromise. "No one wanted to be seen together," recalls Jones. But they kept a sense of humor: "One time, Stuart Altman showed up with Ted Cooper [the assistant secretary of health] ... and he had a six pack."[92]

The president encouraged the talks. Likely at Weinberger's urging, he gave a national radio address from his Key Biscayne home on May 20. Democratic plans such as the Kennedy–Mills plan had merits, said the president, and he was willing to compromise, so long as they conformed to core principles: protect patients' freedom to choose physicians, build on the private system, and offer all parties a stake in the program. Inevitably, the president recalled his brothers' illness and death. Two days later, Nixon followed up with letters to Senate Majority Leader Mike Mansfield (D-MT) and House Speaker Carl Albert (D-OK), repeating the "Administration's desire to reach mutually satisfactory health insurance legislation."[93]

Over the course of the late spring and early summer, Stuart Altman (representing the administration) and Bill Fullerton (representing Wilbur Mills) hammered out a plan. After Kennedy's break with labor, his influence waned. The meetings produced a modified CHIP plan—the financing provisions were rewritten to give the Ways and Means Committee (meaning Wilbur Mills) sole jurisdiction. Then, Mills being Mills, he simply waived hearings on the new plan—the committee had already heard enough about health insurance, he explained.

On the morning of the committee vote, Fullerton happened upon his boss in a men's room near the committee conference room. Standing at the urinal next to him, Mills turned to Fullerton and said, with a sigh, "Bill, we don't have the votes. Maybe next year." In fact, the committee approved the Nixon–Mills proposal by a 16–15 vote—the first time that the Committee on Ways and Means of the U.S. House of Representatives had ever approved a comprehensive health insurance program. But the always cautious Mills demanded a decisive majority before taking controversial measures to the floor. One vote was not enough. The resistance came from the Republicans. Mills implored them to support their president—after all, this was an administration bill—but they refused.[94]

The real problem was that by the early summer of 1974, President Nixon was a dead politician walking. On June 6, the *Los Angeles Times* broke the blockbuster story that the Haldeman and Erlichman indictments had named Richard Nixon as an unindicted coconspirator. On

July 24, the Supreme Court ruled that the president had to release all remaining White House tapes—including the one from June 23, 1972, that recorded Nixon colluding in the Watergate cover-up. The president resigned on August 8—tearfully recalling his mother's sacrifice and his brother's death as he said good-bye to the White House staff.

When Nixon announced his resignation, Altman and Fullerton were meeting over a revised Nixon–Mills plan that might lure some Republican votes. Now, Wilbur Mills had lost his partner. Gerald Ford stepped into office with other things on his mind—not the least calming the Watergate storms. Even had Ford been interested in pursuing the alliance, a pathetic scandal ended any hope for this rare bipartisan collaboration.

Two months later, on October 8, police in Washington, D.C. stopped a car driving at night without headlights. Out jumped an intoxicated woman, who darted off to plunge into the Tidal Basin, a Potomac River pool by the Jefferson monument. The police fished her out and discovered a local stripper known as "Fanne Foxe, the Argentine Firecracker." Back in the car sat a very drunk Wilbur Mills and two companions. The squalid episode humiliated Mills—he became a national punchline—but his Arkansas district faithfully returned him to Congress the following month. It began to seem that this consummate politician might survive—perhaps even retain his chairmanship. But a month later, in December 1974, the now-notorious Fannie Fox appeared in a wispy silk gown on the stage of a strip joint in Boston's combat zone and announced breathlessly that she had a surprise. "I'd like you to meet somebody," she told the audience. "Mr. Mills, Mr. Mills! Where are you?" Wilbur rose to join the Argentine Firecracker on stage. He told a quick joke and got a peck on the cheek. But as he groped his way back to his seat, his political career was over. He retired in 1976, after thirty-eight years in the House.[95]

Even had the principals been in their political prime, the Nixon–Mills–Kennedy partnership would have been a long shot. The Senate Finance Committee, with its skeptical chair, Russell Long, still posed a formidable obstacle. Small businesses would likely have fought the mandate to provide insurance to employees. But advocates of health insurance—Ted Kennedy among them—would later regret that they had failed to seize the chance that Nixon offered them. The tectonic plates had rumbled ever so slightly apart during the tumultuous summer of 1974. For a Washington minute it seemed that national health insurance might actually pass. Then the political ground shifted again, and the moment was gone. It would be decades before another real opening arose, and by then, health insurance reformers, including Senator Kennedy, would have counted themselves lucky to pass a program as generous as the one that the Nixon administration had proposed.

## NIXON'S LEGACY

Richard Nixon's health care policy was almost as singular as the man himself. Though he might have led a Republican attack on Medicare, Nixon chose instead to learn its deeper lesson: expanding coverage eventually requires increasing efficiency or the program will bust the budget. What might make health care more efficient? Nixon found an old but unfamiliar idea—prepaid group practice—repackaged it as a system of competing HMOs, and introduced it into American health politics.

Even more important, Nixon harmonized universal coverage and private insurance. Eisenhower had been the first to envision a private system that was generous and humane, but his conservative view of government had constricted his policies. Nixon—by his own reckoning "a government man"—broke those constraints and played out the Republican logic of Eisenhower's generous impulse. That logic drove him to propose mandating employer coverage and regulating the private insurance offered by employers. To meet his ambitious public purposes, Nixon would push government deeply into private business. Patrick Buchanan's conservative fears about his boss were fully justified.

Many impulses drove Nixon to his health care breakthroughs: he wanted domestic accomplishments—and started touting health care before his first one hundred days were up. He needed a plan for his 1972 reelection campaign—and revived the issue to meet the need. He faced the crisis (his word) of rising costs and gaps in coverage. He wanted to fend off "dangerous" and "impractical" Democratic proposals. He wanted to whip Kennedy. And he desperately wanted to change the subject from Watergate. But he could have been content with far less. He did not need to opt for a plan that forced employers to offer generous insurance backed by government programs—what Republicans then and now dub compulsory health insurance. Something deeper and more personal led him to insist on covering everyone. And almost every time he talked about the issue—in public or in private—he revealed exactly what that deeper something was.

Richard Nixon always saw health care as a powerful and volatile issue, because it was powerful and volatile for him. It was a part of his past—his most searing childhood memory. He knew what illness could do to a family, financially and emotionally. Stress always seemed to trigger memories of his brother Harold dying of tuberculosis. Memories of his mother, vanishing from his childhood to try to cope with Harold's illness. And memories of financial difficulties piled on top of the emotional ones. National health insurance seemed to address his childhood pain.

Nixon did not always manage the issue effectively. He put it aside for long stretches. During his first term, he failed to push the plan with either the public or Congress. His venomous side (which imagined a nation of hypochondriacs) sometimes eclipsed his charitable side (which remembered pain and need). But when he focused, he was a model of effective presidential policy development. He set clear broad goals. He organized competent management in both the White House and in HEW. He read the option memos, annotated them, and made his choices. He hushed the inevitable chorus of naysaying economists. In contrast to many presidents before and after him, he neither obsessed over the details nor ignored them entirely.

If Nixon cared about health care, why didn't he provide more public leadership on the issue? The answer is that he *couldn't*. Nixon hated going public. He roused himself from his dark fortress when political survival was at stake—or when foreign affairs beckoned. Only at the very end did Nixon seem to emerge, tentatively, to seriously push his health care policies. By then, political survival was indeed on the line. Perhaps—in light of the heavy drinking and intimations of suicide—personal survival was too. By Nixon's own repeated account, health care spoke to both the political and the personal. It was central to his sometime self-image as a compassionate man and understanding caregiver—this was Richard Nixon as his saintly mother's good son.

Nixon's health care policy reflected both the genius and the flaws of a man locked away with his yellow pads. He had the insight to recast the entire concept of national health insurance for a rising Republican era, but not the skill to win it. Even at that, the Kennedy–Mills–Nixon negotiations came closer than any other effort between Franklin Roosevelt and George W. Bush.

Nixon changed the health care discussion in the United States. Today's reformers all stand in his shadow. Ultimately, however, Nixon could not change himself. His health care plans went down with him amid the wreckage of Watergate.

# CHAPTER 7

# Jimmy Carter

*The Righteous Engineer*

Jimmy Carter ran for president as a skeptical outsider come to clean up the mess. The former Georgia governor was so new to Washington that the day after his inauguration he had no idea how to get from the White House living quarters to the Oval Office. "When the elevator reached the ground floor, the security men were waiting," he recalled. "Not certain how to find my office, I said as casually as possible, 'I'm just going to the Oval Office' and followed the lead agent."[1]

Critics thought Carter never really learned the way. His approval ratings dropped below 50 percent after the first year and never recovered. But Carter faced an especially difficult problem: a conservative tide was stirring and the Democratic majority that stretched back forty-five years was coming apart at the seams. A month before the inauguration, pollster and advisor Pat Caddell put the problem crisply: "Governor Carter's political situation is precarious for ... the Democratic Party is in serious national trouble—with a shrinking and ill-defined coalition." Democratic factions disagreed with one another on almost everything. They would finally break apart on the issue of national health insurance.[2]

Carter almost certainly could not have enacted the kind of sweeping reform that the liberals, led by Ted Kennedy (D-MA), demanded—and that Carter himself had reluctantly swallowed during the Democratic primaries to pacify the party base. But this administration made the worst of a bad situation, and offers a vivid warning to future presidents about what not to do when—as so often happens—they find themselves holding a lousy health care hand.

Pat Caddell put his finger on what the Democrats were looking for—"We need a new and broader political coalition that can attract new support"—but he could offer only tepid, though telling, advice on how the new administration might find its way: assertively educate administration members on Jimmy Carter's "goals and his philosophy." Most presidents lead a movement or a party or at least a faction to power; this one needed to instruct its appointees about what the president stood for.[3]

And what lay at the heart of Carter's "goals and philosophy"? Not substance or ideology or passion. Rather, President Carter placed an engineer's emphasis on efficiency, detail, procedure, reducing governmental waste, and streamlining bureaucracy. As political scientist Steven Skowronek sums it up, Carter offered a "passionless vision of reorganizing the old [Democratic] order without challenging any of its core concerns."[4]

Health reform, as Carter painfully discovered, was critical to the Democratic coalition. But the factions arrayed themselves along a very wide policy spectrum: some obsessed about deficits, others dreamed of national health insurance. Managed badly, with neither passion nor skill, the health care issue would sunder the few remaining ties that bound Democrats together.

JIMMY CARTER

Carter's personal style reflected his philosophy. The president eagerly found symbolic ways to portray himself as a regular citizen. He was a just-the-facts, no-fuss kind of guy, who knew how normal people lived: he carried his own luggage, wore cardigan sweaters instead of suits, and (temporarily) stopped the Marine Corps Band from playing "Hail to the Chief." He purged rhetorical flourish from speechwriters' drafts. The common touch was no affectation—it went right to Jimmy Carter's core.

*Bedbugs and Jim Crow*

Jimmy Carter grew up in a simple, one-story house without electricity or plumbing. His father, Earl, farmed peanuts on three hundred acres—a lot of land around Archer, Georgia (right near Plains), where most families scraped by on twenty five acres. "Jesus and even Moses would have felt at home on a farm in the Deep South during the first third of the twentieth century," Carter later observed. The work was done by mule, muscle, and black farmers in virtual serfdom.[5]

Jimmy feared and adored his father. "It was not natural for my father to admit a mistake," wrote Carter, "and as a child, I was inclined to consider him omniscient and infallible." Earl was a successful farmer, a harsh southern disciplinarian—Jimmy remembered every whipping— and an enthusiast about local politics. In Jimmy's young world, there was always a right way and a wrong way.

The Carter family saw politics through southern eyes, and the Civil War and Reconstruction seared their pride: "My grandfather Gordy was thirteen years old," Carter later wrote, "when what he saw as the Northern oppressors finally relinquished political and economic control of the state in 1876." Jimmy's mother was the only one in the family who would defend Abraham Lincoln—and no one ever mentioned slavery. In the Carters' Deep South story, the Yankees caused the Great Depression. Though Earl was a Democrat, he hated Roosevelt with a passion. Young Jimmy drew a cautionary lesson about well-intentioned big government programs from watching New Deal agricultural policies in Plains. "I ... learned from tenant farmers themselves how little help the New Deal assistance programs provided, and how often they created additional problems." In stark contrast to Lyndon Johnson, who idealized Roosevelt and his policies, Carter grew up thinking that "the New Deal had become a curse, not a blessing" for the poor, black Georgia farmers scraping out a living under the blazing southern sun.[6]

Under Earl's firm but—in Jimmy's view—fair hand, blacks managed the Carter farm and did most of the hard work. Jimmy fished, hunted, explored, and wrestled with their children. He ate at their tables (usually fatback, greens, and bread), slept in their shacks, got bitten by the same bedbugs, and watched poverty take its toll on their bodies and souls. At puberty, Jim Crow rules and unwritten taboos separated Jimmy from his friends and playmates—black and white adults lived separate lives. For southerners who rose above the racism—as Carter did—this child-hood intimacy with African Americans engendered a passion for civil and human rights that few northern Americans could match.

## Evil Tastes and Smells

Being close to the land in early-twentieth-century Georgia meant hard, often brutal work and frequent danger. Jimmy worked with his father at the forge and anvil, making horseshoes and repairing plows. He fetched water from springs, milked cows, slaughtered chickens, rendered pigs, plucked geese, and picked cotton in the Georgian heat. Like all southern boys, he had to keep an eye out for poisonous water moccasins and rabid dogs.

Carter suffered the infectious illnesses that were endemic to the rural South. When he was three, he nearly died of "bleeding colitis"—probably dysentery, still a leading cause of childhood mortality in poor rural areas around the world. Later, he wrote, the most common ailments were "ground itch, ringworm, boils and carbuncles, sties in our eyes, plus the self-inflicted splinters, cuts, abrasions, wasp or bee stings.... We didn't worry much about red bugs, or chiggers, but Mama made us check for ticks.... Almost everyone was afflicted from time to time with hookworm." Hookworm, a parasite now largely eradicated in the developed world, is contracted by going barefoot on land contaminated by human feces carrying the hookworm larva. Like all boys in the rural South, Jimmy and his friends ran barefoot pretty much from March to October. But Jimmy's mama was a nurse, and "she put medicine between my toes which prevented the parasites from migrating over time into my lungs, then my throat, and from there in to my small intestines. Untreated, millions of tiny worms consumed a major portion of the scarce nutrients within the bodies of our poorest neighbors."[7]

Carter's childhood experiences shaped an ambivalent relationship to health care and medicine. Carter's mother Lillian was a nurse and gave Jimmy some medical security (such as it was it was in those days), as well as a glimpse at the local medical profession. Lillian worked at the Wise Sanatorium in Plains. Founded by three physician brothers, sons of a former mayor, the sanatorium was the source of enormous local pride. "We were firmly convinced that our hospital was the best, even compared with the famous ones in Atlanta and farther north," recalled Carter. "The best not only in surgery, but in anesthesiology and in radium treatment of cancer and other tumors." And the doctors were way ahead of their time in "minimizing the use of medicines" and stressing "diet, exercise ... and prevention of disease." As an adult, Carter would tout the same gospel of disease prevention that he saw practiced at the famous local hospital.[8]

The Sanatorium doctors were at the top of the Plains social hierarchy. They enjoyed, said Carter, "extraordinary respect, almost as super humans." Since diseases "were frequently fatal, it seemed that our very lives were constantly in their hands.... They were always on call." The

Carter family, however, took a more skeptical view of the rest of the local medical establishment: the "other" doctors were poorly educated, out of touch with medical science, expensive, reluctant to make house calls and "prescribed excessive quantities of expensive prescription medicine."[9]

Around the dinner table, Jimmy heard the internal gossip that punctured romantic myths about the world's second-oldest profession. Besides, each treatment seemed less pleasant than the last. Jimmy later surmised—half-joking—that the people who mixed and peddled patent medicine had all concluded that "only evil tastes and smells were effective in combating germs—Castor oil, milk of magnesia, 666, and paregoric all met the test. And hot poultices and iodine burned enough to be respected on croupy chests or open cuts and scratches."[10]

Carter would always have a love–hate relationship with the medical profession. Joseph Califano, Carter's secretary of Health, Education, and Welfare, would later recall how angrily Carter rejected a proposal to raise payments to rural physicians as a way to increase their numbers: "Wait, you're going to pay these guys in Americus [Georgia] *more?* I don't want to pay any doctor more." The Georgia Medical Association no doubt sharpened his skepticism by fiercely opposing his bid for governor in 1970.[11]

During his White House years, Carter would campaign against waste, excess, and profits in the medical care industry. He was far more passionate on that topic than he was about expanding coverage for health services that he thought were overused. His contempt for the medical establishment could sound vituperative. As he later put it: "We have an abominable system in this country for the delivery of health care, with gross inequities toward the poor—particularly the working poor—and profiteering by many hospitals and some medical doctors, who prey on the vulnerability of the ill." Because people pay insurance premiums, continued Carter, they don't hesitate to go to the hospital, stay "an extra day or two," accept "the most elaborate treatment," enabling the medical establishment to rack up "enormous profits," out of which they build up still more "unnecessary hospital facilities."[12]

In contrast, his mother, Lillian, was an example of what was right about health care. Carter remembered her nursing the families of black tenant farmers, charging nothing and ignoring racial stigmas. For Carter, she was a lifelong lesson in Christian kindness. Peter Bourne, a psychiatrist and longtime Carter advisor, concluded that Carter's "approach to health care ... was to depend on volunteerism and Christian noblesse oblige." This highly personal view of health care problems, perhaps fed by Carter's ambivalence toward doctors and hospitals, profoundly affected his policies: "He did not see health care as every citizen's right," concluded Bourne, "nor did he think government has an obligation to provide it." Rather, Carter "preferred to talk movingly of his deep compassion and genuine empathy for those who suffered for lack of health care, as though the depth of his compassion could be a substitute for embracing a major new and expensive government solution."[13]

### The Detail of Things

Carter emerged from his Plains childhood as a healthy, obedient, hardworking, religious young man—small in stature, tall in ambition, and firm in his sense of right and wrong. His father had high expectations for his oldest child, who in turn developed the boundless self-confidence that took him far beyond peanut farming. Inspired by an uncle who was a naval officer, Jimmy always wanted to enroll in the Naval Academy. While his father lobbied furiously for the political backing that was the only route to Annapolis, Jimmy attended a local college and then the Georgia Institute of Technology, where he studied engineering. In 1946, he was accepted to the Naval Academy and began a seven-year naval career in which he trained in engineering, served as the engineering officer on a submarine, and studied nuclear physics at Union College in upstate New York.

Carter's training in technology shaped the attitudes that marked his White House years: a fascination with the intricate mechanics of a problem, a faith that each problem had a correct solution, and the knowledge that choosing wrong could be disastrous. "I was trained by [Admiral Hyman C.] Rickover," he later explained. "I'm an engineer at heart, and I like to understand the details of things that are directly my responsibility." Jimmy Carter prepared himself to manage the nuclear reactor of a submarine hundreds of feet under the sea—an approach to problems that stuck for life.[14]

By 1953, the ambitious naval officer set his sights on becoming Chief of Naval Operations, the top operational job in the Navy. In retrospect, Carter would have been admirably suited for the post, and with his intelligence and drive, he might have attained it. But death intervened. His father contracted pancreatic cancer, a virtual death sentence. Jimmy returned to say good-bye to the tough, independent, southern patriarch from whom he had grown distant during his naval years. Now, they reconnected. His father's death was "psychologically traumatizing," suggests psychiatrist Peter Bourne; and it changed the direction of Carter's career. People around Plains flocked to pay their respects to the dying man. Impressed by the reaction, Jimmy gained a new appreciation for life steeped in community and local leadership. Besides, the farm and the family also needed a new captain. Over the fierce protests of his wife, Rosalynn, Carter went home to Plains, peanut farming, and local politics.[15]

Pancreatic cancer would eventually devastate the Carter family. All three of Carter's siblings would die of the disease—only Jimmy escaped it. This pattern strongly suggests a genetic cause, facilitated by an environmental trigger. "The only difference between me and my father and my siblings was that I never smoked a cigarette," Carter said recently. "My daddy smoked regularly. All of them smoked.... Several of my children smoke. It grieves me. I hate cigarettes worse than anything." Carter never took up cigarettes because he promised his father he wouldn't, and Carter, as he repeatedly told the American people during his campaign for president, never broke a promise. Keeping this one may have saved his life. And it may have reinforced the view of medicine that he first saw at the Wise Clinic in his childhood: a healthy lifestyle preserved his own life; but when the rest of his family failed to make the right choices, there was not a thing the doctors could do to help.[16]

## PRESIDENT CARTER

Carter's return to Plains set him on a new trajectory that led to two terms in the Georgia State Senate (where he astonished everyone by reading every single bill that came before the chamber), one term as governor of Georgia, and finally the presidency. Throughout his political career, Carter evinced the same unshakeable traits: an engineer's approach to social problems, hard work, boundless self-confidence, and tenacious ambition. When Carter lost his first campaign for governor in 1966, he grew depressed and turned to religion for solace. After Jimmy was born again, his fervent Southern Baptist faith reinforced his unshakeable convictions about right and wrong.

Of course, the flip side to self-confidence is stubbornness, and Carter freely admitted to the failing: "Once I made a decision I was awfully stubborn about it," he told interviewers after his presidency. "If I could have one political attribute as the cause of my success ... it would be tenacity. Once I get set on something, I'm awfully hard to change. And that may also be a cause of some of my political failures."[17] For LBJ, too, tenacity had been a key to success—but his was focused on a driving vision, the Great Society. Too often, the Georgian engineer got stubbornly attached to the means rather than the ends—the mechanics of policy, rather than its goals.

Carter was a classic southern liberal. He believed in balanced budgets and a small, efficient government; at the same time, influenced by his mother's generosity and his childhood friendships, he fervently advocated human rights, civil liberties, and racial justice. This southern mix would not fit easily with northern liberals. "In many cases," reflected Carter, "I feel more at home with the conservative Democratic and Republican members of Congress than I do with the others."[18]

Nothing in his background prepared him for Washington, D.C. "It's a difficult thing for a Southern politician to come to grips with a Northern way of doing things," reflected Bert Carp, a domestic advisor in Carter's White House.[19] In Atlanta, added Carter, "I could ignore the people ... who were social, business and media leaders." State government officials did not face competing power centers. Carter had no experience with northeastern elites, urban power brokers or the media heavies (such as the *Washington Post,* the *New York Times,* and the influential columnists). He had never imagined all the subtle, unofficial loops that permeate the capital, making and breaking political reputations. "I underestimated [all] that. I don't think there's any doubt about it. It didn't take long to realize that the underestimation existed, but by that time, we were not able to repair that mistake."[20]

## The Outsider on the Potomac

On a cold morning in January 1975, Jimmy Carter left Plains on his first campaign trip for the presidency. It seemed quixotic—he was a one-term governor from Georgia with no support from the party establishment. The standard reaction—a quizzical "Jimmy Who?"—became the campaign's badge of honor. But Carter understood that the party rules now enabled an outsider to win a couple of small states early in the process and, essentially, ride the resulting media wave all the way to the nomination. Typically, Carter would write that from the first day on the trail to the night "when the final election returns from the state of Mississippi told me that I would be the next President, my confidence never wavered."[21]

At his inauguration, Carter began by quoting his high school teacher; he quoted the Bible, announced that "he had no new dream to set forth today," and spoke of his confidence that "we will triumph together in the right."[22] For Jimmy Carter, doing right meant breaking down the old back-scratching politics. He and his inner circle from Georgia "saw the capital city as corrupted and one of his missions as cleaning it up," wrote Joseph Califano, "and failing that, he seemed determined not to get any Washington political dirt under his fingernails."[23]

The White House set the ascetic tone before the inauguration. When Tip O'Neill (D-MA), the powerful Speaker of the House, offered to advise him on congressional relations, Carter stunned him by saying "no thanks"—if he faced opposition in Congress, as he had in the Georgia legislature, he'd take his case to the people. When O'Neill asked for extra tickets to the inauguration, a White House staff member coolly rebuffed him. No more special favors. The slight would come back to haunt the administration when, inevitably, it needed help from the savvy, expansive Irishman from Cambridge, Massachusetts.

In his first month in office, February 1977, President Carter slapped congressional wrists on a grander scale. He cut nineteen large-water projects from President Ford's 1978 budget. Technically Carter was right (as usual). The projects were expensive boondoggles, and the federal budget was running a large deficit. However, the earmarks were important to representatives who prided themselves on bringing benefits to their districts. An infuriated Congress quickly voted to restore the cuts. Rather than working with Congress to build support for paring the budget, the administration simply dropped a bomb into the mix. It took the high ground—and failed.

The next four years would be full of similar high-minded flops. In an effort to get one piece of legislation through the Ways and Means Committee, White House staff members negotiated with Chairman Dan Rostenkowski (D-IL), a Chicago politician of the old school. As Califano told us the story, Rostenkowski wanted one of his cronies named head of the HEW regional office in Chicago. Now, "[t]he guy was incompetent. That's a given." But Califano worked out a deal: Wilbur Cohen's ultra-competent son would be the deputy and do all the real work. Rosty's guy "would be a ribbon-cutter," and they worked it out so that "this guy would leave at the end of the year." The political accommodation would grease the way for the administration bill. When Carter heard about it he angrily nixed the deal. This was old-style, corrupt Washington politics. Rostenkowski, of course, was furious, and the legislation collapsed. As Burt Lance, a close confidant summed it up, "the quid pro quo was just not in him."[24]

Rostenkowski admired most presidents; he used to say we "were gifted in this country" with the men who led—even Republican presidents "represent all the people and are pretty good" (a large concession from a Chicago Democrat). But he made an exception for Carter: "He never impressed me," he told Reagan speech writer Peggy Noonan. "He didn't know how to be president. He should have been a naval navigator and stayed there." Rostenkowski compared Johnson—who was almost "too big, too vivid"—and Carter "whose smallness seemed to come through." Joe Califano, no friend of Jimmy Carter (who fired him unceremoniously in July 1979), echoed Rostenkowski; his contrast of the two presidents he had worked under reflected a kind of Washington consensus: "Johnson was the twentieth-century virtuoso in moving legislation and manipulating power elites in politics, business and labor—and loved every minute of it." In contrast, Carter simply "did not understand the multicolored threads of power inside the beltway and neither liked nor respected [the] legislators, news people, or lobbyists ... who found satisfaction weaving those threads."[25]

The slaps at Congress might have been forgotten if Carter had possessed a greater talent for politics or charm. After all, Tip O'Neill developed a deep affection for Ronald Reagan, despite the huge political gulf dividing them; they spent hours together in the White House family quarters swapping Irish tall tales. But, as Carter himself put it, "it has never been in my nature to be a hail fellow well met, or to be part of a societal, cocktail party circuit ... it's just not me."[26]

One veteran Congressman, Al Ullman (D-OR), who shared Carter's centrist views, once told Carter in frustration: "The difference between you and me, Mr. President, is that you live in a world of enchantment and I live in a world of reality."[27]

Carter's inner circle of Georgians reflected and reinforced their boss's style. Hamilton Jordan, Carter's former executive secretary as governor, architect of his electoral victory, and closest advisor, positively recoiled from politics-as-usual. He was unavailable to congressmen and senators. Tip O'Neill (who called him Hannibal Jerkin) met with him just three times during the Carter presidency. "He never returns a phone call," sighed Rostenkowski. Cabinet members had the same complaint: "We can move government forward by putting phones in the White House Staff offices and the staff using them," suggested Secretary of Housing and Urban Development Patricia Harris during a stormy Cabinet meeting.[28]

Frank Moore, Carter's choice as legislative liaison for the White House, was widely regarded as ineffective—like his boss, he did not know how to work the legislators. "Every time he comes up here," Rostenkowski warned Califano, "he costs us votes." "Frank Moore ... just tore it with the Speaker and most of the Democratic leadership," Califano told us. "He really tore it." Califano illustrated the point with a bit of gossip. Democratic House leaders—Tip O'Neill, Al Ullman, and Tom Foley (D-OR)—were eating lunch in the speaker's inner office while Frank Moore sat outside. As Secretary Califano approached the suite to join the group, the speaker's secretary intercepted him and told him to go in the back way. "That guy's not coming near this lunch," O'Neill told Califano. Yes, it's another catty Washington story. But it is impossible to imagine Larry O'Brien, the savvy legislative liaison for Presidents Kennedy and Johnson, cooling his heels in an antechamber while the House bulls cursed him out over navy bean soup.[29]

## Organization

Carter created a domestic policy process that reflected his straight-shooting, engineering approach to problems. Stuart Eizenstat, a highly regarded Georgia lawyer, ran a technically superb, apolitical operation that never communicated effectively with the political side of the White House operation.[30]

Carter relied heavily on his Cabinet—a throwback to the Eisenhower administration. He aimed to roll back the changes of the Kennedy, Johnson, and Nixon administrations and restore power to the Cabinet. His governmental ideal involved appointing strong managers and delegating authority to them. When the wheels were coming off the administration, however, in July 1979, the president called his Cabinet together and blasted members for disloyalty—for letting him and the nation down. He fired five members—the secretaries of the treasury (Michael Blumenthal), transportation (Brock Adams), energy (James Schlesinger), HEW (Califano) and the attorney general (Griffin Bell, who was leaving anyway), precipitating a minor national crisis and pro-jecting the public impression of an administration that had lost control of events.

The tension with the Department of Health, Education, and Welfare was especially strong and stretched back to before the inauguration. One memo to the president-elect prophesied difficulty from the start: "In view of your desire to delegate primary responsibility for administration of the federal government to your cabinet officers ... you might want to focus on the critical issue of whether, in fact, the concept of the HEW agency is workable."[31] Within months, a White House memo announced that "[t]he spirit of détente with HEW seems to have broken down."[32] Carter aides recall bitterly how Califano instructed his staff to have no dealings with the White House without informing him first. For his part, Califano told close colleagues how he himself had run roughshod over Cabinet secretaries when he was in the White House, and how he was going to be damn sure the same thing did not happen to him. The deeper problem, however, was that the well-connected Califano viewed Carter as naive, self-righteous, small-minded, and incapable of playing in the Washington big leagues. Nor did he trust the other Georgians who surrounded Carter. As one former HEW official remarked to us in an interview, "It was an open question whether the Cabinet or the White House was in charge."[33] Regardless of who was to blame for the friction, it complicated the process of fashioning policy.

Still another bad decision compounded the organizational problems. For his first two-and-a-half years, Carter had no chief of staff. In this, he was continuing a cherished Democratic tradition—Roosevelt, Kennedy, and Johnson had all tried to do the job. But Carter was not aiming for the creative chaos of his Democratic predecessors; rather, he was exorcising the demons of the Nixon administration—the fresh memory of Robert Haldeman and John Erlichman, the dominating aides, who isolated President Nixon both from his subordinates and from the public. As Carter put it, "I have never wanted a person under me to whom all of my chief advisors had to report and then [to] have that one person report to me." The whole idea was "absolutely incompatible with my concept of governing."[34]

However, when tough judgments were required, Carter's aides would come to lament that there was no one around the president who could translate the results of long, wandering, sometimes contentious meetings into crisp directives. And there was no one who could help reign in (or negotiate differences with) a headstrong Cabinet secretary such as Califano; and like many presidents, Carter was reluctant to do so himself. Joe Onek, a key White House health aid, would later recall an emergency White House meeting in June 1978, when the national health insurance debate was coming to a head. White House staff and Califano disagreed on how aggressively the administration ought to push the issue. Both sides came away thinking that Carter had supported them—but there was no one except the president who could resolve the impasse, and he had moved on to the next issue. A chief of staff could have clarified and implemented. Without one, everyone kept on fighting till the president came back to the issue—again.

## The Book of Promises

True to character, Jimmy Carter felt honor-bound to keep all his campaign promises, and to do so at once, from the very start of the administration. Presidents promise many things to many audiences on the way to the White House, but no modern resident has ever hewed to those utterances as literally and stubbornly as the righteous engineer from Georgia. Carter had Stuart Eizenstat assemble a "Book of Promises" cataloguing campaign commitments.[35] In his first year, Carter served up dozens of bills as if he were checking off items on the political shopping list: welfare reform, tax reform, inflation reduction, job training, government reorganization, hospital cost containment, environmental protection, energy—and the list went on.

The administration gave little strategic thought about how to win the items it blithely piled into the congressional hopper. The sheer volume choked the Carter agenda. Congress—and especially its key committees, such as House Ways and Means and Senate Finance—reeled under the onslaught of tough issues and choices. "I remember our chief lobbyist coming back," recalled Joe Onek, "and saying, 'I go to a meeting and I'm trying to break somebody's arm [to win a vote], and he said, Look, what do you want, my vote on energy or cost containment?'"[36]

Carter himself later admitted that this may have been a strategic mistake. Still, Carter was proud of his legislative record—he won 69.3 percent of his important votes, just behind Reagan (69.9), Kennedy (70.5), and Johnson (72.2).[37] But many others pointed out that there was a problem deeper than the sheer multiplicity of programs and promises on the Carter checklist: the president seemed to have no overarching vision, no ability to set priorities, nothing big to achieve. Speechwriter James Fallows summarized the conventional wisdom when he observed: "Carter believes fifty things, but no one thing." Always the engineer, "He holds explicit, thorough positions on every issue under the sun but has no large view of the relations between them."[38]

Among the avalanche of proposals that Carter dumped on the Washington establishment, national health insurance was nowhere to be found. It appeared in his Book of Promises, for Carter had committed to it during his campaign. But he remained vague and noncommittal about it—speaking of eventual enactment as revenues permitted. Carter's hesitancy about national health infuriated the left side of his base and helped create divisions that sealed his fate—a one-term president swept out in a landslide.

In fact, Jimmy Carter was often correct on the substance. He was remarkable in his study of the details. The problems he assaulted wholesale in the first year of his administration were real problems. He was intelligent, well organized, and hard-working. He won his share of victories—notably in foreign affairs. And he was right to see that his own conservative approach was closer to the popular tide that would bring Ronald Reagan to power in the next election. But he had no coherent philosophy or approach to offer. He was a weak communicator—and, of course, spurned suggestions that he work with a speech coach to improve his delivery (that would be political artifice). When it came to the pressing issues of the day—including health insurance—his background, experience, temperament, philosophy, and style of governance did not match up to the challenges he faced. The results were indecision, delay, and stalemate.

## NATIONAL HEALTH INSURANCE?

National health insurance made it into the Book of Promises thanks to one grudging campaign speech Carter made on April 16, 1976. The dark-horse southerner needed backing from organized labor to clinch the Democratic primaries. He entered negotiations with the United Auto Workers, which was pushing hard for a bold national health insurance plan. The UAW generally backed Senator Ted Kennedy's ambitious proposals (although, as we saw in chapter 6, it rejected his effort to compromise with Wilbur Mills [D-AR] and the Republican administration in the waning days of the Nixon presidency). For Jimmy Carter, the price of a UAW endorsement was a commitment to national health insurance. Carter's health care task force tortuously negotiated the language. As Bourne recalled, Carter himself was so insistent on the phrasing that he woke up after midnight "to approve last-minute wording before the final speech was typed. Sitting up in bed in his underwear, he continued to reject overly specific language, sleepily insisting, 'If I do what you're asking, I'll have George Meany [President of the AFL-CIO] knocking on the door the first day I'm in the White House making demands on me I cannot meet.'"[39]

The final speech, delivered before the Student National Medical Association, the association of African American medical students, was a policy masterpiece: balanced, subtle, comprehensive. It looked at the health care system holistically, called for comprehensive health system reform, and saw health insurance for what it was—only part of the solution to improving the nation's health. Carter talked about prevention, about redistributing physicians, about efficiency in health services, and in the end cautiously edged up to national health insurance: "We must achieve all that is practical while we strive for what is ideal," he said, before very lightly touching labor's bottom line. "The accomplishment of comprehensive national health insurance will not be quick or easy. It requires a willingness to seek new solutions, to keep an open mind. The problems are obvious, the solutions less so."[40]

The engineer had spoken. History would prove that he was correct in many areas, and the speech was enough to win the UAW nod. The press blew past all the nuance and simply credited him with embracing national health insurance. But Carter had parsed his words carefully, and privately never committed to—or felt any enthusiasm for—the idea. This was clear from the earliest moments of the Carter administration.[41]

*The Die Is Cast*

During the transition, Carter sent Stuart Eizenstat, his chief domestic policy advisor, a summary of Senator Russell Long's views on health issues. Long (D-LA), who chaired the Senate Finance Committee, expressed deep concern over waste and abuse in Medicare and Medicaid. He supported an "incremental approach" to national health insurance, starting with expanded coverage for the poor and catastrophic insurance for the middle class. At the top of memo, Carter penned: "To Stu: These ideas are very important, and almost all good ones. Use this. J."[42]

Budget problems reinforced Carter's instinct to go slow. Pat Caddell, the president's pollster, pointed out that the first few months would be crucial. Carter needed to seem in control, to set out clear priorities, to be well organized and forceful. Then the bad news: the budget deficit, which stood at $66 billion (or 3 percent of GDP) and the inflation rate (between 7 percent and 8 percent) left "little, if any, overall increase in current policy expenditures." In other words, be forceful, avoid defeats, and don't spend money.[43]

The politics and economics of the new administration were almost ideally aligned with Carter's own predisposition to avoid dramatic new health care initiatives and to concentrate, instead, on purging the waste from the health care system. This is exactly what his advisors recommended—a forceful effort to control health care costs. Another transition memo pointed to the direction the administration would follow for its first two years. "Cost containment is the most important immediate health policy issue facing the administration." The administration might introduce "modest new health benefits," but such benefits—along with any speculations about national health insurance—would have to await "an evaluation of their conceptual, political and administrative compatibility with the Administration's cost containment strategies."[44]

The administration poured its political capital into a bill designed to contain hospital costs. The idea was to limit increases in hospital prices and capital spending from all sources—not just Medicare and Medicaid, but private insurers and individuals as well. The federal government would tame inflation by regulating all hospital revenue. Naturally, the idea aroused bitter opposition from the hospital industry.

Even before Carter's inauguration, Secretary of HEW–designate Califano testified before the Senate Finance Committee that national health insurance would, of course, be a major priority of the new administration—but that hospital cost containment and welfare reform would come first. The old political hands knew precisely what that meant. The next day, the *Washington Post* quoted a cheerful Dan Rostenkowski, chairman of Ways and Means: "Jimmy Carter [had] talked of pushing national health ... 'as revenues permit.' 'I could see it getting further away,' said Rostenkowski. Rostenkowski believes that Congress must move step-by-step—not all at once—toward the universal ... program ... called for by the party platform."[45]

Califano's reference to welfare reform was another nail in the coffin of national health insurance. If there was one domestic policy issue that Carter felt passionate about, aside from deficit reduction, it was welfare reform. As governor, he had seen the effects of the welfare system, and he ardently believed that Washington's good intentions were backfiring in American communities. His view of welfare reflected his longstanding faith that the New Deal had only made things harder on the poor tenant farmers in Plains. Carter would toss aside his cautious step-by-step approach when it came to welfare. During the transition, the team totaled up the economic and political costs of comprehensive welfare reform and warned about the long history of welfare reform train wrecks in Congress. "But the presentation came at the end of a long meeting," reported two Carter strategists, and "the President-elect somewhat testily concluded that he would have nothing of incrementalism: the system needed a complete overhaul, and he would propose one."[46]

Carter had committed his administration to two domestic initiatives that he cared most about—hospital costs and welfare reform. He made the choices before his inauguration and, in the case of welfare reform, with almost no consultation or analysis. There was no discussion about how difficult the issues would be, how they would affect other domestic initiatives—such as health insurance—the politics of actually winning, or the consequences of losing. What soon became clear, as Bert Carp told us, was that Congress would not have the bandwidth to process these major reforms alongside other programs. And by the time the administration finally got around to health insurance, it was "bruised by the lack of success in doing welfare reform." By then, Carter was "out of money and credibility."[47] Arguably, national health insurance died even before Carter took the oath of office, as a result of rushed transition decisions, when his inexperienced team had not begun to fathom the challenges that awaited them. Later, we will see how decisions made during the transition of another southern Democratic governor, Bill Clinton, would reverberate through his effort to win health reform in the 1990s.

When Carter sent his Hospital Cost Containment bill to the Hill on April 25, 1977, the *New York Times* summed up the administration's mindset: "White House aides have stressed lately that Mr. Carter's paramount domestic goal is balancing the budget by 1981. This might be all but impossible if national health insurance ... were enacted." The decision Carter himself had made in January was now in the public eye: "Welfare reform [has] supplanted national health insurance as the Carter Administration's main social innovation."[48]

Carter' first months in office illustrated enduring themes for presidential politics generally and health reform in particular. First, the crucial question for every candidate: what's the issue in his or her gut? In the hurly-burly of capital politics, a new administration only gets to lay a few issues on the agenda. Carter seized on the things he cared most about. His choices were a fateful signal that keen Washington observers instantly understood—better even than Carter himself. Second, the importance of the transition: Carter sealed the future of other programs—and especially national health insurance—when he put it aside during the heady, politically insulated days between his election and inauguration. Third, the importance of understanding the great political machine: this southern engineer made decisions about what to try—and what, essentially, to cast aside—when he had no Washington experience, no feel for the difficult congressional process, and almost no one

in his inner circle who understood the long, formidable political consequences of the decisions he was making.

## The Coalition Strains

When Carter put aside national health insurance, he left a gaping hole
in his left flank. The attack came fast. Senator Edward Kennedy fired
the first shot in May 1977, five months after Carter's inauguration, at
a UAW convention in Los Angeles: "The American people should not
tolerate delay on health by Congress simply because other reforms are
already lined up bumper to bumper."[49]

Senator Kennedy's remarks set off a lively debate within the administration. Kennedy and the labor leaders wanted to meet with Carter,
remind him of his campaign commitment, and extract a pledge that he
would promptly introduce a national health insurance proposal. Most
domestic policy staff did not even want to meet, but that would have
been a declaration of war. And national health insurance *was*, after all,
in the Book of Promises. On June 16, Carter met with Kennedy and
Douglas Fraser, the president of the UAW, and reassured them of his
commitment to the cause. No one followed up, and the issue slipped
from sight.

On August 1, Peter Bourne, a strong insurance advocate in the
administration, sounded an alarm in a memo to Hamilton Jordan, the
president's most trusted aide:

> I want to raise again my concern about the progress or lack of it in the
> area of National Health Insurance.... At the present rate I am very pessimis-
> tic about our ability to have a comprehensive package on the hill by early
> next year as we had promised [in the June meeting with Kennedy].... The
> President not only talked repeatedly during the campaign about National
> Health Insurance as his top domestic priority, he also said specifically that
> he would submit comprehensive legislation during his first year in office.... I
> believe that if we give this issue adequate attention now we can avoid being
> embarrassed, but it is essential that we move quickly. What is necessary is a
> tighter direct control from the White House, with someone who can devote
> a substantial part of their time to staying on top of the work that is being
> done in HEW.... I do not want to be an alarmist, but I see terrible problems
> looming down the road that I feel can be avoided.[50]

White House aides were beginning to chafe over Joseph Califano's
power under Carter's Cabinet government regime. Califano was preoccupied with welfare and hospital cost containment, yet as secretary

of HEW he controlled national health insurance and—in their view—rudely cut the president's immediate advisors out of the issue. The White House, reflecting the president's ambivalence, was itself divided over this campaign promise. Carter's economic advisors—James McIntyre (head of the Office of Management and Budget), Michael Blumenthal (secretary of the treasury), and Charles Schulz (chairman of the Council of Economic Advisers)—were uniformly aghast at the idea of NHI; as always, the dismal scientists saw a budget-busting, inflation-fanning proposal that would do little to improve American health care. Peter Bourne fiercely supported the reform. Domestic policy advisors Stuart Eizenstat and Joe Onek hovered somewhere in the middle.

Politics exacerbated the stalemate. In November 1977, Califano sent the president a somber warning: "To enact national health insurance will not only require the sensitive drafting of an imaginative and sound proposal with meticulous attention to detail, but also a sustained commitment to a massive political effort—*probably extending over several Congressional sessions.*" Califano then spelled out what he meant by sustained commitment: "You will need to draw on all the resources of your own skilled advisers and staff in orchestrating this initiative. The timing of NHI will need to be carefully considered in light of the schedule of your other legislative programs."[51]

Those other legislative programs were in trouble. By the fall of 1977, Carter was acquiring the reputation of a naive small-timer flailing in the big leagues. In a statement of the emerging Beltway consensus, *Washington Post* reporter Robert Kaiser commented on an October 1977 presidential press conference: "An angry and defensive Jimmy Carter faced the press yesterday to revive his dismembered energy bill, the centerpiece of an embattled political program that has suffered this year as much or more than Carter's declining standing in the polls." The administration had burned through a fifth of its first term, continued Kaiser, and "the President is still looking for a major accomplishment. Thus far, his has been a presidency of initiatives—lots of them—but not results."[52] The last thing Carter needed was another ambitious long shot.

Internally, administration members talked about pushing national health insurance off until 1979, after the midterm elections. Kennedy and labor, however, would have none of that. They lobbed another warning at the administration, this one through *New York Times* columnist Tom Wicker: "The Carter Administration's apparent intention not to send national health insurance legislation in 1978," he wrote, "could mean waiting for years to come." Wicker hinted that the delay might result in the unions throwing their support behind Kennedy for the 1980 election. Here were the first intimations of a major break within the Democratic party over national health insurance.[53]

While the Democratic left pushed for action, center-right Democrats pushed back. Representative Al Ullman snapped, "If Carter sends an NHI bill up here, it will destroy his presidency because it seems so counter to his fight on inflation.... You tell the president that I will have to publicly call the act of submitting a proposal to congress this year a major disaster." And Dan Rostenkowski bluntly described the bottom line: "Where are you going to get the dollars?"[54]

Over the next year, the administration scrambled to manage its disintegrating coalition. The president and his staff kept meeting with Senator Kennedy and labor leaders. In these private meetings Carter would generally reaffirm his commitment to fulfill his campaign promise and would dispatch aides to work with the Kennedy group on a national health insurance proposal. The machinery would crank up briefly, and the process would generate a new round of lengthy, well-crafted policy analyses that dissected the technical, financial, and administrative options for comprehensive health care coverage. Legions of smart advisors kept their bosses' inboxes full. And of course Carter diligently drained his to the last memo.

For example, a flurry of activity followed a meeting between Carter and Kennedy on April 6, 1978. The president promised again to introduce legislation before the end of the year. Kennedy went away pleased, although Carter, acting on the advice of aides, rebuffed the senator's proposal to set up a joint White House–Kennedy working group on NHI.

Within weeks, Peter Bourne was wringing his hands again over the lack of action. "One consideration overrides all others on this issue," he wrote in another memo to Ham Jordan. *"[T]he President has been irrevocably committed to National Health Insurance since early in the campaign and is committed to sending legislation to the Hill this year."* He tried the usual warning: any faltering now will hurt the president. But Bourne knew that he was fighting an uphill battle. "There is a lack of commitment to National Health Insurance within the Administration.... We need to get everyone on board." And that included, first and foremost, the skeptic-in-chief. "The President has not made a speech on health since he assumed office."[55]

The administration faced a series of tough choices: go with a narrow plan, or a broad one? Launch now, or wait until after midterms?

The answers to these questions could not be computed on an engineer's slide rule; every choice would infuriate someone important. A targeted plan such as the one that Carter himself had commended in Senator Long's preinaugural memo might provide all Americans catastrophic coverage and expand insurance for the poor, but for the Democratic left this half-measure was a sellout, a repudiation of Democratic faith. The left pursued the old dream: guarantee every American health insurance. Kennedy wanted the administration to stop dragging its feet, put a plan on the record before the 1978 election—and let the voters choose. This idea, in turn, exasperated everyone else. The Council of Economic Advisors and the Office of Management and Budget, reported Eizenstat, feared "that the announcement of *any* NHI initiative—broad or targeted—could discredit our current efforts to combat inflation and to construct a credible, coherent economic policy. In this respect they may very well be correct." Moreover, Eizenstat thought that most congressional leaders sided with the economists: "[T]hey fear our proposal may run counter to the anti-inflation, anti-regulation mood of the electorate."[56] Meanwhile, over at HEW, Califano favored a go-slow compromise: float a set of principles in August 1978—in time for the November election—and craft a full plan in February 1979.

Eizenstat agreed: principles in the summer of 1978, full plan the following year. "Let Kennedy hold hearings on our principles but do *not* send a detailed plan up until immediately after the elections," he advised the president. The chief domestic aide went straight to the heart of the matter. "It is one thing to honor a commitment. It is quite another to have the UAW and Kennedy dictate the date on which you send this proposal up. As President and head of the Democratic Party you have the right to help Democrats get elected.... It is folly to make them bite the bullet in this conservative climate just before the election."[57] On June 1, Carter signed off on Eizenstat's suggestion.

Eizenstat and Carter ducked the more fundamental issue: what should the plan look like? In fact, the entire White House debate had a strange quality that marks the sad state of the Democratic party. To Carter and most of his aides, this was not a program they believed in— some were appalled by the whole idea. Rather, this was a defining issue for one wing of a party they were trying to hold together. For Truman, Kennedy, or Johnson, extending health insurance was the unfinished task of the beloved New Deal. By the late 1970s, a band of Democrats still kept the faith. Others thought it an atavistic entitlement that no longer spoke to national needs and problems. For the apostates, the

issues were about managing the left and maintaining power. All political eras eventually run down. The New Deal Coalition was cracking
up—and the liberal health care dream was one of the major issues.

   In fact, the administration and partners across the Democratic spectrum were about to get swamped by the next great political wave. On
June 6, 1978, California voted for "Proposition 13," which sharply
limited property taxes. The great Republican tax rebellion had begun.
The vote, said Joseph Califano, fell like "a bombshell" on Washington,
D.C. The most powerful populist movement of the last quarter of the
century—the force that would give the Republican party its fire and pro-
pel it into the majority—had crashed onto American politics. Everyone
immediately knew that this was big. President Jimmy Carter—immersed
in policy details, full of dry, good government reforms, presiding over a
broken coalition—had no answer for the hot, antitax, antigovernment,
anti-Democrat tide rolling in from the west.[58]

## Carter's Choice

Carter had to decide. He couldn't put Kennedy off indefinitely. In June
1978 he focused on the issue, arguably for the first time since his late-
night editing session during the election campaign two years earlier. By
now, both the economy and the administration's faltering public image
severely restricted his freedom of action—Carter's approval ratings had
fallen into the dark territory below 40 percent, a thirty-percent decline
during his first year-and-a-half. An Oval Office meeting between Carter
and his most senior aides on June 15 vividly captured Jimmy Carter's
approach.

   Vice President Walter Mondale, the liberal stalwart, began with
a gloomy assessment of the political climate. "The national mood,"
Mondale said, "couldn't be worse. Inflation and taxes are on everyone's
mind. Proposition 13 is a national fever." How, Mondale wondered,
could they announce a health insurance program that would cost a minimum of $30 billion in new federal spending? They had to be cautious
and buy as much time as possible.

   Carter then chimed in—in high-efficiency expert mode—and
said that they had to "spell out inflationary aspects of the present
situation and laws ... Delineate those things that are truly cost effective ... cost containment [should] be the *major emphasis* ... the need
for cost constraints ... How can we make the present system more
*efficient?* ... what aspects of the new program would *cost more but*

*be very cost-beneficial* ... we can't proceed with the high cost items
at present."

Eizenstat suggested phasing in a plan and tying each new piece to a
set of cost triggers. If expenditures got too high in one phase, the next
part of the NHI proposal would be delayed or cancelled. "Kennedy
would *probably accept*" this, Eizenstat speculated wanly. Kennedy, they
soon discovered, would accept no such thing.

Carter then plunged deep into the details. He insisted that they
"face the controversial issues"—such as patient cost-sharing (the issue
on which labor had broken with Kennedy during the negotiations
with Mills and Nixon). This, continued Carter, "must be [a] federal-
state-private plan.... I'm personally inclined to think we need *private
insurers* ... increased use of HMOs ... also make PSROs work." Was
there another president who had parsed the details finely enough to
know what a PSRO was (a Professional Standard Review Organization, or a physician panel designed to review Medicare cases for
excessive cost and poor quality)? Finally, Carter repeated the decision
he had made the previous week: "State comprehensive principles but
*flatly delineate* that we are *not proposing* the comprehensive features
at present."[59]

Carter had studied the health care issue—absorbing all those memos
that were flying around the White House—and mastered its intricacies at an astonishing level of detail. Only one other modern president,
Bill Clinton, would understand the health system as thoroughly. Carter
thought he knew the right, proper, and courageous thing to do: fix the
health care system, purge the waste, reengineer the entire enterprise.
All his instincts, reinforced by the national mood and the precarious
standing of his administration, argued against introducing a comprehensive health care plan now—or perhaps ever. And if and when the
administration produced a plan, it would feature all the mechanisms
of efficiency—cost-sharing by consumers, competing HMOs, quality-
assurance programs, and a strong role for private insurers. He knew,
despite Eizenstat's wishful thinking, that all this would send the left
straight up the wall. But Carter also knew—or believed he knew—what
the United States needed. No matter whether that forced a confrontation with Kennedy—it was a price which he was willing to pay. Carter
would likely have been mortified to know that his health care analysis
precisely mimicked that of the predecessor he most spurned: Richard
M. Nixon. Both were brilliant analysts; each was also, in his own way,
a flawed political leader.

## GOING NOWHERE: THE CARTER ADMINISTRATION PLAN

With the course now charted, the administration's policy development process began to grind out the principles Carter had called for. Aides crafted memos, and Carter read each one, adding comments and edits. The memo traffic grew so voluminous, the meetings so frequent, the small points so detailed, that Carter scribbled plaintively at the bottom of one of his briefing documents: "We seem to do this every week!"[60]

Carter kept a tight health care focus: He wanted system reform—preventive medicine, cost containment, efficiency. His administration would not emphasize increased coverage and would never promise luxurious health care. Next to one draft principle that promised all Americans "high quality care," he scribbled, "We can't promise everyone first class private hospital rooms, resort rest periods, private duty nurses, etc. Change to 'adequate' or some equivalent descriptive word."[61] Finally, he sought to distance himself from the issue. "I'm not looking for a lot of publicity," he wrote on a July 22, 1978, memo from Eizenstat. The principles would be released by Califano, not the White House. Carter would not be seen touting this tired old liberal ideal.[62] He was getting that monkey off his back.

### Built-in Self-Destruct Buttons: The Party Cracks Up

The ghost haunting the White House process was Ted Kennedy and his liberal faction. The differences with the president finally erupted into a full break on July 28, 1978. In the morning, Carter and Kennedy met with their staffs to discuss the administration's final draft statement of principles. The argument turned on Carter's unwillingness to introduce a comprehensive plan. Instead, the administration stuck with Eizenstat's triggers, each phase contingent on the financial consequences of the previous one. Kennedy may have been clinging to a lost cause, as the Carter team insisted. But he knew how things worked on the Hill and insisted on "a commitment to a single bill that would enable Congress to deal with the program as a whole, rather than allow it to be divided into separate bills and conquered by the special interest groups." Kennedy forcefully rejected the idea of a proposal that contained "built-in self destruct buttons, to halt the program in its tracks if things go wrong." At a press conference later in the day, he concluded by throwing down the gauntlet: "We intend to proceed now, on our own—with the Administration if possible, without the Administration if necessary—to develop a program of national health insurance that will meet the urgent and basic needs of the people of America."[63]

The meeting went beyond policy difference and crystallized the growing personal animosity between Carter and Kennedy. Senator Kennedy rejected the Carter approach and explicitly warned the White House of a break over national health insurance. For his part, Carter felt betrayed by—what else?—the process. "We shook hands and parted in fairly good spirits," wrote Carter. Kennedy had asked for a few hours to study the statement of principles, continued Carter, and the White House, in turn, had promised not to release the document until Kennedy had time to react. Kennedy then went back to the hill and "held a press conference at three o'clock that afternoon to condemn our plan and to announce that he and his associates would oppose it. There was no prospect of congressional support for his own program, which was announced the following year. It was a tragedy that his unwillingness to cooperate helped spell the doom of any far-reaching reforms of the health-care system."[64]

From Carter's perspective, Kennedy's behavior meant "any hope of cooperation was gone." From Kennedy's side, the administration's plan—as he had clearly told the White House staff—violated the senator's most fervently held principles and Carter's previous commitments. Whatever the truth about who was supposed to say what to the press when, each side thought the other unprincipled and politically naive. The personal animosity and health policy differences exposed a still deeper rift. The conservative, southern Democratic wing of the Democratic Party could not find common ground with the old-line, liberal wing based in the Northeast. Neither would muster a compelling political narrative in the years ahead. The split came to the surface over national health insurance. And now that it was out in the open, speculation grew that Kennedy would challenge Carter for the Democratic nomination and run on the issue in 1980.

Just as the break developed, Jimmy Carter won his most impressive victory. Against the advice of his aides, President Carter invited Prime Minister Menachem Begin of Israel and President Anwar el-Sadat of Egypt to Camp David to revive the stalled peace talks between their countries. It was, as Carter's foreign policy experts pointed out, an enormously risky undertaking. But in a thirteen-day marathon negotiation session, Carter's personal tenacity, missionary zeal, and attention to detail were all on magnificent display. He played a role few presidents have had the courage to take on: personal mediator between heads of state divided by deep mistrust and bloody conflicts. And he succeeded. On September 17, 1978, Israel and Egypt signed a peace treaty. It was the high point of the Carter presidency and the cornerstone of Carter's legacy.

The foreign policy success—which briefly bumped Carter's approval rating above 50 percent—did nothing to quell the rebellion in the Democratic ranks. On December 9, the Democrats held a midterm party convention in Memphis, Tennessee. The highlight of the meeting was a panel on health care featuring Ted Kennedy, Joe Califano, and Stuart Eizenstat. The moderator was a thirty-two-year-old named Bill Clinton who had been elected governor of Arkansas the previous month. Over a thousand delegates packed the hall. Tall, vigorous, and handsome, with a full head of dark hair just turning grey, the Massachusetts senator evoked the memories of Kennedys past. His booming voice filled the room as he spoke his passion: "I want every delegate to this convention to understand that as long as I have a vote in the United States Senate it will be for the Democratic Party platform plan that will provide decent health care across this country, North and South, East and West, for all Americans as a matter of right and not of privilege."

The crowd surged to its feet, many wearing blue-and-white Kennedy buttons that Kennedy's advance team had quietly distributed beforehand. Eizenstat and Califano sat impassively. Kennedy pressed on in that famous Boston accent, evoking memories of the martyred brother who had sailed the waters of New England and the war-torn South Seas: "The hopes and dreams of millions of citizens are riding on our leadership. Sometimes a party must sail against the wind. We cannot afford to drift or lie at anchor. We cannot heed the call of those who say it is time to furl the sail." Kennedy had, as the media reported, "lit up" the lackluster convention of a becalmed party.[65] Bill Clinton, just starting out in politics, could not help but notice the power of the health care issue and its deep roots in the Democratic pantheon of noble causes and revered heroes.

### No Child Ever Benefited from a Rigid Commitment to Principle

The definitive split with Kennedy seemed to liberate the White House. Carter did not want NHI to go away completely. He had to fulfill his campaign pledge, and he had to cover his left wing if Kennedy did indeed challenge him in the primaries. But the White House was now free to find its own path without endless negotiations.

Naturally, Carter took a middle course. Responding to an options memo on January 18, 1979, he decided to introduce a catastrophic insurance plan together with Medicaid and Medicare reforms (back to what he had picked up from Senator Long during the transition). This would be his down payment on national health insurance. He would also introduce a more comprehensive plan, largely for discussion purposes. However, he was holding his nose when he even considered anything ambitious: "The economic and budgetary climate is not conducive to introduction of a multi-billion dollar spending initiative," he wrote in the margin of the memo.[66]

Five days later, the 1979 State of the Union address vividly illustrated what was on Carter's mind. He put special emphasis on health care policy, but on cost control—not coverage: "A responsible budget is not our only weapon to control inflation. We must act now to protect all Americans from health care costs that are rising $1 million per hour, 24 hours a day, doubling every 5 years. We must take control of the largest contributor to that inflation—skyrocketing hospital costs."

Carter touted the same hospital cost containment bill that the administration had unsuccessfully introduced the previous year. He counted up the promised savings—$60 billion over five years—and, by Jimmy Carter standards, grew passionate. "The American people have waited long enough. This year we must act on hospital cost containment." In contrast, insurance got little more than a State of the Union squeak: "This year, we will take our first steps to develop a national health plan."[67]

The Carter administration may have been freer after its break with Kennedy, but it still wasn't fleet. It took another five months for the administration to finalize its health insurance plan. A battle erupted between Califano's HEW, which was now eager to push a comprehensive plan, and White House advisors—especially the economists—who wanted to propose only catastrophic coverage. In February 1979, the White House staff finally brought HEW into line. Eizenstat wrote Carter: "HEW and the [Executive Office of the President] are now in general agreement that the Administration should submit first phase legislation consisting primarily of Medicaid/Medicare reform and enhanced catastrophic coverage." Secretary Califano felt that Carter could not abandon his commitment entirely without outraging the liberals, but Eizenstat suggested a minimalist approach to the problem: "You should lay out ... in general terms your vision of what future phases would look like," he told Carter, "while sending up legislation only on phase I." And, finally, at this late date, the sudden realization came that time was running out: "It is clear that, if we are to influence the Finance Committee proceedings, we must develop an Administration proposal within the next month." The bureaucratic bottom line: produce yet another options memorandum by March 16. Needless to say, the administration would not meet the deadline.[68]

Meanwhile, the political environment for Jimmy Carter grew parlous. By early 1979, the glow from his Camp David Peace Accords had completely faded and the administration tumbled back down in public opinion. Carter fell back to 40 percent approval in January, to the 30s by May, and down into the 20s in June. The economy was flagging and inflation surging—the deadly combination known as "stagflation." Fundamentalist Shiites had swept to power in Iran and were vilifying America as "the great Satan." A sharp rise in oil prices created gas shortages, exacerbating the high inflation rate and the weak economy.

Inside the White House, the health policy process ground on. On June 12, 1979, Carter finally announced his administration's National Health Plan. The timing, just seventeen months before the 1980 presidential election, was reminiscent of Republican administrations, which characteristically address health care coverage issues late in presidential terms—as elections loom. The content of the long-range Carter plan also came from a Republican playbook. Carter proposed a variation on the Nixon plan: it provided all Americans with catastrophic insurance, required employers to cover workers, and introduced a new federal insurance program for the elderly, the poor, and the uninsured (subsuming Medicaid and Medicare). The plan included a raft of system reforms—from promoting HMOs to constraining hospital and physician fees. When Carter introduced his initiative, he remained every bit as guarded as he had been before the Student National Medical Association three years earlier. Carter double-underlined the words he intended to stress (here marked in italics):

Today I am proposing to the Congress a National Health Plan. This *major initiative* will meet the *most urgent* needs of the American people in a *practical, cost-efficient and fiscally responsible* manner. It will improve health care for *millions* of Americans, and protect our people against the overwhelming financial burdens of major illness.... The idea of "all or nothing" has been pursued for almost three decades. But I must say in all candor that no child of poverty, no elderly American, no middle class family has yet benefited from a rigid and unswerving commitment to this principle.[69]

Despite talk of a double-underlined *major initiative,* the administration entered negotiations with Senator Long and the Senate Finance Committee to enact its more modest Phase I: catastrophic insurance and Medicaid reform. James Mongan, a Califano aide—before that a staff member for the Senate Finance Committee—had moved to the White House and led the discussions. For once, the administration had some congressional savvy on its team. A brief flurry of excitement gusted up when the White House thought it might win this insurance expansion out of the Congress. The *Washington Post* speculated that President Carter and Senator Long are "moving quickly toward agreement on a national health insurance plan that would freeze out Sen. Edward Kennedy's more ambitious proposal."[70]

President Carter, for his part, seemed to relish the split with Kennedy, which his staff was spinning as evidence of the same southern conservative grit that had gotten him elected in the first place. At a White House dinner, a guest asked the president about Kennedy's widely anticipated run for president. "If Kennedy runs, I'll whip his ass," Carter replied, and the White House press office was delighted to see the remark reported in *Time Magazine.* Kennedy just guffawed and fired back: "I always knew the White House would stand behind me, but I didn't realize how close they would be." The jousting continued when Califano told the press that Kennedy's comprehensive plan didn't have "an elephant's chance of slipping through a keyhole." Kennedy responded by sending him "an assemblage of small, fuzzy, pink elephants easily slipping through a keyhole in white poster board paper. The scrawled note at the bottom: 'Joe, it looks to me like it fits.'"[71]

In fact, even Carter's stripped down Phase I health care proposal was going nowhere. The Senate Finance Committee toyed with the package, but the initiative stalled. By May 1980, Mongan gave up. The only hope, he wrote Eizenstat, was to focus on "getting some cost containment and CHAP [children's coverage] out of the Finance Committee."[72]

What killed the late effort at health reform? Four factors: all emblematic of the Carter White House, its president, and his attitude toward comprehensive health insurance.

First was a continuing political decline that spilled over into health care both directly and indirectly. In July 1979, Carter tried to face up to his deteriorating political standing. He retreated to Camp David, spent ten days listening to Americans from all walks of life, and then emerged to deliver his most famous speech. The American energy crisis had deep roots in Washington, he said, which had become "an island," "an isolated world," shut off from the American people. "The gap between our citizens and our government has never been so wide," continued Carter. A crisis of confidence was striking "at the very heart, soul and spirit of our national will ... and is threatening to destroy ... America." The talk, later dubbed the "malaise" address, proposed bold initiatives to reduce the nation's dependence on foreign oil—the problem, thought Carter, at the heart of American economic trouble.[73] The speech was well received, but Carter, scrambling to get control, fired four (and by some counts, five) Cabinet members. The move was so abrupt and unexpected that the Washington buzz turned to speculation about the president's emotional stability. Firing Brock Adams (secretary of transportation) and Joe Califano—both widely respected liberals—seemed like cold, mean politics. Moreover, Califano was an experienced, well-connected health specialist; his replacement, Patricia Harris (then secretary of Housing and Urban Development) was new to the issues and networks. Finally, by naming his old assistant, Hamilton Jordan, chief of staff, Carter made it look as if the Georgia gang was circling its wagons. The administration appeared to be shrinking as national problems mounted.[74]

Second, what Jimmy Carter really cared about was always cost containment—good policy, bad politics. Hospital cost containment was a measure only a righteous engineer could relish. It took money out of the health system and gave nothing back in the short term. It was tough medicine, but then, that was the kind of medicine Carter had grown up taking. Kennedy argued that the best way to get cost restraints was to build them into a comprehensive coverage. That way you offered the public some financial relief even as you crimped their revered local hospitals. The administration wanted none of that; hospital cost legislation was, in its view, a necessary precursor to any coverage expansion. You had to eat your spinach before you got your dessert. Carter threw himself into the hospital cost containment effort in 1979, lobbying members of Congress in person and in writing. And despite long odds, he shocked both industry and pundits by winning the bill in the Senate. But the hospital industry descended in force on the House, and the legislation went down again on November 15, 1979. At bottom, Jimmy Carter nurtured a lonely passion. Representative Bill Gradison (R-OH) summed up the national reaction: "I have not received a single letter on [the bill]." The effort was another blow to Carter's fragile political standing and lessened his leverage on the comprehensive health reform he cared about far less.[75]

Third, the fight with Kennedy hobbled the health care reform. Kennedy announced on November 7, 1979, that he would challenge Carter for the Democratic presidential nomination. Carter eventually beat him easily; the Georgia Democrat had the advantage of incumbency and was in fact a formidable campaign strategist. Kennedy turned out to be a weaker candidate than many of his supporters had hoped, faltering badly at the start of the campaign. But the left wing of the party—liberals in Congress, labor, consumer groups—formed the main constituency for health reform. The liberal grassroots were not powerful enough to win insurance expansions, but their defection left no one to support the administration's health plans. To put it bluntly, no one else cared. As the liberal tide ran out, the Democratic party was hopelessly split between a left wing that seemed out of step with the times and a conservative wing that could frame no popular alternative to the rising red-meat conservatives in the other party. A divided party, uncertain of its way, was not likely to win such a big, difficult reform under any circumstance.

Fourth, and perhaps most fundamental, Jimmy Carter did not care enough about expanding health insurance coverage to take any major risks for it. Once his administration produced its much-delayed reform proposal, he hardly invested any energy in the issue. Carter was not averse to risk-taking—indeed, he repeatedly pressed difficult, controversial, proposals on a balky Congress and a skeptical public: welfare reform, energy policy, and the Camp David talks between Israel and Egypt were all risky propositions that many chief executives would have thought twice about taking. Carter's health insurance problem was not timidity. It went deeper: he did not believe in it. In part, this was because his attention was fixed on inflation (which was very high) and budget deficits (which seemed high at the time), but it also seemed to reflect—as his scribbles on so many memos testified—an ambivalence about the value of medical care itself.

## Policy Dysfunction

Kennedy and his supporters saw a deep human need for protection against the cost of illness. Carter saw a broken, inefficient health care system to be reengineered. He saw waste and profiteering in hospitals, poorly trained physicians badly distributed across the nation, and patients who refused to make the lifestyle changes that could save them a trip to the hospital. When Carter focused on national health policy, these were the issues that captured his imagination. At his core, he resembled Dwight Eisenhower, the compassionate conservative, more than Harry Truman, the passionate liberal—although it was Truman whom he professed to admire most among U.S. presidents.

Paradoxically, Carter's ambivalence about the coverage issue only led him to lavish disproportionate time and attention on the problem. Jimmy Carter was a detail man from the start, but the endless, anxious wrestle over health insurance became an extreme case of attention to detail and drew the president into long, circular discussions—all to little effect. The result was a late halfway measure that not even the president cared very much about. He was inordinately stubborn about getting the details right, but the ultimate purpose seemed to get lost in his obsession.

The health debates reveal, in the end, a dysfunctional policy process. The administration itself, like the party, was divided. Liberals (such as Bourne) wanted national health insurance; liberal realists (such as Califano) called for a direct but more tough-minded approach; moderates (such as Eizenstat) wanted to split the difference; the economics team hated the entire mess. Carter's high-minded effort to serve as his own chief of staff meant that the tensions and disagreements fell onto his own desk, where he responded not with strong directives but by reviewing long, dense memos and penciling in small edits, questions, corrections, and sermonettes. Carter translated the great debates raging around him into small, smart points on the paper trail.

Where Eisenhower, Johnson, and Nixon sent a broad direction and delegated, Carter—despite his embrace of Cabinet government—took on the arduous task of scrupulously vetting every policy jot. As the process dragged on, Carter came to seem indecisive—which he was—and even duplicitous. It was as though somewhere in the recesses of the president's mind, his willingness to slave over the details—his commitment to getting policy just right—compensated for his hesitancy and delay in fulfilling a campaign pledge he did not believe in.

Why, with all these problems, did Carter squeeze out a comprehensive reform package at all? Four reasons. First, he promised. However reluctantly and equivocally, he had made a pledge, and perhaps more than any other president in the twentieth century, he fiercely hewed to his promises. He really meant it when he kept repeating his famous campaign sound bite: "I'm Jimmy Carter. I'm running for president. I will never lie to you."[76] Second, the liberal base. He could not go into the 1980 reelection campaign without a health care platform. It was the signature issue for many members of his party. Third, Carter was, fundamentally, a compassionate and caring man, who wanted to relieve the suffering of the sick. He wanted to improve the health and welfare of the American people. And finally, he was an engineer. He believed the package he eventually introduced—with its system reforms, its emphasis on prevention, its efforts to control costs, and its careful phasing in of benefits—would help fix the medical system.

## THE LESSONS OF FAILURE

Did it really matter what Carter did or didn't do about health care? After all, he governed during difficult times—the economy racked by inflation and recession, productivity declining, gas lines winding around the block, and radical Islam rising to complicate the geopolitics of oil.

Moreover, as his chief pollster saw from the very start, the liberal era was over, the New Deal vision (and its later variations such as the Fair Deal and the Great Society) was tapped out, and the Democratic party coalition was at the end of its days. Liberal Democrats had not come to terms with their fall from power: they could strike a deal with Nixon—why not with Carter? The southern Democrats, for their part, offered no new vision or direction; they would not even be able to hold their own region and would watch helplessly as the South turned from solid blue to largely red—slowly tipping the country as it changed.

The great imponderable for the Carter administration was whether a nimbler, more charismatic, or more visionary president might have found a way to rethink the Democratic coalition, possibly even in a way that involved health care reform. Or perhaps, as most political scientists believe, the weight of recent social and economic history was simply too heavy, the tide to the right irresistible.

To get any kind of health reform, Carter would have had to manage the issue brilliantly. Instead, his administration illustrates everything that can go wrong—an almost perfect list of presidential *don'ts*. His administration ironically echoes the Johnsonian lessons for successful health reform by violating every one.

> *Move Fast.* Carter was slow to move on an issue that requires
> speed. "So what happened was that Carter basically screwed up
> in the first year and lost his credibility, and never really recovered
> it," summed up White House advisor Ben Heineman. "By the
> time we got around to national health insurance it was a joke."[77]

*Promote Your Vision.* The president never projected the big picture. Had he announced his ideals early and broadcast them decisively, he might have blunted the cries from the left that he had "furled his sails" and retreated on NHI. There is no getting around it: only a forcefully articulated vision generates popular support.

*Develop Popular Support.* Without a vision or an electoral mandate, it is difficult to win big, complicated, contested changes, or to rally a failing, fractured party. Carter's passion for efficiency and reengineering is typical of fading coalitions; failure to agree on substance leads to emphasis on technique. Ferreting out ways to run things more smoothly is fine, but not for the centerpiece of a party's program.

*Manage Congress.* As LBJ put it, "the only way to deal with Congress is continuously, incessantly, and without interruption." In contrast, Carter blithely assumed that he did not need help from the speaker of the House.

*Don't Focus on the Mousetrap.* Perhaps most important, Carter tried to solve political problems with policy solutions. The coalition was collapsing, but he worked assiduously at finding the right fix— morally right, technically efficient—that would solve the problem. Technical fixes do not solve political problems. Leaders who try are often written down as goo-goos (a derogatory shortening of "good government" that has been aimed at political naïfs since the 1880s). Carter was a true-blue goo-goo. The next Democrat to try health reform would also recruit a goo-goo who tried, calamitously, to fix every political problem using technical wizardry.

*Cut through the Process.* Carter let the process eat him alive. He was always reacting—never leading. His health policy development process was technically excellent but lacked political and strategic guidance. He sweated the details for months, even years—forever scribbling in the margins of memos while he shrugged off a leader's real jobs: set out broad strategic goals, manage conflicts, and come to closure.

*Find a Savvy Chief of Staff.* Carter repeated the classic Democratic organizational mistake when he tried to play chief of staff. As a result, there was no one in the White House to referee conflicts, interpret meetings, or implement decisions. Nor did it leave the lines of communication to the president more open, as Carter had hoped. Cabinet members and congressmen complained bitterly that no one returned their phone calls to the White House. Carter's problems offer a sharp warning to Democrats who seem congenitally predisposed to forget: few appointments are as important as chief of staff. Name a savvy one from the start of the administration, or end up bringing one in later to clean up the mess.

Ultimately, Carter wanted to avoid health insurance. He didn't think it was the right policy. He didn't trust the doctors and hospitals who might cash in on it. He didn't trust the nostrums they plied. His ambivalence seems to have been so profound that almost alone among the many entries in his Book of Promises, he tried to cast this one out—or to sneak something through in obscurity. The result was four years of policy paralysis, an unpopular one-term president, and a lost last chance for the beleaguered Democrats to unite and stem the rising Republican tide.

# CHAPTER 8

# Ronald Reagan

*Socialized Medicine and the Working Stiff*

President Ronald Reagan walked out of the Washington Hilton Hotel after delivering a speech to the construction unions two months into his first term. "Not riotously received," Reagan later scribbled in his journal, although the incurable optimist could not stop himself from adding, "still, it was successful." As he neared his limousine, a reporter began to shout a question about the Solidarity movement sweeping Poland. The president paused—then a series of pops rang out like fire-crackers. "What the hell's that?" asked the president, turning toward the sound. The Secret Service knew. Agent Jerry Parr grabbed Reagan, folded him roughly at the waist, shoved him into the car, and, as the president sprawled on the floor, leaped on top of him and covered his body. Agent Tim McCarthy, who had opened the car door, now stepped in front of the gunman, spread his arms wide, and took a bullet to the chest while the president's limousine spun away.

"Jerry, get off," barked Reagan. "I think you've broken one of my ribs." The president sat up in searing pain. Perhaps the broken rib had punctured his lung, he thought. Agent Parr ran his hands over the president, found nothing, and radioed the driver. "Rawhide's okay, let's head for the Crown." The car sped the president toward the White House. But President Reagan couldn't breathe. He took a napkin from lunch out of his pocket and coughed up thick blood, full of frothy bubbles. "I think I cut something inside my mouth," he said. Agent Parr took one look and told the driver to head for George Washington University Hospital. He called the hospital and told the skeptical duty nurse, "No ma'am, this is no drill."

The napkin and Parr's handkerchief were sopping with blood by the time they pulled up at the emergency room. Reagan—always minding his entrance—stepped out of the car, pulled up the pants of his brand new blue pinstripe suit, buttoned the jacket and walked toward the doors. He struggled to breathe, started to collapse. Two agents, a nurse, and doctors grabbed him, lifted him up, and ran him into emergency room bay 5. Chaos. The president's lungs were filling with blood, his blood pressure falling, his heartbeat weakening. He was going into shock, drifting in and out of consciousness. Reagan was going to die unless they acted fast.

But the trauma team could not find the source of the problem. They slid a tube down his throat, carefully examined his body, X-rayed him, X-rayed him again—and finally found the little, bloodless entrance wound under the arm. The bullet had ricocheted off the car, struck Reagan in the side, hit a rib, flipped, ripped through the lung, and lodged an inch from his heart. They wheeled Reagan into the operating room, put him under, and, after several tries, got the bullet out. The bullet, known as a Devastator, was meant to explode inside its victim, but the assassin, John Hinkley Jr., had fired this one from a cheap gun with a short barrel, and it had not reached the required speed.

Ronald Reagan handled the fear and pain the same way he handled everything else—with cheerful quips and tall tales. To Doctor Giordano: "I sure hope you're a Republican." (The liberal Democrat responded, "Today, Mr. President, we're all Republicans.") To his wife, he recycled Jack Dempsey's crack about losing the heavyweight boxing title: "Honey, I forgot to duck." And to a nurse, he resorted to W. C. Fields: "All in all, I'd rather be in Philadelphia." Ronald Reagan had a quotation or a story for every occasion. He recycled them shamelessly, and listeners could never be sure whether they came from his memories, the movies, old Irish yarns, or last month's *Reader's Digest*. The stories would exasperate both friends and foes looking for a serious policy debate—but now, with the president seriously wounded, they seemed nothing less than heroic.[1]

After a two-week hospital stay, the president emerged from the hospital wearing a red cardigan and a big smile. It was, his team soon learned, an act that he could only sustain in short bursts. For weeks the White House hid the president's incapacity—the public heard about the quips, saw the photo ops, and learned nothing about the slow recovery. Whispers about a caretaker presidency dissipated as Reagan recovered—but later investigations raised the age-old question about presidential illness: what should the public know?[2]

A month after the shooting, on April 28, 1981, a recovering Ronald Reagan stood before a joint session of Congress and a national television audience ready to launch his Revolution. After an ecstatic ovation, the president "digressed" for a signature flourish—defending the United States against the shadow of criticism. The great tide of messages, flowers, prayers, letters, and love that overwhelmed him and Nancy had routed "those few voices ... saying that what happened was evidence that ours is a sick society." A crazy boy with a devastator bullet inspired by a violent movie (Martin Scorsese's *Taxi Driver*) was no match for the "millions of compassionate Americans and their children, from college age to kindergarten," linked through their patriotic goodwill to brave astronauts, fearless police officers, and heroic Secret Service agents—a Reagan variation of Lincoln's "mystic chords of memory." And always the Reagan take-home: sick societies "don't make so many people like us proud to be Americans."[3]

Then, Reagan turned smoothly to his tax and spending cuts. Now, the old actor grew gimlet-eyed and touted up the house. During the third standing ovation, he wrote in his diary, "about 40 Democrats stood and applauded.... It took a lot of courage for them to do that.... Except for that, all the applause came from the Repub. Side. The Demos. Just sit on their hands."[4]

Here is Ronald Reagan, the visionary who changed the course of American history. He won four elections in his political career—all by landslides. He routed the New Deal's social gospel vision, founded a new Republican era, and stands alongside Roosevelt and Johnson as a modern presidential giant.

Here, at the same time, is a man who did not seem to have a clue about the details. "An amiable dunce," said Clark Clifford famously. "[S]leepwalking through history," added biographer Haynes Johnson. A cheerful lightweight, in OMB director David Stockman's view, who had no business proposing the ultimately disastrous economic program that he never understood and that would triple the federal debt; Stockman, the genius behind Reagan's numbers, offered perhaps the most accurate misjudgment: "His conservative vision was only a vision.... He had no concrete programs." Bud McFarland, Reagan's national security advisor, summed it all up: "He knows so little and accomplishes so much." Men such as David Stockman, Bud McFarland, and Don Regan (the second chief of staff)—policy mavens with their eyes fixed on programs, numbers, and detail—left this White House shaking their heads in frustration. In contrast, political visionaries thrilled to Reagan's big picture. "Those who found him 'vague' and impossible to pin down," comments John Diggins, "were looking for his persona"—or his policies—"when they should have been looking at his politics." Or his dreamy vision of America.[5]

## THE REAGAN VISION

It all came back to the vision—his greatest triumph and his most stubborn limitation. The Reagan vision revolved around three fixed verities—all on display in his April 28 address to Congress.

### Fixed Verities

First came a soaring patriotism. Anything that moved Ronald Reagan— a choir, a space launch, an encouraging letter, an old movie—inspired the same thought: "You have to feel good about our country."[6] His America was rooted in nostalgia, inflected with God's benevolence, and bursting with freedom and plenty. In his second autobiography, Reagan imagines taking Mikhail Gorbachev for a helicopter ride to the real America. "Up from the air I would have pointed out an ordinary factory, and showed him its parking lot filled with workers' cars," daydreams Reagan, "[and] then we'd fly over a residential neighborhood and I'd tell him that's where those workers lived—in homes with lawns and backyards, perhaps with a second car or a boat in the driveway.... They not only live there," continued Reagan in his flight of fancy, "they *own* that property." He and Gorbachev land at a random house, knock on the door, and ask the people "how they live and what they think of our system." The homeowners come to the door and talk proudly about individualism and freedom. After hard decades of civil rights, student protests, the Vietnam War, oil shock, and economic malaise, Reagan offered Americans an anodyne celebration of comfort and belonging— of a proud American *us*.[7]

Second: Communism is evil, and we fight for our lives against it. Reagan experienced the Red scare after World War II as an epic struggle for the soul of America. He believed that he had been on the front lines in the battle over Hollywood—a fight, as he saw it, for the very definition of our culture: "I knew from the experience of hand to hand combat that America faced no more insidious or evil threat than communism." He dismissed mutual tolerance. "My theory about the cold war," Reagan told his future national security advisor, Richard Allen, in 1976, "is simple: 'we win, they lose.'" Later—in one of his most famous speeches—he told the national association of evangelicals not to give in to "the demons" and accommodate the Evil Empire.[8]

Reagan's anticommunist impulse ran into a larger Manichean reflex. A simple conflict lurked behind every debate—the good *us* fights a malevolent *them:* patriots versus cynics "who believe ours is a sick society"; honest students versus spoiled protesters; hard-working Americans versus welfare queens; freedom fighters versus dangerous Reds in central America; forty brave Democrats applauding for President Reagan versus glowering liberals playing political games. By raising Republicans to parity with the Democrats (he hosted Democratic converts to the Republican cause in the White House) and wielding his *us* versus *them,* he opened the door to a new era of bare-knuckle party politics. Reagan's rhetoric—with its soaring optimism and gauzy style—softened the clash. The generation of politicians who followed him—repeating "we win, they lose"—never managed that trick.[9]

Finally, Reagan came to Washington pitching a big idea: "Government is not the solution to our problem," as he put it in his first inaugural address, "government is the problem." Roosevelt, Truman, Kennedy, and Johnson had all passionately believed in the power of collective action to raise individual lives; even Nixon had announced, "I am a government man." Not Reagan. Government was no instrument for the common good; on the contrary, it was elitist and tyrannical, a dead weight on the shoulders of the common man. Reagan promised to chop taxes, cut spending, roll back regulations, and shrink the federal government.[10]

Where did health care fit in? The question raises the great puzzle of his administration and illuminates the limits of the Reagan Revolution. Although he entered politics eviscerating socialized medicine during the Medicare debate, President Reagan ended up overruling almost all his advisors and sponsoring the largest expansion of Medicare—in fact, the largest health care entitlement—in almost forty years (from 1966 to 2003). This chapter explains how Ronald Reagan changed, why he expanded Medicare, and what that tells us about the presidency itself.

## The Limits of the Revolution

Ronald Reagan had honed his core beliefs repeating a speech—*The Speech*—for almost a decade. Between 1954 and 1962, he hosted the *General Electric Theater* on Sunday nights; during the week, he visited some of the 139 GE plants to talk about Communism, government, and free enterprise. Late in the 1964 election campaign, a group of conservative businessmen bought national television time and asked Reagan to give The Speech on behalf of Republican candidate Barry Goldwater. That night, a political superstar was born—but the speech, celebrated by conservatives to this day, left President Reagan with his greatest political liability.

The Speech ended with an exuberant attack on Lyndon Johnson's Medicare proposal: "The doctor's fight against socialized medicine is your fight. We can't socialize the doctors without socializing the patients. Recognize that government invasion of public power is eventually an assault upon your own business." Those who refuse to fight alongside the physicians, continued Reagan, just "feed the crocodile." Then the inevitable *us* versus *them:* "If all of this seems like a great deal of trouble, think what's at stake. We are faced with the most evil enemy mankind has known in his long climb from the swamp to the stars. There can be no security anywhere in the free world if there is no fiscal and economic stability within the United States." Reagan insinuated a small slip from Medicare to "the most evil enemy mankind has known in his long climb from the swamp."[11]

Reagan flamboyantly repeated the attack on Medicare. "If this program passes," he warned in a recording he made for the American Medical Association, "behind it will come other federal programs that will invade every area of freedom as we have known it in this country until we wake to find that we have socialism.... You and I are going to spend our sunset years telling our children and our children's children what it was like in America when men were free." He peppered his correspondence with variations on the theme. The bill, he wrote a friend, "serve[s] only as a foot in the door.... To be blunt about it, we can no more have partial socialism than a person can be 'a little bit pregnant.' I have dozens of quotes from socialists ... boasting that [Medicare] is only designed to establish the principle so that socialized medicine can follow." Seventeen years later, running for president, Reagan seemed to be in the same old groove when he assured a supporter: "I am opposed to socialized medicine."[12]

Yet President Reagan tossed aside the old cause rooted in two of his fundamentals—defeating Communism and deflating government—overruled most Cabinet members, White House staff, economic advisors, core constituents, and conservative representatives and championed the largest Medicare expansion in decades. Why?

For starters, those early speeches left Ronald Reagan vulnerable. Medicare (joined by Social Security, which he also criticized in The Speech) was a popular "third rail" of American politics. Democrats constantly hit Reagan on Medicare; Jimmy Carter (in the 1980 election) and Walter Mondale (1984) painted Reagan as a threat to the program. Each election found him reassuring older voters that he meant their entitlements no harm. ("There you go again," he responded in both campaigns, suggesting that harsh cuts were the furthest things from his mind.) When the Reagan administration faced its gravest crisis—as the polls plummeted and Ronald Reagan caught the blues—the president seized on Medicare expansion for relief.

Budget director David Stockman illuminates a more subtle explanation. A real conservative revolution—a genuinely small government—required "draconian reductions ... that would "hurt millions of people in the short run." Only an "iron chancellor" could make such "wrenching changes" stick. "Reagan had no business trying to make a revolution," groused Stockman, "because it wasn't in his bones." Instead, he was "gentle and sentimental." The Reagan revolution failed, concluded Stockman, because hard-luck stories melted his ideology (Reagan's staff assiduously culled hard-luck stories from his mail to stop him from sending small checks to strangers). Somewhere along his political path, Reagan began to talk more about catastrophic medical expenses and less about socialized medicine. By the time he reached the White House, his letters and speeches were repeating the newfound concern.[13]

In short, both Democratic attacks and Reagan's own sentimentality limited the revolution. To be sure, he would turn national politics hard to the right; but he never came close to delivering the small-government idyll that revolutionaries such as Stockman dreamed of. Health care offers perhaps the sharpest contrast between rhetorical record and administration programs. Like every other president,

Reagan could not escape the call for health care coverage; the real surprise is that he had no desire to do so—that he actively sought out a health care expansion. By the last two Reagan years, an unexpected question had arisen: what should a properly Republican entitlement look like?

## LESSONS FROM DUTCH REAGAN'S LIFE

Jack Reagan looked at his baby son in 1911 and blurted out, "for such a little bit of a fat Dutchman, he sure makes a hell of a lot of noise, doesn't he?" The nickname stuck. As he grew up, the young man thought Ronald too prissy and had everyone call him Dutch.[14]

Jack Reagan was a prankster, a storyteller, a sports nut, a dreamer, and an alcoholic. Any little success set him out on a binge. One blustery winter night when Dutch was eleven, he came home and nearly stumbled over his dad, sprawled on his back in the snow, dead to the world and reeking of whisky. The boy was tempted to just pretend his father wasn't there. But how could he? He grabbed the old man's overcoat, dragged him into the house, put him to bed, and never said a word about it to his mother. Perhaps, as many observers have suggested, Reagan developed the traits that often mark the children of alcoholics—genial, quick to please, anxious to avoid personal conflicts. Certainly his tales about Jack always end with a positive spin. Reagan always loved and respected his father, he avers, because his mother, Nelle, "tried so hard to make it clear that he had a sickness that he couldn't help."[15] His father's health troubles never seemed to lead Reagan to any political conclusions. The family's poverty, however, led curiously back to his great political obsession.

Reagan remembered an idyllic small-town all-American childhood full of swimming, fishing, hiking, messing with guns, and occasional fistfights with young bigots who mocked his dad's Catholicism. These were his Huck Finn years, he said fondly, the grounding for the romantic America that infused his politics. Later, he discovered that the family had been "poor." He put the word in quotes because "I didn't know that when I was growing up. And I never thought of our family as disadvantaged. Only later did the government decide it had to tell people they were poor." It would never occur to him, for example, that his mother's oatmeal meat—"the most wonderful thing I had ever eaten"—was "born of poverty."[16] Always the Reagan antinomy: his family living cheerfully in the golden past and an intrusive government threatening happy memory by butting in, defining poverty, finding divisions, and fostering dissatisfaction.

Here is the gut-level contrary to Harry Truman, Lyndon Johnson, and (sometimes) Richard Nixon. They, too, felt the hardscrabble. They concluded that fighting poverty was a noble aspiration and a collective responsibility. For Reagan, government meant intrusive bureaucrats measuring poverty and poisoning the all-American memories of his youth.

Reagan developed the most romantic of youthful résumés: an unlikely right guard on the football team (he should have been too small), a star actor (although he was shy and insecure), and a positively heroic lifeguard on the Rock River ("one of the proudest statistics of my life is seventy-seven—the number of people I saved from drowning").[17] Reagan's autobiographies have precisely the same tone and narrative line as Horatio Alger's books for boys written in the nineteenth century: A virtuous, hard-working boy full of pluck and good cheer gracefully works his way up to success. At every turn, he catches the eye of a benign patron—in Reagan's case, a football coach, a drama teacher, the college president, the owner of a radio station, a Hollywood agent, a group of businessmen. The patrons magically open doors, teaching and boosting. In the early years, the drama stops at regular intervals so our hero can count up the money he has made. A superficial reading might suggest simply that hard work and virtue lead to success. But, like the Horatio Alger books, the deeper moral is not about our protagonist but about America itself: This is a nation of generous communities, full of benign mentors who recognize hard work and stand ready to lend an honest fellow a hand. Here good cheer, hard work, and virtue always earn their just rewards.

It is all most engaging, although there is the nagging little line of questions in the wake of every Reagan tale: is it really true? And, more important, what does it tell us about Reagan himself? Take Reagan's favorite story—he apologizes for repeating it yet again in his second autobiography: After college, Dutch broke into radio as a sports announcer. Broadcasting for WHO in Des Moines, Iowa, he recreated baseball games in the studio while a telegraph operator sat by his side and handed him summaries of each play. In the ninth inning of a scoreless game between the Chicago Cubs and the St. Louis Cardinals, the wire went dead. If he reported the truth, Dutch would lose his audience to the stations broadcasting directly from the ballpark. Instead, he kept right on talking. "I knew there was only one thing that wouldn't get into the score column and betray me—a foul ball." In Reagan's account, the batter, Billy Jurges, fouled off the first pitch; a couple of kids fought over the ball in the stands. Billy missed a home run when his shot tailed foul. Dizzy Dean, the pitcher, walked around on the mound. He pitched—another foul. And another. For seven minutes, listeners heard nothing but foul balls. When the telegraph finally started to work again Dutch discovers that "Billy popped out on the first ball pitched." Well, "not in my game he didn't," quipped Reagan, "he popped out after practically making a career of foul balls." For days people met Dutch on the street and remarked on all those fouls—was it some kind of record?—while he shook his head, agreed that it had been amazing, and never let on.[18]

What to make of this amiable story? For Diggins, this is Mark Twain reincarnated in the broadcast booth. "One reads the passage above with humor and marvels at Reagan as a raconteur." Others, see a "fabulist," always poised to blur the line between fact and fable. Dinesh D'Souza admires Reagan, but all those false fouls leads him to muse, "Reagan may have acquired, from this period, a bad habit that he retained in political life: embroidering news accounts by adding details for effect."[19]

However, this was no meaningless tic or "bad habit"—it went to the heart of Reagan's success and failures. He focused on parables rather than on policies. His airy indifference to the analytical world of evidence, arguments, and ideas freed him to repeat his handful of moral lessons, to impress them on American discourse.

Broadcasting led to the movies and made Reagan famous. Like a good trouper, Reagan taciturnly took direction. When he landed his first role, the studio remade him. His head was too small (new haircut), his neck was too short (special shirts and the big Windsor knots that *fashionistas* would mock forty years later), and his name was all wrong—you can't put Dutch Reagan on a marquee, groused the publicity men. As they bandied names about, Reagan tentatively cut in and suggested the given name he had always ducked. "How about Ronald? ... Ronald Reagan?" Hey, "not bad," they chorused, "not bad at all."[20] Thanks to the studio's publicity men, Dutch became Ronald. Details—What's in a name? Was that a record for foul balls?—never touched the man. But he knew a few things in his bones, and those things were beyond data or debate. Change his name, dress him in a Windsor knot, tell him where to go and what to say—but there was no directing Ronald Reagan away from his verities.

The movies gave him a great lode of parables, memories, and "facts"—he drove critics wild with teary renditions of heroic movie plots presented as actual events.[21] "Reagan was the greatest story teller," reported Representative Dan Rostenkowski (D-IL) years later. "He could drive you crazy [telling] ... the same stories over and over again.... He really made no show whatsoever of listening to arguments.... He saw reality not as a thing to bow to but a thing that could be changed and shaped."[22]

Was it really true that the army bureaucrats back at headquarters granted Reagan's unit permission to destroy a warehouse full of useless files "provided copies are made of each paper destroyed." Who knows? Who cares? The parable is irresistible: government bureaucracies are fatuous; they'll choke the life out of any enterprise. Ronald Reagan's lifetime of parables took a rising conservative movement, turned it sunny (we didn't know we were "poor"), rooted it in a kind of golden Americana (kids endlessly chase Billy's foul balls), injected foolish villains (idiotic government bureaucrats), and cast it all against the terrible international struggle between good (us) and evil (them). This nostalgic America is what we fought for, what made America the last best hope on earth. Reagan's parables conquered American politics and the way we talk and think about it. But skimming cheerfully over details, numbers, and policies set the limits to change.

In 1965, a gang of Republican businessmen asked Reagan to run for governor of California. "I'm an actor, not a politician" responded an incredulous Reagan. "I'm in show business." "While I'm highly honored," he wrote to friends, "I don't think I'm right for the part." As it turned out, he made politics—as one biographer put it—the role of a lifetime. In the 1966 California governor's race, Reagan won by a million votes (almost 58 percent of the votes cast). He won again four years later and in 1975 stepped down as governor and set his sights on the White House.[23]

## REAGAN'S HEALTH

Ronald Reagan had a long series of health care problems that did not seem to directly touch his political views. However, illness shaped the Reagan administration in important ways by compromising Reagan—especially around the Iran–Contra issue that burst into a great scandal and nudged him toward Medicare expansion. Perhaps even more important, health and illness affected the president's image in a presidency that, more than any before it, trafficked in imagery. For Reagan, politics and policy were all wrapped up in visuals and the persona they projected. The pictures of Reagan mounted on horseback recalled the movie star, the attempt on his life made him a genuine hero, and whispers about old age and "senility" threatened both the movie star and the American hero. The constant effort to define this president—to shape his image—meant that real-life medical problems mixed together with movie maladies affected not just his decisions or his attitudes but the all-important picture he projected onto the political screen.

As it happened, Reagan's two favorite films landed him in the hands of the medical profession. And the doctors could not save him either time.

## The Gipper Will Be Happy

Reagan desperately wanted to play the melodramatic role of George Gipp in *Knute Rockne—All American*. He persuaded a dubious producer to try him for the role by slapping yearbook pictures of himself in his Eureka College football suit on the man's desk—Reagan got everyone blurring the line between his life and his films. In the scene that made Reagan an A-list movie star, the Gipper lies dying of viral pneumonia. The football player looks up and tells the legendary Notre Dame coach, "some day when things are tough and the breaks are going against the boys, ask them to go in there and win one for the Gipper. I don't know where I'll be but I'll know about it and I'll be happy." Inevitably, Reagan turned the movie into a parable. "Eight years went by ... before Rock revealed those dying words, his deathbed wish," Reagan told the Notre Dame seniors at a 1981 commencement address (just two months after the assassination attempt). Rockne saved the story for a team that was torn by dissension, and factionalism. "The seniors on the team were about to close out their football careers," continued the Reagan exegesis, "without learning or experiencing any of the real values that a game has to impart." The Gipper's story so inspired them that "they rose above their personal animosities ... joined together in a common cause and attained the unattainable."[24]

Reagan himself often slipped into this old trope. "Do it for the Gipper" he urged the 1984 summer Olympic team. "Win those races for the Gipper," he rallied Republican voters, and—casting himself as the dying player—added, improbably, "Wherever I am, I'll know about it, and it'll make me happy." His followers cheerfully picked up the image. "Lately, I've been hearing … win one for the Gipper … by Congressmen who are supportive of [my] program," said Reagan. Even the headline writers at *USA Today* cheerfully took up the Gipper tag.[25] Ronald Reagan's presidency turned not so much on specific policies as on the image of a man who embodied the familiar all-American values. His movie death—with its moral about rising above faction and joining in a common cause—became shorthand for rebuilding the patriotic American community. It was as much a part of the Reagan presidency as any idea, policy, or program.

A second movie casts medicine in a malevolent light. In *Kings Row*— which Reagan considered his finest role—a sadistic doctor amputates both Reagan's legs at the hips for dallying with his daughter while carrying on with another woman. Reagan's character wakes up in bed, looks at his half-body, and screams to his new wife, Randy, "Where's the rest of me?" The line stood, in Reagan's mind, for "that first moment of accepting responsibility," the moment of growing up. He used it for the title of his first autobiography. Reagan seemed to use *Kings Row* as the dark version of the Gipper's story, drawing, effectively, the same moral about rising above immaturity and setback. In real life, however, Reagan never seemed to fathom the dark side. Reagan takes *Kings Row*—a twisted, gothic drama in which one doctor poisons his abused daughter, a second uses surgery to punish the wicked, and a third (Reagan's best friend) almost commits a woman to an insane asylum to stop her from talking about the doctors—and describes the movie as "a slightly sordid but moving yarn about the antics in a small town, something I had more than slight acquaintance with."[26] Ronald Reagan's America was all sunshine—always menaced by shadowy forces, always triumphant over the challenge.

## Age

In real life, President Reagan's most persistent health question was his age—and, more pointedly, whether the oldest man to step into the Oval Office (at sixty-nine) was touched by dementia. Reagan took the issue on directly. He told reporters that his mother had been "senile"—Reagan still used the old word—"for a few years before she died" at age eighty and he promised to resign if his physicians found any signs of senility while he was in office. *New York Times* health correspondent Lawrence Altman, a doctor, discussed the issue several times with Reagan and later wrote that he saw no signs of impairment.[27]

Still, the age issue kept creeping up. Reagan sometimes seemed old and foggy—his misfires were legendary: he failed to recognize his secretary of Housing and Urban Development, Samuel Pierce (mistaking him for a black mayor), he went to Brazil and called it Bolivia, he fell asleep at meetings, he could not recall crucial decisions. He seemed—to some observers but not others—completely innocent of basic policy matters. And then there was his easy schedule. His office once tried to hush the whispers by putting together a jam-packed "average White House working day" for the media; reporters subverted the effort by gibing that his handlers had put together an "average Reagan month."[28]

The issue became front-page news in the reelection campaign of 1984. During the first debate, Reagan seemed confused and, well, old. The low point came after he trotted out his trusty (old) line: "There you go again." In 1980, the jaunty phrase had reassured voters that he posed no threat to Medicare. This time, Walter Mondale, the Democratic nominee, was primed: "Do you remember the last time you used that line?" "Yes," responded Reagan. Mondale pounced: he accused Reagan of breaking his pledge and trying to rip $20 billion out of Medicare— Medicare, always Medicare. The Gipper had no answer and simply dropped his eyes—"the only time I've ever seen him do that," wrote Lou Cannon, who had covered Reagan his entire career.[29]

The *Wall Street Journal* leaped in with a piece entitled, "Fitness Issue—New Question in Race: Is the Oldest US President Now Showing His Age? Reagan Debate Performance Invites Open Speculation On His Ability to Serve." The networks began running the aging clips. The president nodding off at the Vatican, the president rambling, the president drawing a complete blank on a question during a photo op and dutifully repeating the answer that Nancy Reagan whispered in his ear: "We're doing everything we can."[30]

Reagan masterfully spiked the controversy during the next debate. "I will not make age an issue of this campaign," he said. "I am not going to exploit, for political purposes, my opponent's youth and inexperience." That took care of the issue—and of Mondale. But the question still remains, and it took on new significance when the Mayo Clinic diagnosed Reagan with Alzheimer's six years after he left office (in 1994). His physicians insist that there were no signs of dementia during his presidency. Still, "no one can be absolutely certain," concludes Lawrence Altman, precisely "when Mr. Reagan's Alzheimer's began." President Reagan "experienced many ailments" in office; he was slow to mend and made some of the crucial decisions of his presidency while convalescing.[31]

Part of the problem may have been compromised hearing. Aides got used to standing directly in front of the boss and talking loudly. Reagan deployed his signature maneuvers—vague headshakes, offbeat responses, and tangential tall tales—when he could not hear what others were saying. Of course, the boss used all the same moves when a subject did not interest him or to smooth over conflicts or deflect an argument he did not want to hear.

## Cancer

In July 1985, physicians performed a colonoscopy and discovered a cancerous tumor—a villous adenoma. Nancy Reagan consulted her astrologer and learned that it would be preferable to put the surgery off a week, but the president overruled her. No way he wanted to go through the colonic preparation another time. In an operation that lasted almost three hours, physicians removed two feet of Reagan's colon. "I woke up confused," wrote the president in his diary. "I was laced with tubes and very much a patient for a stay." As always, Reagan took a sunny view. "His cheerful mind," recalled chief of staff Donald Regan, "never worried about the possibility of recurrence and he asked few questions on the subject." From his hospital bed, he watched a television reporter saying the president has cancer. "The President had cancer," corrected Reagan in his diary. "It has been removed." He remained puckish. One set of visitors walking into the hospital room were jarred to find Reagan lying still in bed, a rose plucked from one of the bouquets clutched in his hands, which lay across his chest—the old joker was playing dead.[32]

This hospital stay, however, had a deep political echo. While the president was recovering, his national security advisor, Bud McFarland, came by to brief him—over Nancy Reagan's vociferous objections—on a proposal from two Iranian officials; they suggested entering negotiations to free seven American hostages held in Lebanon. Reagan discussed the initiative that would metastasize into the Iran–Contra scandal, the most difficult event of his presidency. Sixteen months later, recovering from still another operation, the president only fed the uproar when he could not remember what he had heard or approved when he was lying in his hospital bed in the summer of 1985.

The president remained in the hospital for more than a week and seemed to recover slowly. In order to cheer up the White House staff and demonstrate that the president had bounced back, Don Regan organized a gathering in the East Room. Ronald Reagan was his old self—eyes twinkling, head shaking, talking the cheerful talk. "It almost worked," recalled speech writer Peter Robinson. But then he noticed that "the president had lost so much weight that his shirt collar was two sizes too big." Robinson drew an arresting conclusion: "If you ever need proof that someone who seems larger than life is human after all, look at the gap between his neck and his collar after he's had a bout with cancer."[33]

Robinson was onto something important. Reagan's presidency was different, in part, because he was larger than life—the projection of a few fiercely held ideas thrown up onto a national screen. His own health episodes—a bullet lodged an inch from his heart, two feet of colon removed, fears of aging, compromised hearing—did not seem to touch him or his presidency any more than the philosophical arguments or the policy details that he fended off with charming, well-worn stories. His real-life health episodes seemed no more important—in fact, they were less central to his political image—than his death as the Gipper or his lost legs in *Kings Row*.

Reagan was less like other presidents—a man grappling with his mortality as he faced the problems of the Oval Office—than he was a man with a simple image, a seductive dream about America and its place in the world. That dream had power; it would overthrow the old New Deal Democratic order and replace it with an individualistic, antigovernmental, anticollective, robust Republican vision. The Reagan idea—thrilling to proponents who called him the Great Communicator, infuriating to skeptics who found no one home to duel over the facts— seemed to rise above every detail. It was larger than the president's own health, bigger than the details of his history. It reshaped every policy issue. Indeed, it remade American politics.

### Prostate

The administration's tortured Iran policy began while President Reagan lay in the hospital recovering from colon cancer. As the scandal peaked, in January 1987, Reagan underwent another surgery, this time to remove an obstruction from his prostate. As always, Reagan chirps at how his medical team is "pleased as all get out at my recovery." But, in truth, recovery was slow.[34]

Shortly after returning to the White House, Reagan faced harsh questions from the John Tower commission investigating the Iran– Contra scandal—and he shocked observers from both parties with his rambling confusion. That week, at the low point of his political career, the president umpired the largest health policy conflict of his administration: should he champion a great expansion of Medicare? The president's health wove itself, willy-nilly, around the president's policies.

## THE $44 BILLION ASTERISK—AND A HIDDEN HEALTH CARE REVOLUTION

As Reagan stood before Congress on April 28, 1981, and launched his revolution, the Democrats knew they were in trouble. House Majority Leader Jim Wright (D-TX) wrote that Reagan's "demeanor under the extreme duress of his physical ordeal" created "the aura of heroism" that made him and his program irresistible. "We've just been outflanked and outgunned." Tip O'Neil, the speaker of the house, agreed. "The President has become a hero. We can't argue with a man as popular as he is."[35]

### Cut!

Reagan pushed a program of tax cuts, budget cuts, and deregulation. But how much? How revolutionary? The administration squeezed what seemed like astonishing figures out of Congress: a $750 billion tax cut and more than $35 billion in domestic program reductions. The administration removed 400,000 people from the food stamp program, closed the public health service hospitals (which dated back to 1798), eliminated grants to HMOs, cut funding for social science research, and combined twenty-one separate grant programs into four large black grants that reduced both federal discretion and budget commitment. The budget roared through the House on May 7 (63 Democrats crossed the aisle to vote aye) and the Senate on May 12 (70–28). The rout left House majority leader Jim Wright lamenting that the administration had stripped control of the budget away from Congress, "dictat[ing] every last scintilla," and "every last phrase."[36]

But that was supposed to be just the start. The Reagan budget promised $44 billion more in "unidentified savings"—the shadow cuts became known, in Potomac parlance, as the Reagan budget's "magic asterisk." Where would the phantom $44 billion come from? No one in the White House figured out, gloated David Stockman, that "future savings to be identified later … was nothing more than a euphemism for 'we're going to go after Social Security." After all, that's where the money was. Besides, thought Stockman, Social Security had become "closet socialism"—the only way to end Big Government was to confront its "original sin." Stockman secretly dreamed of carving still another $110 billion out of the program (which totaled $645 billion in the 1982 budget).[37]

Administration officials gathered on May 9, 1981, and devoted an hour to discussing the Social Security cuts. This might not seem like much time in which to weigh a radical change, purred Stockman, "but since only three people in the room ... understood the issues, I assumed that an hour would probably do it." (The three in the know were Stockman, his ally economist Martin Anderson, and Secretary of HHS Richard Schweiker.) No one else had paid much attention to the artfully incomprehensible Stockman memo, confident that the White House staff would gather after the meeting and change or bury any troublesome proposals.

However, the revolutionaries outflanked the politicos. In an inspired political move, Martin Anderson lobbed the president a bouquet (or was it a grenade?): "You'll be the first president in history to honestly and permanently fix Social Security. No one else has the courage to do it." Reagan became so enthused at the prospect, that rather than follow the usual procedure and take the proposal under advisement, he approved it on the spot. "It represents everything we've always said should be done," gushed the president. "Let's go forward with it." He had no clue about the details, clucked Stockman. And now he had cut off his political advisors, who could not reverse an enthusiastic presidential decision.[38]

As soon as the *New York Times* announced the plan, all hell broke loose. The biggest cuts targeted workers who retired early at age sixty-two. Under existing law, the program paid them 20 percent less than retirees who waited until they were sixty-five; the new proposal jumped the penalty up to 45 percent, starting—here, the normally adroit administration slipped up—not in the distant future but the following year. Workers who had already told their companies they were retiring in nine months would suddenly get a letter explaining that the Social Security benefits they were expecting would be slashed from $650 a month to $450.

The reaction was murderous. Even conservative members of Congress screamed. "My phones are ringing off the hook," one furious Republican from South Carolina told Stockman. "I've got thousands of sixty-year-old textile workers who think this is the end of the world. What the hell am I supposed to tell them?"[39] President Reagan's approval rating plunged 16 percentage points. The Democrats came to life, thrilled by the unexpected gift. The administration could not capitulate fast enough to stop the House (405–13) or the Senate (96–0) from stomping on the dead proposal. The administration retreated to the safe ground of a bipartisan National Commission on Social Security.

"From that day forward," lamented Stockman, "Social Security, the heart of the US welfare state, was safely back in the hands of actuaries who had kept its massive expansion quiet over the decades." Without hard discipline over entitlements, the budget grew and red ink flowed— this administration tripled the national debt and saddled the government with a great deficit spending "albatross," as Lou Cannon put it. Small-government conservatives thought the Social Security rout meant the end of the Reagan Revolution.[40]

However, all that borrowing had political consequences. The Reagan administration had found a powerful brake against spending programs. While Democrats skewered Reagan's fiscal record—quite suddenly discovering their own fiscal probity—the red ink swamped new spending programs before they could be floated. After all, new programs would mean even higher deficits or new taxes. Senator Daniel Patrick Moynihan (D-NY) accused Reagan and his administration of intentionally creating the fiscal chaos in order to subvert government programs. After all, he reasoned, Reaganomics never added up. Even David Stockman, who had designed the program, half agreed. Without taking on Social Security, the tax cuts could not generate enough revenue to avoid the massive deficits. But while Stockman slammed the old man for not being tough enough to slash, he impatiently absolved Reagan of cynicism. Ronald Reagan knew, in his sunny bones, that cutting taxes would raise revenues, because he had A Story that told him so: During the war, the IRS imposed limits on income. Movie stars made four films a year, hit the income ceiling, and went home. When the war ended and the IRS removed the limits, the stars took more roles, enjoyed bigger paydays, and paid more taxes.

The story misled the Gipper—his administration's tax cuts never generated big enough paydays to balance the budget. However, if small, fiscally sound government proved impossible, the Reagan revolution managed the next best conservative thing: they built limits into the national government. New liberal programs would be difficult to fund.

The budget barriers that had hemmed in the Carter administration became far more formidable.

When the Democrats—through a bit of policy effort (budget packages designed to shrink deficits and reduce long-term interest rates) and a lot of luck (the great high-tech and dot-com boom of the 1990s)—managed to slip the Reagan administration's fiscal shackles, the George W. Bush administration went right back to the old Republican playbook, cutting taxes, growing deficits, and locking the Democrats into the deficit straitjacket.

## The Hidden Health Care Revolution

Meanwhile, the National Commission on Social Security, rounded up after Stockman's debacle, unwittingly enabled a tectonic change in American health care. The commission, led by Alan Greenspan, included a bipartisan group of Washington all-stars. Members laid down their ground rules at the start: they would operate by consensus; Congress would vote the entire proposal up or down without amendments from the floor; and Medicare was off the table—the commission focused entirely on keeping Social Security solvent.[41]

The Greenspan Commission released its plan in January 1983. As it glided through Congress, Representative Dan Rostenkowski, chairman of the Ways and Means Committee, ignored the ground rules and slipped a Medicare provision into the package. The administration approved the maneuver, which received almost no notice or discussion. The reform changed the way Medicare paid hospitals which, in turn, sparked a revolution in health care financing.

At the time, hospitals treated patients and then submitted a bill. Federal regulations—originally written to reassure providers that government would not meddle in the health care business—weakly stipulated that the hospital's charges be "reasonable." Naturally, the more health care services a hospital performed, the higher the bill it submitted. Medicare's blank check exacerbated the health care cost crisis lamented by every presidential administration. Congress now proposed changing the payment rules. Medicare would pay a fixed fee, set in advance, based on the patient's diagnosis, regardless of how many days the patient spent in the hospital or how many services the hospital performed. The new payment rules, known as Diagnosis Related Groups or DRGs, flipped all the financial incentives. With the Medicare fee now set in advance, hospitals could enhance the bottom line by providing less care to elderly Americans.

Jimmy Carter had fought tooth and nail for his Hospital Cost Containment and managed to squeeze the reform out of one chamber before it got buried. Now, a variation of the same reform flew right through Congress. The proposal landed in December 1982, breezed through committee by January, won an official White House endorsement on February 28, 1983, got through both chambers by March, and was ready for the Rose Garden signing ceremony (along with the rest of the Social Security package) in April—the legislative equivalent of the speed of light. Even Lyndon Johnson, fretting over those dead cats stinking up the porch, had never managed so large a health care change with so little fuss.

Why did the change go down so easily? For starters, the proposal got lost in the glare of Social Security reform—the big, bipartisan story built out of the Reagan administration's most spectacular political pratfall. The Medicare provision, in contrast, was a boring, technical change—who could possibly explain Diagnosis Related Groups to a lay audience? Opponents in New Jersey, where the system had first been tried, tagged the system *Son of Gobbledegook*. By the time DRGs reached the federal level, however, most opponents had peeled away. Congressional leaders had grown exasperated with the hospital industry's failed voluntary efforts to contain costs—which vanished as soon as the threat of Carter's reform disappeared. Many hospitals did the math and discovered they would prosper under the new pricing scheme. And Congress sweetened the package for the hospitals most likely to be hurt. For instance, teaching hospitals—with more expensive cases—received double the ordinary DRG rates.[42]

Perhaps a Democratic administration might have touched off hard questions about bureaucracy and regulation. But Ronald Reagan's celebrated verities—markets are good, government regulations bad—gave the health care technicians an extra layer of cover as they stealthily transformed the American hospital system. President Reagan's broad, conservative rhetorical framework facilitated a federal intrusion into hospital practice. Proponents dubbed the new Medicare pricing system "competition" and praised the incentives it gave hospitals to be efficient—after all, they would prosper as long as they did not lavish too many resources on patients. There was just enough truth in these fibs to lend them a veneer of verisimilitude. But the bottom line remained: the federal government—not the hospitals—would set the price for medical services to Medicare beneficiaries.

The great Republican innovation lay in focusing only on Medicare costs. Previous efforts—such as Jimmy Carter's hospital cost containment—had applied to all payers. Now, Medicare would control its own costs—and the devil take Blue Cross or Aetna. Hospitals would try to keep up their income by shifting the costs from payers that effectively reduced their hospital payments (such as Medicare) to those that failed to squeeze (the private insurance companies).[43] The other payers scrambled for their own ways to control hospital payments. The American hospital system entered a new era of shifting costs (from payer to payer), competition (between payers), and bargaining (between payers and the hospitals).

The new pricing scheme also shifted power relations in the hospitals. The era of the totally autonomous physicians—prescribing whatever they thought best—came to an end. Lavish testing, multiple procedures, and long hospital stays (which had traditionally brought in big revenues) now all cost the hospitals money. For the first time, hospital administrators began overseeing physician behavior. The quiet change in payment methods introduced a cascading set of changes—dramatically shorter hospital stays, fierce competition among health care payers, and new limits on physician autonomy.

Three years later, the Reagan administration came up with an even bigger health care surprise.

## CATASTROPHIC!

The most remarkable event of this health care presidency was the entitlement Reagan sponsored against the vociferous objection of most advisors. Why would Ronald Reagan, who had so fiercely opposed Medicare, endorse the largest expansion in its history? Most observers put it down to political expediency—he needed a win at the lowest point of his political career. But there was also something more profound going on: Reagan's views had evolved—perhaps more markedly in health than in any other domestic field.

The Reagan arc begins with the fierce rhetoric at the heart of The Speech—Medicare as a leap into tyranny and darkness. By the 1970s, however, a fresh note slipped into his thinking. "While I am opposed to socialized medicine," he wrote a supporter in 1979, "I have always felt that medical care should be available to those who cannot otherwise afford it." He pointed, in particular, to "the problem of insurance for those catastrophic cases where the medical care goes on for years at a tremendously high cost. I proposed a form of government insurance for that in California when I was governor, but we couldn't get any legislative support for it." Writing privately to a conservative supporter in 1979, a year before his election to the Oval Office, Reagan carved out an exception to his revolt against the state: "[T]his is a particular problem which must be faced and where government could have a hand."[44]

After a tough 1982 midterm election, Reagan returned to the theme. "In the coming year," he announced in his State of the Union address, "we will ... submit legislation to provide catastrophic illness insurance coverage for older Americans." Nothing happened; even more than most presidents, Reagan relied on his Cabinet and staff to fashion concrete policies out of his high-flying philosophy; there was no one on his team to run with this issue in 1983. He was for it, as one Cabinet official later put it, "but he didn't know how to get it done." The first term merely signaled a Reagan soft spot for catastrophic health costs.[45]

The issue landed squarely on the national agenda in 1986 when Otis Bowen—"Doc Bowen," as the President called him—became the administration's third secretary of Health and Human Services. Doc Bowen was a savvy former governor of Indiana who kept a prescription pad on his desk and cheerfully dispensed cold remedies to staff and press. Bowen's wife had spent three months in a hospital before dying of bone cancer; he arrived in Washington brandishing a plan to address catastrophic health care costs for the elderly. In November 1985, even while he was negotiating the confirmation rituals, a hospital journal featured an article coauthored by Bowen and his chief of staff, Tim Burke, titled "A Cost Neutral Catastrophic Care Proposal for Medicare Recipients."[46]

Bowen and Burke addressed a simple problem: Medicare limited hospital coverage to sixty days. That was plenty for most elderly Americans, but a small number ran past the allotted benefit and faced ruin. This was not the only—nor the largest—gap in Medicare coverage; the program offered only limited coverage for prescription drugs and almost none for nursing homes and long-term care—by far the biggest and most expensive problem facing people over sixty-five. Bowen and Burke, however, focused on the more tractable matter of hospital benefits.[47]

As soon as he took office, Secretary Bowen pitched his favorite reform. Each Cabinet Agency submitted proposals for the State of the Union address—a feverish, annual contest for presidential attention and air time. Just two months after his appointment, Bowen won a place in the 1986 State of the Union address. "After seeing how devastating illness can destroy the financial security of the family," said Reagan on February 4, 1986, "I am directing the secretary of Health and Human

Services, Dr. Otis Bowen, to report to me by year end with recommendations on how the private sector and government can work together to
address the problems of affordable insurance for those whose life savings
would otherwise be threatened when catastrophic illness strikes."[48]

Bowen had aimed to win an outright endorsement for his program
but only managed the requested study. Most administration officials
expected a report with multiple options that prominently featured a
private sector plan. Bowen established the usual committee and, a para-
gon of fairness, did not even attend its meetings so as not to taint the
careful scrutiny of issues and options. Then, in October 1986—three
weeks before the report was due—he uncorked his fastball: Bowen
directed the committee, composed of his subordinates, to evaluate his
own proposal.

On November 19 Secretary Bowen went before the White House
Domestic Policy Council—a committee of Cabinet members from
the relevant departments that framed domestic policies in the Reagan
years—with the fruits of his labor: the very same catastrophic insurance
plan he had published a year earlier. Medicare would pay for all hospital and physician costs that went beyond $2,000 a year; the increase
would be financed by a flat $4.92 monthly premium on all Medicare
recipients.

The Reagan White House had returned authority to the Cabinet
Agencies. Programs were proposed by the Cabinet Agencies and vetted by a standing committees made up of the department secretaries.
Health issues were hashed out in the Domestic Policy Council (DPC),
which was chaired by Attorney General Ed Meese, a longtime Reagan
stalwart. The DPC greeted the plan, as Bowen would later put it, "with
stunned silence which grew into vocal opposition." Led by Meese, Beryl
Sprinkel (who chaired the Council of Economic Advisors), and James
Miller (director of the Office of Management and Budget), they heaped
objections on the Bowen plan: the whole point of the Reagan revolution
was to shrink government—not to grow it. Worse, this government plan
would harm private insurance plans marketed to seniors. And it would
end up costing a fortune; the liberal Democrats, starved for domestic programs after six years in the political wilderness, would add on
every program they could imagine and—in the standard Washington
metaphor—"light up the proposal like a Christmas tree."[49]

Bowen took the pummeling and then casually sidestepped his powerful critics. He had already scheduled a press conference for the next day.
The others, as the *New York Times* later reported, were "outraged."

They knew very well that canceling the press conference would set off a media frenzy. Bowen had outwitted the White House controllers, who had no choice but to let Bowen announce the proposal they hoped to bury. Peter J. Ferrara, a Washington lawyer who had been a staff member for the first Reagan year, called the Bowen plan "the exact opposite of what the Reagan Administration has been saying for six years."[50]

Democrats cheered Bowen when he unveiled his plan the next day. Senator Ted Kennedy (D-MA) urged his Republican colleagues to "listen a little more" to Doc Bowen and "a little less to the insurance lobby." Eight separate catastrophic insurance proposals landed in the House hopper in the next two months.[51]

Normally, the boss and his aides would have adjudicated the differences that arose in the Domestic Policy Council. However, Ronald Reagan had missed that first DPC meeting (there would be six) on catastrophic care, for he had run into the hardest days of his presidency—perhaps of his entire political career.

### Dark Days

Republicans had seized control of the Senate on Reagan's coattails in 1980. Two weeks before Bowen announced his plan, in November 1986, the Democrats snatched the chamber back. Although President Reagan had campaigned long and hard, only five of the eighteen senators he stumped for won. Now, his pollster showed him the bad news: elderly Americans had voted against the Gipper and had grown critical of his administration.

Reagan met his Cabinet two days after the defeat. His was full of resolve and exhortation: "[H]istory is replete with stories of lame ducks," said the president, "I won't be added to that list. We have so much to do ... we have so much to do." Then Reagan got down to specifics: "Otis, as a doctor you know that in publicly funded health care, as well as in private care, we as a Nation must have the best health care at a reasonable cost." And a bit later, "Otis Bowen is finalizing his proposal on catastrophic health insurance.... I am anticipating reading it and truly hope it will protect citizens from economic destitution that can arise from a severe illness." A lot of Cabinet time for Doc Bowen, but, of course, he offered one concrete answer to the president's political problem—his lost seniors.[52]

But there was worse just ahead. The press "are off on a wild story built on an unfounded story," wrote Reagan in his diary the next day.

The Iran–Contra scandal was about to burst. "Irresponsible press bilge," fumed the president, before expressing his usual reflex: "I laid down the law.... I want to go public personally and tell the people the truth."[53] Reagan tried. But there was a flaw in his counteroffensive: he did not know or did not remember what exactly had happened. On November 19—as Bowen was wrestling with the Domestic Policy Council—Reagan was fighting the press at a formal press conference. "They were out for blood," but—always the positive spin in the old trouper's mind—"our gang seems to feel 'I done good.'"

His gang spared him a more candid assessment. His chief of staff explained what television viewers had seen: "The President, overbriefed but underinformed, uncertain of the facts, concerned with keeping secrets that had already bubbled up onto front pages all over the world, lacked his usual cheery demeanor." Worse, "a written clarification had to be issued twenty minutes after he had left the podium." Anyone watching the difficult press conference knew the president had not "done good."[54]

A week later, Attorney General Ed Meese and Chief of Staff Don Regan had finally connected the Iran–Contra dots and briefed the president. The United States had sold $30 million dollars worth of arms (roughly two large planeloads) to Iran in exchange for Iranian influence in getting American hostages released from Lebanon. Eighteen million dollars from the arms sales had been funneled through Israel to the Contras fighting in Nicaragua—directly violating a congressional prohibition against financing the war in Central America. "This may call for resignations," sighed the president, as he prepared to go on national television and eat crow.[55]

President Reagan's approval rating plunged. He had enjoyed 64 percent positive ratings in October. On December 2, a front-page *New York Times* story announced a 21-percentage-point fall—the largest single-month drop ever recorded in a president's approval rating. By February, he would be down to 40 percent. Worse, a majority of the public told pollsters they thought he was lying. "For the first time in my life," wrote Reagan afterward, "people didn't believe me." "He never had his integrity questioned before," Nancy Reagan told reporter Lou Cannon, "and that really bothered him." For once, concludes Peggy Noonan, Reagan "lost his sunny disposition" and gave way to the blues. Reagan hit his emotional bottom, concluded Cannon, in the last two months of 1986 and the first two months of 1987. Even stalwart Ed Meese fretted about impeachment.[56]

To add to the gloom, the president underwent another operation (on January 5, 1987)—a colonoscopy followed by surgery to remove an obstruction in his prostate. "The day and night stretch out," he wrote in a rare complaint, "when you are hitched to an intravenous plus an ongoing irrigation of the bladder." Reagan recovered slowly. He dutifully listened to his briefings and signed his papers. But he appeared, wrote his chief of staff, "to be in the grip of lassitude. He seldom if ever emerged from his office and wandered down the hallway.... The quick humor and curiosity ... operated at a much lower level of intensity."[57]

All this trouble surrounded the administration precisely as its members debated the health plan; Doc Bowen launched his proposal in November and Reagan himself decided the issue in February 1987—on the day before his most pathetic Iran–Contra moment. The Reagan administration debated the largest health care entitlement in thirty-five years as scandal, illness, and depression washed over President Reagan.

### The Debate

The debate raged within the administration. Ed Meese tried to ambush Bowen at one DPC meeting by inviting representatives of the insurance industry. Current law prohibited private insurance policies from offering more than 365 hospital days to patients who had exhausted their Medicare benefits. If the administration lifted the limits, reasoned the conservatives, there would be no need for Bowen's program. The maneuver backfired when the private insurance people reported they had no desire to enter this small and costly new market—the premiums would be too high to make the new benefit profitable.

At a full Cabinet meeting, Beryl Sprinkle floated another market alternative to the Bowen plan (which he had been developing with the conservative Heritage Foundation). Why not offer Medicare beneficiaries vouchers with which they could buy catastrophic insurance on the private insurance market? In response, Bowen grabbed a magic marker and began to diagram the voucher plan. Money would flow, said Bowen, from the government (he drew a line) to the individual, then to a private insurance company (another line), then to the hospital, back to the individual, back to the government—line, line, line. "The lines went all over the page," chuckled Bowen later. "I exaggerated a little but it worked very well." He framed his Rube Goldberg with a question: "How would an Alzheimer's lady of 90 handle a voucher?"[58] By the time Bowen was finished, he had covered the sheet of paper with lines and arrows and had everyone in the room, including (especially) President Reagan laughing at the complexity of the Sprinkle vouchers.

Still, the conventional wisdom ran against Bowen. Conservatives believed that Reagan's people would steer the president clear of this un-Republican entitlement. Meese would look him in the eye, they thought, and sink the catastrophic insurance plan. The president himself, however, continued to express sympathy. "I think [it] has promise," he wrote in his diary after the December Domestic Policy Council meeting. He went further and added an odd hope that "we can [also] find something for those working stiffs." There was not much about health care for "working stiffs" on the administration's radar—but the line reveals which way Reagan was leaning. A week later, as the decision loomed, Reagan sounded like a schoolboy facing a tough final (perhaps reflecting the high feelings on all sides): "It's my decision to make—I've got a lot of studying to do."[59]

Most White House advisors, most Cabinet members, most of the Domestic Policy Council, and most conservatives in Washington opposed the enterprise. As the debate went on, the acrimony grew. The members of the Domestic Policy Council "did everything they could to derail it," recalled Bowen. Then again, thought Bowen, most of them had never been elected to anything. He looked around at one Cabinet meeting and counted just two other men who had ever won an election: Ronald Reagan and Secretary of Labor Bill Brock. Bowen concluded that most of the others just didn't get the political force of the issue.

Two weeks before the administration's final decision about whether to proceed with catastrophic insurance (on January 28 and 29), Bowen made a triumphant tour of congressional committees in the House and Senate. Senator Ted Kennedy, now in the majority, announced that if the administration did not introduce the bill, he would. Bowen's well-timed testimony to Congress put still more pressure on the White House.

But it was hard to get to Reagan himself. He had cut way back on an already light schedule—generally heading back to private quarters after lunch. And the conservative members of the DPC—Ed Meese, Don Hodel, Beryl Sprinkel, Jim Miller, and others—were all keen to keep Bowen from making the case directly to the president. The only chance Bowen found to shake off the plan's opponents was at Cabinet meetings when he sidled up to the president and tried to do a bit of persuading—although every Cabinet member had the same goal. Donald Regan finally insisted that the plan go to the president—"you've done all this work," he told Bowen. "[W]e're going to make sure the president gets to hear it."[60]

On Sunday, February 6, President Reagan lugged briefing books on three weighty matters to Camp David: the Anti–Ballistic Missile treaty with the Soviet Union, the "Star Wars" antimissile shield, and, at the bottom of the stack, a decision memo for the catastrophic insurance program. On February 11, 1987, the members of the Tower Commission investigating Iran–Contra came to the White House to interview the president. John Tower asked the president about the discrepancies that had emerged about Reagan's role. Don Regan, the chief of staff, had insisted that Reagan knew nothing about arms for hostages. Robert McFarland, his national security advisor, claimed that Reagan had given the green light from his hospital bed back in July 1985. When the commission first asked Reagan himself, the previous month, he had agreed with McFarlane. Now he was not sure. As they politely questioned the president, he got up, walked over to a table, picked up a note prepared by his lawyer, and read it verbatim: "On the issue of the TOW shipment ... you said you were surprised to hear that the Israelis had shipped the arms. If that is your recollection, and if the question comes up at the Tower Board meeting, you might want to say that you were surprised."

The members of the commission were gobsmacked—stunned. The president did not seem to understand what he was reading. Lou Cannon later interviewed the participants and summarized their thinking: Reagan was "mentally confused" and "devoid of any independent recollection;" his "recollections were worthless" and simply reflected "the last person he had talked to." There did not seem to be anyone home.[61]

The following day, February 12, the White House announced that the Reagan administration would sponsor Bowen's health care bill. The administration released a fact sheet on the new proposal and, two days letter, the president devoted his Saturday radio address to the new plan. He began by putting aside his last painful days and mimed control over events: "This afternoon I'd like to spend a few moments discussing a decision I made this week." He described the problem in broad terms: "A catastrophic illness can strike anyone—the young, the old, the middle-aged. The single distinguishing characteristic is simply this: whatever form it takes, a catastrophic illness costs money—lots of it." Reagan offered a simple proposal for people over sixty-five—a limit on out-of-pocket Medicare expenses. For "the young," "the middle-aged," or (recalling his diary entry) "the working stiff," there were only hazy promises to find solutions. Reagan bridged this awkward difference with the familiar Gipper move—offering himself, a victim of colon cancer, as an emblem of how people over sixty-five faced particular challenges: "The problem has grown in recent years as we've achieved medical breakthroughs enabling Americans to live longer lives. Come to think of it, I myself have already lived some twenty-two years longer than the life expectancy at the time of my birth."

While Reagan placidly imagined "peace of mind for some 30 million older Americans," the furious backroom editing of the short radio address offered a more accurate window on the politics of the program. The original draft promised to "provide direct assistance to Americans 65 and over who find themselves in need of medical care." Beryl Sprinkle, still implacably opposed to this entitlement, scratched out "assistance" and scrawled in the margin, *"assistance is incorrect. The insurance is supposed to be self-financed."* Reagan's address followed the economist's instructions and promised to "make available catastrophic medical insurance."[62]

Sprinkle's change signals something distinctive about the proposal: classic social insurance redistributed wealth. Young and old, sick and the healthy all chipped in to fund the benefits that the unlucky—those who fell ill—would need. Not this time. Medicare beneficiaries would fund their own benefits. The Reagan revolution aimed to put an end to cross-subsidies running from one group to another. And the looming deficits—now running $200 billion a year—frightened the Democrats out of their traditional social insurance faith; any benefits would have to be paid for by the beneficiaries themselves. The new program was, as Sprinkle had penned in the margin of Reagan's draft radio address, "supposed to be self-financed."

*Lit Up like a Christmas Tree*

Democrats scoffed at Reagan's paltry offering. "A hoax," jeered Representative Henry Waxman (D-CA). "The administration has come upon a car wreck and changed only a tire."[63] As conservatives had warned, Democrats leaped onto the proposal and added benefits. The administration's plan addressed the narrow problem of catastrophic hospital expenses; Congress added prescription drug coverage (which the American Association of Retired People [AARP] was pushing hard to win), skilled nursing facilities, hospice care, home health services, and more.

Even after all the Democratic add-ons, Medicare still failed to address long-term nursing home care—perhaps the single biggest worry for elderly Americans. Enter Representative Claude Pepper (D-FL), the legendary eighty-seven-year-old who was a fierce, unabashedly liberal champion of people over sixty-five. He lined up 150 cosponsors and 90 organizations to support his bill ensuring long-term care for the elderly. Leaders of both parties resisted this popular budget-buster. Congress voted down the Pepper additions, but Claude Pepper himself remained in the political mix, constantly prodding Democrats with his plan.

The Democratic amendments managed to unite the Republicans. Secretary Bowen wrote House speaker Jim Wright and warned that even he would counsel the president to veto legislation with a drug benefit. The House brushed aside the threat and voted through a catastrophic insurance package with the drug benefits intact. The House was groping back toward the social insurance principle. Rather than simply charge Medicare recipients a surcharge, as the Bowen plan proposed, the Democrats would use general revenues to pay for the (now vastly increased) Medicare benefits. Four days later, on July 25, President Reagan was back on the radio charging that Congress had taken his "sound, sensible program," "more than tripled the costs," and "threatened ... the entire Medicare trust fund."[64]

Conservatives in the White House pushed hard for a veto, working their connections on the Hill and spraying memos to allies around the administration. They all knew the troubling bottom line—leaders in both Congress and the White House wanted to win a Medicare reform. Domestic policy advisor Bruce Bartlett wrote to White House colleague Gary Bauer reviewing the state of play after Congress returned from its summer recess. "There are good reasons to veto the catastrophic health bills." He repeated a popular conservative talking point and raised the danger that the prescription drug benefit would force elderly Americans to subsidize AIDs patients (through the disability entitlement). But, continued Bartlett, "the basic problem that we have to deal with" was that Senate Republican leader "Bob Dole [R-KA] strongly supports it [a catastrophic illness benefit]. The danger," he concluded, was that "someone like Dole may be able to fashion a compromise which is not quite bad enough to veto."[65]

Sure enough, the Senate passed a version of the bill that edged closer to the administration's proposal. The Senate bill was entirely self-financed by a surcharge on Medicare premiums. The White House then negotiated with Senator Lloyd Bentsen (D-TX), a fiscal hawk who also insisted on returning the package to budget neutrality. In late October, the White House announced a bipartisan compromise.

The final bill gave seniors full coverage for hospital stays after deductibles of $560 (for hospitals) and $1,370 (doctor bills); they also got 80 percent of their prescription drug costs after a $600 deductible, 150 days of skilled nursing care and 38 days of home health care.

Beryl Sprinkle and others tried one last time: "The Council of Economic advisors cannot recommend that the President sign this bill." At the OMB, officials focused on the fine print and found that Congress had sneaked through all kinds of technical changes that "the administration has long been fighting."[66] Conservative congressmen lined up behind their administrative allies and echoed the call for a veto: "This bill is a fiscal time bomb," wrote Jim McCrery (R-LA) and Clyde Holloway (R-LA), two newly elected House Republicans. "A huge tax increase," complained Representative Herbert H. Bateman (R-VA). "The largest single tax increase for older Americans in the history of the nation," added Representatives Larry Craig (R-ID), Peter DeFazio (D-OR), and others. Bateman tried the same wedge issue that was floating through the White House memos: "[S]enior citizens might even have to subsidize thousands of dollars in life-prolonging drugs for … AIDS patients."

Citizens across the political spectrum echoed the congressional critics. The vice president for personnel at Ohio State wrote the White House complaining that his faculty and staff retirees already had these benefits and should not have to pay for them all over again. The Committee to Save Social Security and Medicare and the Pharmaceutical Manufacturers Association both stood in opposition. "This … stinks," added a Florida man who urged the president to pass real national health insurance on the Canadian model.[67]

Of course, the deal was done. President Reagan had always leaned toward catastrophic insurance. He raised the issue in letters, lamented his failed efforts to win a catastrophic insurance program as governor of California, dropped the idea into his third State of the Union address, featured it at the painful Cabinet meeting that followed the 1986 midterms, and endorsed the Bowen plan over a chorus of objections. Reagan and Bowen had drawn the line at the add-ons in the House bill, but they had hammered out a compromise with fiscal conservatives in the Senate—conceding prescription drugs but holding firm on self-financing. The only real question inside the administration was how to spin the final result.

T. Kenneth Cribb, Reagan's top advisor for domestic affairs, suggested that Reagan's remarks during the signing ceremony "should distance the president" from the legislation that was "essentially forced upon the President."[68] Reagan followed the advice and delivered a gloomy address as he signed the catastrophic benefit into law. He warned that "if future Congresses aren't diligent, these new benefits could contribute to a program we can't afford." Because "the program ... is to be paid for by the elderly themselves," concluded Reagan, "this could be more than a budget problem; it could be a tragedy."[69]

Liberals were no happier. Their ideas had been blocked by the budget hawks in their own party. Why did seniors have to bear the full costs of their program? This, they insisted, marked "a dangerous departure from the social insurance principles." Medicare was turning into a program, said Henry Waxman, financed by "our most vulnerable citizens." And all this for a benefit that ducked nursing homes—the real catastrophic danger for most elderly Americans.[70]

Bowen's original proposal had been self-financing—a monthly fee of $4.92 a month, $59 a year. Now, with prescription drugs and all the rest, the surcharge rose to $400 a year for seniors making $40,000 and as high as $800 a year for seniors in the top tax brackets. That burden would make the program a political liability—precisely as President Reagan warned while signing the bill.

The legislation was shot full of ironies. A conservative Republican administration introduced and won a large health care entitlement. Each political side treated the final program with disdain, thinking it had conceded too much in the process. The result—the largest expansion in Medicare history—would not survive the next Congress. "On the list of Good Ideas That Bombed," concluded the left-leaning *Washington Monthly,* the catastrophic care act ranks near the top.[71]

## CONCLUSIONS

Ronald Reagan launched his political career with fierce blasts against Medicare—the path, he said, to darkness and tyranny—and ended up championing the largest expansion in the program's history, over the vociferous objections of most of his advisors. What changed? Most Reagan watchers assume that there is a hard-luck story lurking behind the conversion—although if so, we never found it and even Otis Bowen never heard it.

In fact, the most elaborate and important stories come from Reagan's own experience in the health matrix. Reagan suffered through a long list of maladies—an assassination attempt, aging, colon cancer, and (later) Alzheimer's. The direct effect was a weakened presidency marked by confusion, blunders, and hazy recollections. The White House team badly needed a political win by the time Otis Bowen came touting his health plan. The indirect effects, however, went even deeper. Reagan repeatedly offered his own health as a metaphor for the larger body politic: "Thanks to some very fine people, my—my health is much improved," Reagan told the Congress and the nation after his assassination attempt. "I'd like to be able to say that with regard to the health of the economy." Or, explaining why the catastrophic coverage focused on the elderly: "Come to think of it, I myself have already lived some 22 years longer than the life expectancy at the time of my birth." Disease and cure, illness and health offered a grand trope for a president posing as a revolutionary.

Movie images were even more effective. Viral pneumonia infected George Gipper, played by Ronald Reagan. The Hollywood football hero fused with the Republican president and memorialized his grand aspiration: squabbling, selfish individuals recall the Gipper, "join together in a common cause, and attain[] the unattainable." The image has everything: the handsome hero, a fatal illness, a great sob story, a pious lesson, and a killer political application.

Reagan's private diary touches the same mix of corniness and savvy: "I'm concerned ... as to whether we can find something [a health plan] for those working stiffs." What might, at first glance, seem a hackneyed pose signals something significant. Everything in Reagan's universe rested on the same inevitable canon: government is bad, Communism is evil, America is the golden land of patriots. Somewhere on Reagan's path to the presidency, health care slipped out of the communist night and took root in the sunny, small-town idyll of patriotic America.

Still, this administration pushed the nation toward the right even when it was expanding Medicare. For starters, the administration tried to bury the idea of social insurance. The Republicans aimed to smash the great web of cross-subsidies that marked New Deal and Great Society programs. There would be no subsidy from young to old or (if the Reagan team had had its way) from rich to poor. Beneficiaries paid for it all.

Reagan could make the assault on social insurance stick thanks to his economic program. Democrats gazed at the massive deficits and sourly pledged fiscal responsibility—they acquiesced to a budget-neutral entitlement (a true oxymoron in the liberal lexicon). Some conservatives, led by Beryl Sprinkle, tried to push the new benefit further into the conservative realm by offering vouchers and promoting markets. That proposal was not yet ready for the political rough-and-tumble—Bowen reduced it to a laughingstock—but it would develop into a solid fixture of Republican health policy.

The catastrophic insurance proposal, as it wended its way toward law, exposed the administration's strengths and weaknesses. Jimmy Carter had been too entangled in the details, Ronald Reagan did not tangle with them enough. From Stockman's Social Security cuts to Bowen's catastrophic insurance proposal, Reagan pitched the big idea and then waited passively while the people around him came up with proposals. Reagan would have liked a catastrophic insurance program earlier, but, as Bowen noted, no one offered him one. President Reagan was a visionary who was weak, even indifferent to detail—precisely the reverse of Jimmy Carter, who was all detail and no vision. Any ranking of the presidents demonstrates which Americans value more.

Timing always has big political consequences. The Reagan team rolled right over Congress in its early days. By year seven, the administration was negotiating from weakness; much of the catastrophic insurance program, as advisor Kenneth Cribb put it, "was essentially forced upon the President." Still, from start to finish, the Reagan team offers a model for working with Congress. They steamrolled the opposition when they could and negotiated when they had to. A savvy administration is one that knows how and when to be flexible with Congress. Lyndon Johnson got more ambitious as the Democrats' power waxed, and Reagan retreated as his waned. Both won big programs.

Finally, Reagan faced down his own economists. As an institutional matter, overruling economists became more difficult in each successive White House. Lyndon Johnson could breezily insist on going the extra billions for coffee and sugar, education and health care. The Nixon administration made it harder by inaugurating a new fiscal manager—the Office of Management and Budget. The Reagan administration raised the technical ante in health care still higher when it endorsed DRGs. Future debates would revolve around arcane formulae on a new level of complexity. Although the Reagan administration did not design or sponsor the DRGs, the Reagan brand—deregulation, government-bashing, cheers for markets—helped this regulatory intrusion slip through Congress and into the doctors' world.

In short, Reagan offered eight dizzy years of continuity and change. He served up both the predictable (cut programs! slash taxes!) and the startling (a new Medicare entitlement). But he, too, underscores many of the lessons that have emerged in past chapters: move fast for the things you care about, project the big picture, learn to be flexible with Congress, master your bureaucracy, hush your economists, and—most dramatically amid the great Reagan right turn—there is just no escaping health policy.

# CHAPTER 9

# George Herbert Walker Bush

## *Stick to the Running Game*

In early February 1992, President George Herbert Walker Bush ducked from the warm Southern California sun into the thronged waiting area of the maternal and child health clinic at Logan Heights Family Health Center in downtown San Diego. Jacketless, sleeves rolled up, fresh from enthusiastically working crowds, the tall, trim, energetic president looked momentarily puzzled. His slightly crooked campaign smile began to dim. Low-income mothers—brown, black, Asian, white—clutched squirming infants and chased their toddlers. Newly immunized babies screamed in hurt protest. Secret Service agents hustled about. Cameras flashed.

"Why am I doing this?" murmured the president of the United States, loud enough for nearby reporters to record his words.[1] Why, indeed. The answers were obvious: because he had just announced a "comprehensive" health plan that his pollsters and advisors hoped would blunt swelling charges that the president didn't care about health care or other domestic problems troubling American voters; because he was trying to "sell" his plan with a series of carefully staged health events such as this one; because his handlers wanted Americans to know that this "kindler, gentler" conservative cared about the millions of poor, uninsured clients who relied on community health centers such as Logan Heights; because he wanted some good press to stanch his bleeding poll numbers.

But it wasn't working. And perhaps the president knew why. His heart wasn't in it. Actually, his heart wasn't in the whole battery of domestic initiatives—trade, education, research and development, crime, drug abuse—that he had laid out before the Congress during his recent State of the Union address. Bush was going through the motions, and he couldn't hide it—from the public, from his staff, or from himself. To some health aides, the diagnosis was as clear as the San Diego weather. When the subject was health, Bush would arrive late, never touch the briefing book, kill fifteen minutes talking about sports, and wrap up the meeting early. He just wasn't very interested.

George H. W. Bush was warm to friends and family. He worked hard and prided himself on his competence. He was honest and patriotic. His feel for foreign policy was sure and strong. He battled persistently and often effectively against a hostile Congress. But Bush did not care about health care. The White House process that produced his health care positions suffered from presidential inattention and resulted in a health care presidency that eerily resembled Jimmy Carter's: drift, confusion, and missed opportunity. They all helped make Bush, like Carter, a one-term, second-tier president.

## GEORGE H. W. BUSH

Few American presidents have had a better résumé than George H. W. Bush. A distant cousin of Queen Elizabeth II, Bush epitomized the venerable Protestant aristocracy. He was born on June 12, 1924, amidst the sprawling, gabled affluence of Milton, Massachusetts. He grew up among the baronial estates of Greenwich, Connecticut—one of the wealthiest communities in the United States, discretely hiding its opulence behind hedgerows, fences, and long, sloping lawns.[2]

### From Andover to Odessa

Bush descended from solid, wealthy Republican stock: fiscally conservative but civic-minded. One grandfather was the first president of the National Association of Manufacturers, which still represents the interests of big business in Washington. His father, Prescott, earned his money in investment banking, joining George Herbert Walker, his father-in-law, at W. A. Harriman and Co., where Walker was president. Later, Prescott became a partner at Brown Brothers Harriman when Harriman and Company merged with their Wall Street rival. Prescott's family always affected a sort of genteel poverty—after all, they had only three in help, nothing like the platoons that served some of their neighbors. Nevertheless, even during the Great Depression, Prescott's son, the future President Bush, left his shoes outside his bedroom door each night so that Alec, the chauffeur, could give them a good shine before school the next morning.[3]

Prescott Bush was active in Greenwich politics, moderated the Greenwich town meeting, and became head of the Connecticut Republican Party. A tall, stern, imposing, and disciplined man, he was anti-Roosevelt, anti–New Deal, and antitax. But with old Yankee noblesse oblige, he also raised money for the United Negro College Fund and supported birth control (which was illegal in Connecticut until 1965). A strong backer of Dwight D. Eisenhower, Prescott was elected to the Senate in 1952, where he took positions typical of moderate-to-conservative Yankee Republicans, a now virtually extinct breed. Prescott's service in the Senate made George H. W. Bush the only president in the twentieth century who was the son of an elected federal official.

Home life for the young George Bush was suffused with discipline, expectation, duty, and obligation. Children wore coats and ties to dinner. You didn't brag about accomplishments, but you always aimed to win. You went to church on Sunday. You gave to your community. You didn't talk about yourself. You played sports. You studied hard. You made something of yourself.[4]

George first attended Greenwich Country Day School, a private school organized by his parents' contemporaries for wealthy Greenwich offspring. Then it was off to Andover, the elite Massachusetts prep school, where well-bred children got strong classical educations before they decamped to Harvard, Yale, Princeton, or Dartmouth. Bush's stay at Andover was briefly interrupted by an arm infection—which, in preantibiotic days, could have been life-threatening. The young man spent several weeks at the Massachusetts General Hospital in Boston but recovered fully, and returned to school. He stayed back a year but seemed otherwise unaffected by his brush with illness.

In his senior year at Andover, Bush was heading for Yale, but the attack on Pearl Harbor intervened. Despite his parents' opposition, he enlisted in the Navy as soon as he turned eighteen. Here, George Bush first showed a rebellious and adventurous streak that would enable this purebred Yankee to bridge, however imperfectly, the old Republicanism of his forbears and the new, aggressive, socially conservative Republicanism emerging in the Sunbelt. Bush became a Navy fighter pilot and was assigned to an aircraft carrier in the Pacific Theater, where he saw combat over the Marianas, Guam, and the Philippines. He was shot down twice and the second time had to bail out. He was rescued by a U.S. submarine, but his two crew members were both killed. The air war was less harrowing than combat on the ground—there were no wet foxholes, no shattering bombardments, no bloody assaults on exposed beaches, no hunger, no frostbite—but the young Bush saw his share of suffering and loss. He knew war first-hand, and it undoubtedly changed him.

But war did not slow George Bush down. Discharged just after VJ day in September 1945, he sped through Yale in two-and-a-half years, was invited into the super-secret Skull and Bones Society, majored in economics, captained the Yale baseball team (he played first base), and graduated Phi Beta Kappa. Barbara Bush, his wife of eighteen months, gave birth to George W. Bush in July 1946 while his father was charging through college.

The former pilot kept adding spice to the standard New England recipe of wealth and privilege. After his graduation, Bush declined to enter the secure world of Wall Street finance. Instead he followed the scent of oil and money to the new economic frontier in Texas. The competitiveness, ambition, and gambler's streak that shone through this decision would eventually lead him into politics.

Money eased his entry into the rough and dusty world of Texas oil. He went to work for Dresser Industries, a drilling supply company whose president was an old friend and client of his father's at Brown Brother's Harriman. Later, when George decided to start his own drilling supply company, his connections to New York finance ensured him the capital that he needed.[5]

Still, Texas was a long way from Greenwich. The drilling company sent him to Odessa, an isolated hamlet of trailers, sheds, and shacks in the hot Texas midlands. There, two future presidents and a first lady shared a small single-story house—and just one bathroom—with a mother–daughter team of hookers.[6] The Bushes moved from place to place in Odessa before their patrons at Dresser Industries transferred George to California and, later, the less rough-and-tumble town of Midland, Texas.[7]

Texas connected George H.W. Bush with a different side of America: a raw, tough, blunt, individualistic, conservative frontier. The Sunbelt unabashedly embraced wealth, ostentation, and a not-so-subtle racism.

There was nothing genteel about George Bush's new crowd—his ability to make friends and excel in this tough new circle boosted his political appeal.

## A Book with Many Pages

The young businessman first dipped his toe into politics to advance a Texas visit by vice presidential candidate Richard M. Nixon during the 1952 campaign. He ran unsuccessfully for Senate in 1964 and won a seat in Congress in 1966. Bush tacked hard to the right in his 1964 statewide campaign and then veered to the center two years later in his run for Congress, winning a substantial portion of the Hispanic and black vote in what had been a Democratic district. His father, Senator Bush, lobbied Wilbur Mills (D-AR) and Minority Leader Gerald Ford (R-MI), and helped his son secure an unprecedented plum for a freshman representative—membership on the House Ways and Means Committee. Congressman George Bush was soon presiding over tax breaks for his friends in the oil patch.[8]

The person who put George H. W. Bush on the path to stardom was that connoisseur of raw political talent, Richard Nixon. Because Bush had made it in the bruising world of Texas politics and business, Nixon looked past his roots in the despised soil of Andover, Yale, and privilege and saw the promise in the handsome, fiercely competitive, pragmatic Bush. Here was a possible weapon in Nixon's campaign to rip the Sunbelt from the Democrats and construct a permanent Republican majority. Nixon and his team convinced Bush to run for the Senate against Ralph Yarborough, a weak Democratic incumbent; he had beaten Bush in 1960 but Nixon knew he was too liberal for the changing Texas electorate. The Republicans' plans were upset when Lloyd Bentsen, a tall, wealthy, silver-haired conservative defeated Yarborough in the Democratic primary and soundly whipped Representative Bush in the general election.

As a consolation, Nixon appointed Bush ambassador to the United Nations, where he began his long education in diplomacy and foreign policy. Later, Nixon made Bush head of the Republican National Committee, where he proved loyal to a fault, supporting the president long after most of Nixon's other allies had abandoned him. Under President Ford, Bush served as head of the U.S. liaison office in Beijing, where he learned how a rival nation saw America. When he tired of that remote posting, President Ford brought him back to Washington to run the Central Intelligence Agency. The Texas Yankee was accumulating an impressive foreign policy résumé.

After Jimmy Carter's election in 1976, Bush returned to Texas, made money, and plotted his own run for the White House. Four years later, he lost the Republican nomination to Ronald Reagan and then ran as Reagan's vice president. Once again, he faithfully served his boss. In 1988, Bush routed Massachusetts governor Michael Dukakis in a ruthless presidential campaign. On the issues, he promised fidelity to Reaganomics: "My opponent won't rule out raising taxes, but I will. And Congress will push me to raise taxes, and I'll say no, and they'll push, and I'll say no, and they'll push again. And I'll say to them: Read my lips. No new taxes."[9]

Bush would do whatever it took to win. He relentlessly attacked Dukakis for being unpatriotic (Dukakis refused to ban flag burning or to require school children to recite the Pledge of Allegiance), soft on crime (a member of the ACLU) naive about race (while Dukakis was governor, a black prisoner named Willie Horton had been furloughed only to murder again), out of touch with real Americans (he was from Massachusetts), and weak on national defense. Dukakis was, by his own account, unprepared for the ferocity of the national campaign; he thought the public would be offended by the outlandish personal attacks—on his patriotism, for example—and refused to dignify them with a response.[10]

Worse, he submitted to an ill-advised photo op clumsily organized to burnish his credentials as commander in chief: Dukakis, helmet perched unconvincingly on this head, peeked out of the turret of an army tank as the vehicle crashed across the ground. The image backfired. Dukakis looked completely out of place—a summer camper trying to steer the *Titanic*.

The Bush who emerged from his long journey—through Greenwich, the South Pacific, Odessa, Midlands, Houston, Beijing, Langley, and on to the White House—combined old Yankee noblesse oblige, Texas oil-country tough, and impressive foreign policy savvy. Once past the nasty political combat that got him into office, Bush proved a serious president. He rejected Reagan's hands-off White House style. He preferred substance to stage management. The old Bush family values ran deep: one never boasts or calls attention to oneself or indulges in public displays—these standard political reflexes always made Bush uncomfortable. Instead, let your accomplishments speak for themselves. His physician, Dr. Burton Lee, would later comment: "I don't think anybody could have possibly worked harder at his job than President Bush, studying every issue in almost Carter-like fashion. At Camp David on the weekends he was up at 5 o'clock in his library studying these issues."[11]

Reagan avoided unscripted interactions with the press, but Bush sought them out. He gave 280 press conferences in four years—more than Reagan held in eight. He was substantive but not bold. He accepted the call to service with the seriousness of the well-bred. But he was serving not to change but to preserve; where change was necessary, he believed, it ought to be deliberate and slow. George Bush loved sports—he took hyperactive vacations and dashed from jogging to fishing to golf to horseshoes—but the long jump was never his forte.[12]

Bush's critics, especially those on the right, bemoaned his emphasis on competence. "What was lacking," complained Bush's conservative domestic aid, Charles Kolb, "was a sense of purpose and direction. There was no focus."[13] "Ronald Reagan ran ... on ideas and promises," added conservative columnist Charles Krauthammer. "George Bush did not. Bush had no agenda. He promised only to be an adequate steward for the country.... George Bush does not believe in very much. He never pretended to."[14] Bush himself famously admitted his deficit in "the vision thing."

If a vision had descended on him, how could this buttoned-up, self-effacing old Yankee have communicated it? Right from his inaugural address, Bush drew the line on the vivid leadership and oratory of the Reagan years. "Some see leadership as high drama, and sounds of trumpets calling, and sometimes it is that. But I see history as a book with many pages, and each day we fill a page with acts of hopefulness and meaning." Bush shrugged public leadership aside, and in doing so crippled his own administration.[15]

He dramatically downsized the White House public affairs staff, cutting the number of speechwriters and—in a symbol of reduced status—canceling their coveted White House mess privileges. During his first month in office he gave his speechwriters a list of things to avoid: lofty language, broad themes, macho talk, Rambo posturing.[16]

President Bush preferred foreign policy—perhaps more so than any twentieth-century president. He developed a unique and effective style of personal diplomacy that suited his proclivity to work behind the scenes, building on personal relationships with foreign leaders whom he had gotten to know as UN ambassador, CIA director, and vice president.

These skills were all on display in his adroit management of the international coalition that mobilized to expel Iraq from Kuwait during the first Gulf War.

Domestic matters were usually a different story. The president fidgeted and "became visibly bored.... The interest and engagement ... when defense or international issues came up relative to any domestic issue were so apparent," recalls Gail Wilensky, a key health policy aide during the last eighteen months of the administration.[17] The contrast was so dramatic that *Time Magazine* named the "two George Bushes" the 1990 Men of the Year: one went to the foreign policy master, the other to the domestic politics mediocrity.[18] In many ways, George Bush was the mirror image of that other Texan in the White House, Lyndon Baines Johnson. LBJ excelled in domestic policy, but stumbled abroad. Bush did just the opposite.

Bush diligently tackled some important domestic issues. He bit the bullet on the budget deficit inherited from the Reagan administration, even though doing so violated his memorable "read my lips" pledge and infuriated conservatives. He spent time and energy on education policy. The landmark *Americans with Disabilities Act of 1990* owed a great deal to his advocacy. And his Yankee Republican side overcame the Texas oilman in him when he firmly supported strengthening the Clean Air Act.

### We Need Someone Who Is Afraid of Frogs

But one issue that never grabbed him was health care—although he had plenty of personal experience with health and medicine. In the spring of 1953, the Bushes' second child, three-year old Robin, developed lethargy and skin bruises. She had been a plump, happy, active, little girl with curly blond hair. A local pediatrician in Midland, Texas diagnosed leukemia. The bruises likely reflected the failure of Robin's bone marrow, which, because of a spreading cancer, wasn't producing enough normal platelets—blood cells vital to clotting. At that time, leukemia—now mostly curable among children—was a death sentence and the pediatrician who gave George and Barbara the bad news suggested that they take the little girl home and let her die peacefully. But George's uncle, Dr. John Walker, was the president of one of the nation's foremost cancer hospitals, Memorial Sloan-Kettering in New York City, and he advised them to come back to New York to consult some specialists. "You could never live with yourselves unless you treat her," he said. The Bushes flew to New York.[19]

Experimental treatment—exactly what type is unclear—enabled Robin to survive another seven months. Barbara and Robin spent much of that time at Memorial Sloan Kettering. George Bush commuted to New York on weekends, leaving the boys, George W. and Jeb, with neighbors. In her last hours, Robin began to bleed internally. Although there was little chance of success, Robin's physicians wanted to operate. Barbara agreed, saying, "Where there's life, there's hope," but the little girl died after surgery. George Bush, who was on his way back from Texas, returned to the hospital the next day to thank the staff.[20]

The Bushes gave her body to Sloan-Kettering "for science." Presumably, this means they allowed an autopsy, useful for teaching aspiring physicians and learning about the effects of disease. The parents also agreed to donate their own organs at death. Without the little girl's body, the family did not hold a funeral, and George and Barbara returned to Texas, where their two boys awaited them. Months later, George's parents buried Robin in Greenwich.[21]

The loss of a child, in this case an only daughter, is a shattering experience for any family. It can destroy marriages and change lives. Hard-charging executives sometimes turn their careers on a dime and dedicate themselves to conquering the illnesses that ripped away their offspring. Robin's loss did not have this kind of dramatic effect on George H. W. Bush, but she clearly stayed in his thoughts. In 1958, he wrote his mother, Dorothy:

> I like to think of Robin as though she were a part, a living part, of our vital and energetic and wonderful family of men and Bar. [By then, the Bushes had four sons.] ... This letter is kind of like a confessional ... between you and me, a mother and her little boy—not so little but still just as close, only when we are older we hesitate to talk from our hearts quite as much. There is about our house a need.... We need some starched crisp frocks to go with all our torn-kneed blue jeans and helmets. We need some soft blond hair to offset those crew cuts.... We need a legitimate Christmas angel.... We need someone who's afraid of frogs.... We need a girl. We had one once.... But she is still with us.[22]

Forty-two years later, in a 2000 interview with reporter Hugh Sidey, the wound still sounded fresh: "We lost our daughter and that was a tough experience.... Dear God, why does this child have to die? [She was] the epitome of innocence to us, beauty, everything else, and there was no explanation. But all these things contribute to your life, maybe your character, to what you stand for.... It hurt badly."[23] That same year, the Bushes quietly moved her grave from Greenwich to the designated family resting place on the campus of Texas A&M University in College Station, Texas, site of the George H. W. Bush Presidential Library.

President George Bush never publicly referred to his only daughter when discussing health issues. Perhaps the experience was too painful. But it also seems likely that sharing grief—or any personal feelings—was simply not the Bush way. One shouldered on and did one's duty. In this reaction to personal suffering, George H. W. Bush is reminiscent of Franklin D. Roosevelt, who made his enormous disability into a self-improvement project and never discussed it publicly. FDR's inspiration, in turn, was his "Uncle Ted," who, weakened by asthma as a child, beat the disease with rough physical exploits—fighting, riding, and hunting. Theodore Roosevelt, Franklin Roosevelt, and George Bush all shared the same Yankee Brahmin code. In contrast to Eisenhower, Kennedy, Johnson, and Nixon, neither FDR nor Bush seemed to translate their personal experiences into health care policy. They buried their pain and tried not to look back.

A flawed policy process also deflected Bush from health care issues. Domestic issues were dominated by Richard Darman, a shrewd, blunt, and ruthless bureaucratic operator with a taste for power. Darman was the director of the Office of Management and Budget and, predictably, saw issues through a budgetary perspective. He focused the president on reducing the budget deficit—an important goal, but one that was diffi-cult to reconcile with major health initiatives. The head of the Domestic Policy Staff, Roger Porter, a Harvard professor who had been a White House aide in the Ford administration, deferred to Darman on money matters. "Roger Porter and others in the White House may have had big titles," wrote Charles Kolb, "but by mid-1990 all the power was effectively flowing in Dick Darman's direction."[24]

Porter did not think health policy was ready for presidential attention—it was, in his estimation, a "maturing" issue that should be deferred. Health care and other big-ticket domestic policies never get much of a hearing unless policy advocates find a way to countermand the budget analysts; but in the Bush White House, there was no one to balance the money men.

Ultimately, of course, the disarray in White House domestic policy reflected one overriding factor. Unlike Eisenhower and Nixon, this pres-ident did not care enough to organize a robust policy process for domes-tic affairs. Charles Kolb described Bush's approach to domestic policy with a kind of puzzled amazement: "[P]olicies became Administration Policies not because Bush chose them but because they just sort of happened. They welled up from below instead of issuing from some governing philosophy or ideology." The White House process even dulled the president when he ran for reelection in 1992. The issues he campaigned on, reflected Kolb, "weren't felt passionately; they were merely on a list handed to him by someone." He ran as he governed: without "zeal, enthusiasm, or conviction" about domestic matters.[25]

George H. W. Bush was competitive, took risks, and befriended leaders around the world. He was a masterful foreign policy president. But on the home front, he never projected the leadership that the modern presidency demands. He seemed bumbling, detached, and always a step behind events. Jimmy Carter and George Bush could not have come from more different places: Carter from the impoverished swamplands of the preindustrial South, Bush from the manicured lawns of old New England money. They joined very different U.S. navies: Carter hunkered in claustrophobic nuclear submarines while Bush touched the sky. But their presidencies developed an eerie resemblance: good, serious, smart men, full of substantive interests, concerned with competence, aspiring to the right thing; yet each lacked vision, direction, an ability to move the public, or any gut feeling for health care issues and why they matter to the people.[26]

## WAITING FOR HEALTH CARE TO MATURE

President-elect George Bush inherited Ronald Reagan's fiscal mess. Reagan's tax cuts had never generated sufficient gains from economic growth—supply-side theory notwithstanding—to offset losses in revenue. By 1989, federal deficits exceeding $150 billion a year stretched into the future as far as anyone could see. To complicate matters, the Democrats controlled both houses of Congress, and Bush's brawling campaign tactics against Dukakis had inflamed partisan tensions.

Even before his inauguration, Bush and his White House team made it clear that they would not rock boats or engage in wild talk about the first one hundred days. The federal budget, they believed, ruled out any domestic policy drama. A preinaugural memo in January 1989 surveyed the grim political landscape and laid out an ultracautious White House strategy:

*Premises*
1. Virtually no money.
2. Deficit will dominate discussion.

3.  Congress may or may not be nasty but it will definitely vie for
    control....

*Technique*
  1.  Minimize intensity—do not set up 1989 as a dramatic or break year
      for the Bush Presidency.
  2.  Manage the process—keep objectives limited. Don't go for a long
      bomb when a running game will do.
  3.  Institutionalize the Bush approach of cooperation and consensus—
      don't be afraid to share credit with Congress.[27]

It looks like the prescription for a caretaker presidency. Nothing in
the president's initial approach to health care altered that impression. He
made his first comments on the subject, in March 1989, when he swore
in Dr. Louis Sullivan, an African American hematologist/oncologist, as
his secretary of Health and Human Services. Bush spoke of the need
to get "better value for health care dollars, targeting effective services,
finding ways to contain escalating costs.... Work to sustain programs
like AFDC ... and Head Start."[28] Like Carter, Bush focused on cost and
inefficiency.

Bush's most important health care decision of 1989 was to stand
aside while Congress repealed the Medicare catastrophic insurance
amendments that Ronald Reagan had signed into law a little more than
a year earlier. The financial logic of the reform—that it would be self
financed by seniors—now came back to haunt it as more affluent beneficiaries rebelled against the $800 annual surcharge for benefits that
many already enjoyed anyway. The federal government subsidized
farmers and bailed out the entire savings and loans industry, argued
the program's liberal critics; why should seniors carry the entire catastrophic insurance burden?

The rebellion got its defining media moment on August 16, 1989,
after Representative Dan Rostenkowski (D-IL) met with disgruntled
senior community leaders in his district. After the meeting—with news
cameras rolling—a crowd of seniors blocked his car, pounding on the
windows and banging on the hood. Rostenkowski slipped out of the
car and walked away as several dozen people trailed after him, shout-
ing, "liar," "impeach," and "recall." Rostenkowski had nothing to say.
His colleagues soon filled the silence. "The elderly were ungrateful,"
said Representative Henry Waxman (D-CA), "so let them stew in their
own juices." The pictures of elderly Americans attacking Rostenkowski
made the cover of *Time*.[29]

The program's architects hoped President Bush might find a way to salvage something. But the only comments from the Oval Office fretted about deficits (the accounting rules meant deficits would rise with repeal). "I hate to place the blame," recalled Otis Bowen, Reagan's secretary of HHS who had designed the plan, "but ... President Bush remained totally silent" while Congress scratched the program in November 1989.[30]

At the time the repeal of a health care program was a minor historical footnote compared to the epic events in Germany. The Berlin Wall— the front line and bleak symbol of the Cold War—fell. After more than four decades, the United States and its partners had quite suddenly triumphed over Communism. Two months later, George Bush delivered his 1990 State of the Union address and declared "the beginning of a new era in world affairs." The president—mindful of the contrast between inspiring international events and the sputtering economy at home—used the context to suggest ways to "invest in human capital to maintain 'our competitiveness'" and "the spirit of American ingenuity." Deep in the speech, he announced that he had asked Secretary of HHS Sullivan to conduct a study of the U.S. health care system—actually, he called it a study of existing studies (there were several national panels conducting reviews). He concluded with the health issue that really spoke to him: "I am committed to bring the staggering costs of health care under control."[31]

The emphasis on costs continued when, the next month, President Bush spoke at Johns Hopkins University with Sullivan at his side. "Today over 11 percent of our gross national product goes to health care," Bush intoned, "and we rank number one in the world in per capita health-care expenditures. Yet we do remain behind other industrialized countries in life expectancy. And in the developed world, we rank twenty-second in infant mortality rates." His prescription: support maternal and child health by fully funding Medicaid and supporting community health centers (Bush was, after all, a kindler, gentler conservative); invest in disease prevention; bring the malpractice system to heel. By now the health care themes of the first two years of Bush's presidency were set. Cost control, prevention, malpractice reform, and maternal and child health—a true running game: small, safe advances that might improve health and that would not tax the budget. Without Ted Kennedy (D-MA) rattling the rafters about coverage, Jimmy Carter might happily have seized on exactly the same set of issues.[32]

But Carter had pushed an aggressive hospital cost containment agenda; the Bush administration instead took a passive approach. Internal White House memos noted that the Sullivan study, which the president had called for in the State of the Union, was drifting—it lacked leadership and purpose, it failed to get to the roots of the problem, it was focusing too much on health care delivery (the old paradigm, in Bush White House lexicon) and not enough on prevention (the new paradigm). But in health care, drift was just fine by the White House staff.[33]

Roger Porter advised the president that there was no urgency concerning health care issues. True, health care costs were increasing 10.4 percent annually, and the number of uninsured had grown from 31 million to more than 33 million between 1988 and 1990. But the repeal of catastrophic coverage showed that Americans were not interested in more "social welfare spending." Health care was still, in Porter's view, a "maturing issue," not ready for prime time or for presidential engagement. As to rising costs, he recommended easy conservative nostrums: use the presidential bully pulpit to advocate prevention (get people to stop smoking). When he turned to the quality of health care, however, Porter injected an innovative note: there was much that medicine could learn by studying the methods of continuous quality improvement used in industrial settings. In this, Porter and his staff showed that their cautious approach to health care did not exclude out-of-the-box thinking. As we shall see, the innovativeness of the ideas that circulated in the Bush administration on some health care topics stood in stark contrast to its passivity on policy. Creative thinking just underscored the Bush years' lost opportunities.[34]

By late 1990, however, many observers outside the administration thought the health care issue was considerably more "mature" than the Bush Domestic Policy Group. The country was in a recession, and the public was looking to government for a response. Job loss threatened people's health insurance. On December 17, 1990, two respected congressmen from the House Ways and Means Committee, Bill Gradison (R-OH) and Nancy Johnson (R-CT), wrote Bush Chief of Staff Sununu to sound an alarm. The Democrats, they warned, would make health care a major issue in the next session of Congress "because of growing public concern about the availability of affordable health care and the ramifications for our economy of continuing health care inflation." They urged Bush to "take the initiative and set the terms of the coming debate.... The President can [stand] for many health reform policies that do not have serious budgetary implications. He can, for example, help smaller employers obtain or retain affordable insurance coverage. He can support policies to promote managed care or coverage with sufficient deductibles and coinsurance to contain costs without government regulatory intervention."[35] In other words, conservatives needed a health care agenda of their own that could blunt the force of a coming Democratic attack.

The Gradison–Johnson overture was not well timed. Four months earlier, in August, Saddam Hussein's Iraq had overrun oil-rich Kuwait. George Bush knew the Arab world like few American presidents, because his drilling supply company had serviced Arab clients during the 1950s and 1960s. He also had one of the world's thickest Rolodexes of foreign leaders—including many intelligence chiefs (after all, he had run the CIA). Working through the United Nations, the president gathered an international coalition with enormous legitimacy and crushing military superiority. The congressional health care alarm went off just as military forces were massing in Saudi Arabia; a month later, on January 16, 1991, allied jets would launch.

John Sununu, Bush's truculent and domineering chief of staff, shot Gradison and Johnson a curt, dismissive note. In Bush's State of the Union address, delivered on January 29, 1991, less than a month before Allied land forces stormed into Kuwait, he naturally focused on the stakes in the Middle East. He made only the briefest reference to health and clung to the familiar script: "Good health care is every American's right and every American's responsibility. And so, we are proposing an aggressive program of new prevention initiatives—for infants, for children, for adults, and for the elderly—to promote a healthier America and to help keep costs from spiraling."[36]

Neither Bush nor his staff were prepared to even discuss health care with sympathetic outside groups. On January 7, 1991, domestic policy aide Johannes Kuttner recommended that his boss, Roger Porter, decline a request to meet with the Health Insurance Association of America, then the Washington representative of U.S. health insurers: "Given the state of development of our thinking on access to health care," Kuttner wrote, "I do not believe such a meeting should be a priority for your time"—an unusual brush-off toward a friendly group.[37]

The Sullivan study, which Bush had requested thirteen months earlier, remained paralyzed. "HHS needs guidance on what product is expected in response to the President's directive for a 'study,'" wrote Kuttner on

April 16, 1991. "It has no such guidance right now, and as a result, very little work is being done."[38]

Gradison and Johnson's warning, however, proved prescient. By spring 1991, Republicans and Democrats alike were tossing health care coverage proposals into congressional hoppers. Republicans generally proposed reforming private insurance markets to make policies cheaper and more accessible; Democrats aimed for more comprehensive health reform. On May 15, 1991, the *Journal of the American Medical Association,* the influential scholarly publication of the American Medical Association, editorialized: "An aura of inevitability is upon us. It is no longer acceptable morally, ethically or economically for so many of our people to be medically uninsured or seriously underinsured."[39]

The media jumped on the editorial and gave it wide circulation. The Sullivan study was no longer diverting attention from the leadership vacuum at the top of the Bush administration, a problem that Roger Porter candidly admitted in a memo to the president: "Health issues continue to be the subject of public debate." While "others urge immediate action," he warned, "Administration officials ... are cast as individuals voicing caution.... The Administration is often portrayed as not meeting the challenge at hand. The most frequently stated perception of the Administration's health policies is that we have no health policy.... Until we say more, the tone of commentary ... is likely to remain unchanged."[40]

George Bush was not inclined to "say more." In June, he addressed the conservative organization of small business, the National Federal of Independent Businesses, and stuck to familiar themes: "Health care costs have become a major factor for many businesses. Although some people think it makes sense to establish our own brand of federally mandated national medical care, I disagree strongly. And we have offered reforms to hold down medical costs without reducing the amount of available care. Some encourage people to take care of themselves. Others encourage people to resolve disputes with doctors instead of hauling everyone involved off to court."[41]

But popular pressure to confront the issue continued to grow. In July 1991 Republican pollster Robert McInturff passed a warning to the president's political aides that found its way to Sununu's inbox. Soon the president's most senior advisors, including the redoubtable budget director, Richard Darman, were discussing how to address the comprehensive reform proposals pending before the Congress. They trooped up to Kennebunkport to brief the president during his August break, and eventually, on September 25, 1991, Bush and his staff held a quasi-summit on domestic policy, including health care, at Camp David.

According to reports in the *Washington Post,* Bush's advisors remained uncertain about how seriously to take this troublesome issue. The consensus was that the White House needed to address health care—but also that there was no rush. Democrats remained divided, the prospect for a bill moving through Congress was remote, and health care was always a losing issue for Republicans. A dissenting minority disagreed. "That notion [that health care is a Democratic issue], in the view of some within the GOP, is outdated and should be abandoned. They believe the White House has become a 'lagging indicator' on the health care issues." One leaker concluded that the president was "still getting his legs" on the subject of health care.[42]

He would need those legs sooner than he thought. In early November 1991, President Bush traveled to Italy for a summit meeting of NATO heads of state. He was there on November 5 when news broke about a special senatorial election in Pennsylvania.

Senator John Heinz (R-PA) had died in a flying accident; former Governor Dick Thornburgh stepped down as Bush's attorney general and entered the race to replace him as a prohibitive favorite—three months before the election he had a 40-percentage-point lead in the polls. During the first debate, Democrat Harris Wofford waved a copy of the Constitution and launched his celebrated slogan: "If the Constitution guarantees criminals the right to a lawyer, shouldn't it guarantee working Americans their right to a doctor as well?" Thornburgh stuck to the Bush administration playbook. He campaigned with Secretary of HHS Louis Sullivan and—echoing President Bush—blasted the Democrats' folly: "a massive, federal bureaucracy to run a centrally directed health care system." When Wofford won by 10 percent of the vote, national health insurance shot to the top of the nation's domestic policy agenda.[43]

### FINALLY A PULSE AT THE WHITE HOUSE

After nearly three years of virtual indifference, President Bush became a sudden convert to health care reform. At a press conference in Rome on November 8, reporters peppered the president about whether he would respond to Wofford's victory with a "comprehensive" reform plan of his own. He replied: "I'd like to have a comprehensive health care plan that I can vigorously take to the American people. We're moving forward with certain portions of health care now, as you've heard from Secretary Sullivan. It's a matter of concern. And I think the answer to your question will be, yes."[44]

As if to ratify the president's change of heart, on November 25, 1991, *Time* devoted its cover story to health care. The front page promised "10 Ways to Cure the Health Care Mess." The story's inside headline blared: "Condition Critical. Millions of Americans have no medical coverage and costs are out of control."[45]

Politics and the fierce glare of the media spotlight had forced the White House to confront an issue it would have preferred to avoid, but unfortunately for President Bush, neither his gut nor his policy process had caught up with his political needs. "The critical nature of the problems ... were not understood by the President," recalled Wilensky. "The comfort level really wasn't there relative to other domestic issues.... It wasn't that he didn't care ... it was just not his issue."[46]

Now that health policy mattered, OMB director Richard Darman took charge. Bypassing HHS and the normal domestic policy apparatus, he assembled his own group of experts to hammer out a health care plan. The group had begun meeting over the summer, but Thornburg's debacle now sped up the schedule. The byword was "comprehensive": the proposal had to be credible as a counter to the sweeping national health insurance plans touted by Wofford, his Democratic allies, and even some moderate Republicans. The plan had to control costs and improve access to health care, but it also had to reflect Republican principles. That meant reforms that relied on market mechanisms.

Darman did not have much time. Any funding for a new proposal had to be included in the 1993 federal budget, which had to go to the printer early in the New Year so that it could be introduced in early February 1992. What is more, the president had to talk about the plan in his January 28 State of the Union address, so the key outlines had to be hammered out by then. That gave the health care team about six weeks to birth a complicated policy on a topic with which Republicans had little expertise. As Gail Wilensky readily admitted, "Domestic policy strength was much scarcer in Bush 1 than in the Clinton Administration."[47]

At the same time, the sudden presidential focus on health care also created a tremendous opportunity. Not since the Nixon administration twenty years earlier had Republicans seriously tried to put their stamp on health care. The Cold War was over. The political battleground for the next decade and beyond looked to be on domestic terrain. Here was a chance to create a GOP approach that might steal an issue from the

Democrats and heal a troubled health care system with conservative medicine. This, in effect, was what Gradison and Johnson had been asking the White House to do a year earlier.

Unfortunately, the Darman group made a miscalculation that severely damaged the Bush proposal from the start. To extend access to uninsured Americans, the White House decided to rely on tax credits to help low- and middle-income Americans buy private health insurance. This would become a Republican standard. President George W. Bush and Republican candidate John McCain would embrace the same approach. Although less expensive than Democratic proposals, the Darman plan would nevertheless cost the treasury tens of billions of dollars in forgone tax revenues. The Darman team at OMB needed to find the money, and the solution they hit upon was to cut the tax breaks (dating back to the Eisenhower administration) for employer-sponsored health insurance. This was elegant policy—long advocated by economists and OMB policy-wonks of both political parties. But the politics were fatal.

Under the Sununu regime, the Bush White House had not done much consulting with Congress on its health care program, but the amiable Sam Skinner, who replaced Sununu as chief of staff on December 5, 1991, was more open. The day that the Bush budget went to the printer, he invited Representative Bill Gradison to the White House to discuss the president's health proposal. Gradison was extremely knowledgeable on health care issues and had graduate training in economics. The gracious and soft-spoken Ohio Republican did not relish confrontation. But when he heard about the financing plan, he was appalled. Limiting the deductibility of employees' health insurance would outrage large swaths of the working population, including many Reagan Democrats on whose votes Republicans depended. The idea would be dead on arrival, would embarrass the White House and its congressional allies. When White House officials heard that, they literally stopped the presses on the 1993 budget. The offending provisions were snipped out. As a result, the administration missed its budget submission deadline by a day—a delay that went unexplained at the time. Although the administration avoided a political pratfall, it now had a problem: it had released a health plan without explaining where the money would come from. Without a financing mechanism, of course, no one would take the proposal seriously.[48]

No one knew about this problem as the State of the Union address approached. Expectations were high. Even the business community, or at least the press that covered it, anxiously awaited the conservative retort to the Democratic oratory about universal coverage that was getting almost daily coverage as the presidential primaries in New Hampshire and Iowa drew near. On January 20, 1992, *Business Week* ran a story entitled "Health Care: Finally a Pulse at the White House." It went on to comment: "With poll after poll finding that health care has become a top voter concern, President Bush knows he has to offer an election-year response to Democratic cries for action."[49]

That response finally unrolled in two parts. In his State of the Union address, Bush glided over the specifics and outlined the familiar conservative principles—markets would be far more efficient than government. "Really there are only two options. And we can move toward a nationalized system, a system which will restrict patient choice in picking a doctor and force Government to ration services arbitrarily. And what we'll get is patients in long lines, indifferent service and a huge new tax burden. Or we can reform our own private health care system, which still gives us, for all its flaws, the best quality health care in the world. Well, let's build on our strengths."[50]

Details followed, in early February, during a two-day nationwide health care tour with stops in Cleveland, Las Vegas, and San Diego. The trip was meant to sell the Bush plan as a serious, comprehensive response to the Democrats. In Cleveland, on February 6, Bush laid out the four elements of the Bush plan:

- First, tax deductions of up to $3,750 to help low and middle-income Americans buy private health insurance.

- Second, local networks of insurance purchasers would help individuals and small groups to buy cheaper private plans with less administrative overhead. The plan would reform the insurance markets so that insurers could not deny coverage to people with pre-existing illnesses; people would be able to take their plans with them when they moved from one job to another. These insurance market reforms would later become a standard feature of Democratic proposals.

- Third, the Bush plan promised cost savings through malpractice reforms, the elimination of state mandated health insurance benefits, and the use of information technology to improve the efficiency of insurance claims processing. Bush's focus on health information technology continues to the present and reached a new level of emphasis in the Obama administration.

- Fourth, the plan would allow states greater flexibility in their Medicaid programs. Some elements of the Bush maternal and child health proposal would eventually find their way into the State Child Health Insurance Program later in the 1990s.[51]

A February 14 memo from the White House's public affairs and political outreach groups—much atrophied from Reagan-era golden days—sketched the considerable challenges facing the president's proposal: "Until several months ago, the Administration basically avoided becoming involved in the health care debate. Until that time, Public Liaison activities and communication with health care constituency groups revolved around photo opportunities and proclamation signing ceremonies." Now that the president had put a serious plan on the table, the public relations shop had to promote the Bush plan and discredit the Democrats. With the Democrats in control of Congress, the White House public affairs staff braced for the worst-case scenario: "We will need to be prepared in the event that one of the Democratic health care reform bills actually gains momentum.... We do not want the President to be forced to veto a health care reform bill."[52]

The administration's sales team faced more obstacles than merely starting from a dead stop. The press (no doubt alerted by Democratic critics) immediately jumped on the lack of a financing plan and concluded that the Bush plan was mostly about politics—a kind of strategic defense initiative to intercept incoming Democrat plans—rather than a serious attempt to address serious health care issues. The *New York Times* story of February 7 was typical: "President Bush moved today to plug a gap in his election-year domestic plans by proposing several tax incentives and other changes in the law that he said would make quality medical care more affordable." Then, inevitably, it focused on the hole in the plan. "White House aides estimated the plan would cost about $100 billion over ... five years.... Asked today how he would pay for the program, Mr. Bush replied, 'We'll figure that out.'" The headline in the *Baltimore Sun* summed up the standard media spin: "Bush Vague on Financing for Health Care Proposal."[53]

Bush did not help his cause by turning defensive whenever he discussed his proposal. His Cleveland speech spent as much time attacking Democratic proposals as it did promoting his own plan. Of course, blasting big government was a lot simpler then describing his arcane four-point plan Lamented a White House memo, "... the public remains confused and unconvinced that its concerns are adressed in a meaningful way."[54] But it also looked more like a political strategy than a serious proposal because the president treated it like a political strategy. On the other side, the Democratic Congress was not about to cede Bush any quarter on health care—which Democrats considered their issue—during an election year.

Within weeks of the roll-out, the sales team was worried. A March 2 memo from an HHS official to the Bush campaign staff fretted: "We all know that the President's health care reform proposal is right for America. The problem is many Americans don't know yet that the President's plan is right for them.... How do we cut through the clutter and give the President's plan a fair public hearing?"[55]

There was an obvious answer: the president could keep the issue in the public eye. But Bush's interest was waning. As the Washington winter drifted into spring, the staff in health care boiler room expressed frustration over trying to keep their boss's attention on the issue.[56]

It could not have been encouraging for the president's team to hear his response to AP reporter Helen Thomas during an April 10, 1992, press conference. The provocative Thomas asked the president whether his failure to specify financing mechanisms showed that he had given up on health reform. "What does this say," she needled him, "about your leadership and your really caring about these people?" Bush replied patiently that he thought he had a serious plan, that they were working on the financing, but then: "If you're asking me, do I believe a health care program, given the political nature of this year, can get through this year, I'd have to agree with many of the Democratic leaders that it's unlikely."[57]

By early May, public affairs personnel charged with selling the president's plan were complaining to Gail Wilensky, now the White House point person on the health reform initiative, that the president had only given one speech on his plan. We "need to insinuate ourselves into this debate" they told Wilensky. "[It will be] helpful both for reminding the public and POTUS [the president of the United States] about what this means [and for] getting POTUS comfortable with arguments." The frustrated spin-doctors reminded her about the power of the presidency: "The press will write whatever George Bush says. Give them a lead!"[58]

While the public affairs offensive foundered, technicians kept on drafting. Between May and July, the White House staff, with HHS support, produced discrete legislative proposals—on insurance market reform, on malpractice reform, and on promoting health information technology. The strategy of introducing multiple bills—rather than one comprehensive plan—reflected an administration calculation that some proposals were more likely to pass and should be sent up to the Hill first. Moreover, time was short—Democrats were moving their own plans, and Congress would adjourn early for the fall election.[59]

But breaking up the "comprehensive" proposal into multiple pieces made the plan seem less bold and, well, less "comprehensive." Even more damaging to the package, however, was the administration's failure to introduce the most popular part of the reform: expanding access to insurance. Why? Because it could never find a satisfactory financing package. It could not raise taxes without outraging conservatives. It could not cut Medicare or Medicaid without alienating elderly voters and undermining its commitment to maternal and child health. It could not use deficit financing, because the budget deal of 1990 required that any increase in federal outlays be matched with a revenue source—the so-called "pay-as-you-go" (or "pay-go," to the insiders) budgeting rules. The administration ended up with a fragmented and incomplete set of provisions that floated up to Congress between three and five months after the president's February 6 call for comprehensive health care reform.

At Darman's urging, and with the polls showing health care to be a live issue, Bush returned to it in the spring and summer of 1992. On May 13, he went to Johns Hopkins University for, in his words, a "kind of second unveiling of our program."[60] The circumstances were very different from February 1990, his last appearance at Hopkins, when he had almost offhandedly sent Louis Sullivan off to study existing health care studies—thus keeping the whole mess out of his hair. Now, he said without equivocation: "In the greatest, most technologically advanced Nation on the face of the Earth, there is no reason that one of seven Americans has no health insurance. And what we must do is clear. We must guarantee every American access, access to affordable health insurance."[61]

He again spoke to the country on health care in a radio address on July 3. The administration had failed to gain any traction on the issue and by now decided the best way to handle health care reform was to blast Congress for inaction.[62] Bush used the fall of Communism to hit the Democrats: "The biggest story of our time is the failure of socialism and all its empty promises, including nationalized health care and government price setting. But somehow this news that shook the world hasn't seeped through the doors of the Democratic cloakrooms on

Capitol Hill. And that's why I am asking your help. Let's get them the message."[63]

Bush followed up by inviting interest groups that supported his plan to the White House. He and his staff met with congressional leaders, especially Republicans, to broker common positions on health care issues and to urge movement, especially on health insurance market reforms. But the administration was not getting results, either in Washington or with the public. The problem became painfully evident during an August 4 briefing on health care, when Gail Wilensky found herself reminding the press that the president *did* have a comprehensive health proposal before the Congress. A reporter immediately shot back: "Why is it that six months after the comprehensive proposal was made, legislation enabling all of this hasn't been submitted? Why are there any pieces not filled in?" Kevin Moley, the deputy secretary of Health and Human Services, gamely (if not entirely convincingly) blamed the Congress: "I think we have agreed ... that if we believe the Congress were serious by virtue of passing those parts of the President's plan that are before them now ... we would, in fact, tomorrow meet with them on other parts of the President's plan. But they need to act."[64]

For his part, the president never seems to have internalized the details of his own plan. Nor did he ever develop his own "vision" for the nation's health care. This became stunningly clear in the nationally televised presidential debate of October 11, 1992, when moderator Jim Lehrer asked President Bush to respond to Bill Clinton's health proposal. Bush bobbed, weaved, and—barely coherent—finally stumbled back to the solid ground of malpractice:

> Well, I don't have time in 30 seconds or one minute to talk about our health care reform plan. The Oregon plan made some good sense, but it's easy to dismiss the concerns of the disabled. As President, I have to be sure that those waivers which we're approving all over the place are covered under the law. Maybe we can work it out. But the Americans for Disabilities Act, speaking about sound and sensible civil rights legislation, was the foremost piece of legislation passed in modern times. So we do have something more than a technical problem. Governor Clinton clicked off the things: You've got to take on insurance companies and bureaucracies. He failed to take on somebody else, the malpractice suit people, those that bring these lawsuits against—these frivolous trial lawyers' lawsuits that are running costs of medical care up by $25 billion to $50 billion. He refuses to put anything—controls on these crazy lawsuits.[65]

One can imagine Bush's health care team cringing in front of their televisions. Given a shot at putting his administration's health care ideas before a huge and attentive audience, Bush reacted like a deer in the head-lights. We do not know whether his management of health care reform—on October 11, 1992, or in the preceding four years—contributed to his defeat. But it seems clear that Bush's stumble in the debate exemplified a larger and more important missed opportunity during his White House years.

## The Lost Opportunity

Both Eisenhower and Nixon offered the nation a Republican vision for making a flawed health care system more equitable and efficient. Each rejected the Democrats' reliance on regulation and government-sponsored health insurance; each aimed to make private insurance more affordable and the health care delivery system more efficient. George Bush, the kindler, gentler conservative, might have carried this legacy into a new era by bridging the traditional Republican attitudes of his native Northeast with the more ardent conservatism of his adopted Southwest. The health care system had deteriorated since Nixon's time, and the rightward tide in national politics had turned Nixon's approach—mandating employer insurance—into a Democratic strategy that was now unacceptable to Republicans. The GOP needed a new approach. Bush seemed well positioned to construct that synthesis and equip his party with a new health strategy.

To be sure, Bush faced serious obstacles: big deficits and Democratic majorities. But as Bill Gradison and Nancy Johnson had argued in their December 1990 letter to John Sununu, there was much Republicans could do to improve the health care system without spending a lot of money. Besides, history was running the Republicans' way: the GOP had won five out of the last six presidential elections. And it would snatch both chambers of Congress in 1994.

In fact, once Bush turned his staff loose to work on health care, some of the ideas that bubbled up proved remarkably prescient. For the most part, the innovative proposals involved ways to make the health care system more efficient. Roger Porter casually mentioned, in November 1990, the possibility of applying industrial quality management approaches to health care delivery. Today the idea enjoys widespread, bipartisan endorsement.

Another briefing document, dated April, 10, 1992, anticipated the potential of health information technology to empower health care consumers and to transform health care systems. "True efficiencies ... will come from automation of clinical information.... The single most important way to improve quality of care is to provide the public with information that allows them to compare the quality of different providers. This will create consumer demand for quality. However, automation of clinical information is needed in order to provide the raw data on which to base a thorough analysis of quality."[66] The paragraph could have been ripped from George W. Bush's 2008 health care playbook. The younger Bush would make health information technology and consumer empowerment major priorities for his administration, harnessing these forces in his bid to rewrite both government health programs and private health insurance markets. And Barak Obama, the first president elected while tapping on his BlackBerry, would pile even higher expectations on the power of information technology to transform medical care.

Still another enduring contribution of the George H.W. Bush administration lay in the idea of reforming individual and small group insurance markets. Both Democrats and Republicans would return to the idea of creating networks that might give small groups more power in negotiating with insurance companies. This idea now enjoys wide bipartisan support, and was a linchpin of the ambitious 2006 Massachusetts health reform.

In fact, observers who took the time to look closely at the ideas that the Bush administration finally sent to Capitol Hill often came away surprised and impressed. On August 2, 1992, even the *New York Times* editorialized that the Bush plan was "smart, in places ingenious," even as it criticized it for not providing universal coverage.[67]

However, despite its innovative ideas, the Bush administration never managed to fully develop, package, or sell its proposal. It began to work on the reform far too late. An earlier start might have given the team time to ferret out the landmines, such as its politically unrealistic financing scheme. The administration was also burdened by an overly insular policy process run by an agency normally preoccupied with budget affairs: the Office of Management and Budget. And, most important, the president never embraced—or tried to sell—his administration's proposal. As we have seen in every chapter, health care reform rarely gets very far without leadership, vision, and passion from the Oval Office.

Richard Nixon, flawed as he was, would likely have appreciated Bush's opportunity—snatch FDR's lost reform from the Democrats just like Nixon himself had grabbed the South from the Democrats or like Bill Clinton would steal welfare reform from the Republicans. But George Bush never grasped the possibility. He was a tactician, not a strategist—fiercely competitive, but without a defining dream. He didn't go for the long bomb in domestic policy; the running game would always do. Yankee to his roots, he didn't like selling. His terrible personal loss never translated into a particular concern about the health care of others. George H. W. Bush would have much preferred to ignore the arcane matter of health care reform. That was always clear to his frustrated aides, and eventually it became clear to the public—and to the Democrats who seized the issue and used it to hammer the president during the election of 1992.

Neither George Bush nor Jimmy Carter moved the ball on health care reform during their single-term administrations. They exemplified a breed of president who, although competent and fundamentally well-intended, regards health care as more trouble than it is worth. To make progress on this issue, presidents need more than intelligence and diligence. They need the full range of political and rhetorical skills. They need to work the Washington machinery and move the people. And, perhaps most important, they need the deep emotional understanding of human suffering that leads them to take big risks and make hard choices when the time for decision arrives.

# CHAPTER 10

# Bill Clinton

*Kicking the Can down the Road*

They'll always have 1993–94. The memories burn deep in the psyches of health reformers: months of soaring anticipation, elation, dread, defeat, and despair. Like a bewitched talisman, the story of Clinton health care reform remains hot to the touch, radiating hope and warning for the next time. In 1993 and 1994, everything was possible. And so was nothing.

At the center of it all stood William Jefferson Clinton, the kid from Hope whose incandescent talent rocketed him from a nightmarish childhood to the Oval Office. This was his story. He promised health reform, he managed the process, and he owned the outcome. Not since LBJ had one man's obsession with health care so arrested the nation. And not since Jimmy Carter had a president failed so ignominiously to deliver.

Of course, the events of 1993–94 reflected forces well beyond the personality, talents, and flaws of a single man. It was all there: the changing nature of the presidency and the Congress, interest groups gorged with money from a bloated health system, a skittish public, a conservative tide in American politics. The fascination of Clinton health care reform stems in no small part from the richness of the story which, in many ways, is the capstone to presidential health care policymaking during the twentieth century. Textured as it is, however, the story and its lessons must start where Clinton health reform began: in the heart and mind of the forty-second president of the United States.

## WILLIAM JEFFERSON CLINTON

Senator Jay Rockefeller (D-WV) had his own take on Bill Clinton: "He's the first person who's ever been president of the United States who was an abused child. If you are an abused child, you can withdraw into yourself, be angry, be vicious. Or you can want everyone to like you. Obviously, he's of the second school."[1]

Actually, Bill Clinton was not the only president who suffered child abuse—Nixon was also a victim, at least by modern standards—but there is little question that Clinton lived a harrowing childhood that powerfully influenced his adult behavior. His early years vividly illustrated the underbelly of rural American life.

### Sin and Redemption

Clinton's mother had terrible taste in men. His biological father, William Jefferson Blythe Jr. (after whom Bill was named), died in a car accident three months before Clinton's birth on August 19, 1946. In June 1993, on his first Father's Day in the White House, the *Washington Post* sent him a memorable gift—investigative reports documenting that Blythe, only twenty-eight when he died, had been married twice before he wedded Clinton's mother, Virginia. Neither mother nor son had any idea. Clinton had two half-siblings he'd never heard of: Leon Ritzenhaler, a retired "owner of a janitorial service" in Northern California, and Sharon Pettijohn, born in Kansas City in 1941.[2]

Blythe grew up dirt-poor in Texas, but he had grand ambitions. He worked hard, resolved to leave farming behind, and became an auto parts salesman traveling the South. He was a natural. His sister remembered him: "I think that's why he was such a good salesman. He never saw a stranger."[3] Hard work, fierce drive, a way with words, a way with women—all traits that would reappear in the son Blythe never knew.

In his memoir, Clinton reflected on the effects of growing up without a father: "My father left me with the feeling that I had to live for two people, and that if I did it well enough, somehow I could make up for the life he should have had. And his memory infused me, at a younger age than most, with a sense of my own mortality.... Even when I wasn't sure where I was going, I was always in a hurry."[4] The feelings are eerily reminiscent of the musings of Richard Nixon's mother about the effect of losing his brothers; he, too, thought he had to live for two (and later three) people. In any case, Clinton grew into an impatient, ambitious man, prone to leaping before he looked.[5]

When Clinton was about a year old, Virginia Blythe left him with her parents while she studied to be a nurse anesthetist in New Orleans. He found himself in another troubled household. He remembers his grandfather as a benign, loving man, but his grandmother, also a nurse, was tempestuous, "full of anger and disappointment and obsessions she only dimly understood. She took it out in raging tirades against my grandfather and my mother ... though I was shielded from most of them."[6] Most but not all. For the young child there was no tranquil haven.

When Virginia returned she came with baggage: Roger Clinton, "a handsome, hell-raising, twice-divorced man from Hot Springs, Arkansas."[7] They married in 1950 and moved to Hot Springs, which was very different from sedate Hope. Hot Springs embodied many of the contradictions that would permeate Clinton's character and behavior—sin and redemption lived in congenial proximity.[8] Named for its sulfurous waters and bathhouses, Hot Springs was a vacation and gambling town with casinos, bars, resorts, prostitutes, and the Mob. For fun, Clinton and his friends would call the local bordello, Maxine's, tying up the line to frustrate "the real customers." At the same time there were the churches, including Clinton's Park Place Baptist Church, where the future president was baptized and regularly attended Sunday School and services.[9] John Harris sums it up nicely: in Hot Springs, "Clinton learned that decent pious people could have all manner of private weaknesses."[10]

Though Clinton remembers his stepfather as kind and loving toward him, he was a binge drinker who turned vicious when he drank. Clinton recalls stories that could have come straight from the police blotter: "One night ... they were screaming at each other in their bedroom.... For some reason, I walked out into the hall to the doorway of the bedroom. Just as I did, Daddy pulled a gun from behind his back and fired in Mother's direction. The bullet went into the wall between where she and I were standing. I was stunned and so scared.... The police were called. I can still see them leading Daddy away in handcuffs."[11]

Like so many children of domestic violence, Clinton eventually had to take a stand. He was fourteen, and large for his age. Typically, he acted partly to protect a younger sibling: "One night Daddy closed the door to his bedroom, started screaming at Mother, then began to hit her. Little Roger was scared, just as I had been nine years earlier on the night of the gunshot. Finally, I couldn't bear the thought of Mother being hurt and Roger being frightened anymore. I grabbed a golf club ... and threw open their door. Mother was on the floor and Daddy was standing over her, beating on her. I told him to stop and said that if he didn't I was going to beat the hell out of him.... He just caved."[12]

If the men in Clinton's nuclear family were dangerous and disappointing, Bill never saw the women that way. Like Richard Nixon, he idolized his mother, whom he saw as strong and loving: "I don't know how Mother handled it all as well as she did. Every morning, no matter what had happened the night before, she got up and put her game face on. And what a face it was. From the time she came back home from New Orleans ... I loved sitting on the floor of the bathroom and watching her put makeup on that beautiful face.... Until I was eleven or twelve she had long dark wavy hair.... I liked watching her brush it until it was just so."[13]

Today, Bill Clinton's childhood of violence and alcoholism might have played out differently—with restraining orders, indictments, imprisonment, shelters, substance abuse treatment. But in 1950s Arkansas, the family was mostly on its own, and domestic violence became Bill Clinton's secret. Virginia divorced her husband in 1962 but then fell for his entreaties and remarried him a few months later.[14] Bill seems to have first confronted the psychological legacy of his early experiences after his half-brother Roger was arrested for dealing cocaine in 1984, when Clinton was governor of Arkansas. Roger had much of his father (Roger Clinton) in him: "a good-times fellow, gold-chained and open-collared ... the gregarious and unreliable 'dude,' surviving on guile and charm."[15] (One might argue that Bill Clinton, too, had sipped from the same cup.) The arrest, according to Maraniss, led to a "period of intense introspection" for Clinton, and his first experience with family counseling together with his brother and mother. He later told a friend: "We learned a lot about how you do a lot of damage to yourself if you're living with an alcoholic and you just sort of deny that behavior and deflect it all. You pay a big price for that."[16]

## Brilliant—and Blind

By the time he confronted his childhood ghosts, Clinton had already transcended them—at least on the surface that he showed in public. He had coped with his early experiences through compulsive, almost maniacal efforts to attract the love of everyone around him—by running for office. And he succeeded, thanks to the Bill Clinton mix: extraordinary gifts, terrific ambition, and raw need.

There was first of all his brainpower. He excelled in school, often effortlessly. His talents won him admission to Georgetown University, then a Rhodes scholarship, and paved the way for Yale Law School, where he mastered the curriculum with a fraction of the effort that his talented classmates expended. In his first semester, he hardly went to class, instead working on the losing senatorial campaign of Connecticut Democrat Joseph Duffy. For exams, he borrowed classmates' notes and performed brilliantly. Said one classmate: "He was very quick. I would love to know how fast he could read. He would get through more in an hour of concentrated effort than just about anybody I've ever seen. And he never slept much. If he slept more than four hours and a half a night, I'd be surprised."[17]

Arthur Schlesinger Jr., who had known many presidents, would later say of him: "He is a man of penetrating intelligence. He has impressive technical mastery of complicated issues. He has genuine intellectual curiosity and listens as well as talks."[18]

The ability to listen was another unique trait. Clinton's Arkansas background exposed him to the tradition of southern storytelling, which helped shape a curiosity not just about ideas and issues, but about people. "All my kinfolks could tell a story, making simple events, encounters, and mishaps involving ordinary people come alive with drama and laughter.... I learned that everyone has a story—of dreams and nightmares, hope and heartache, love and loss, courage and fear, sacrifice and selfishness. All my life I've been interested in other people's stories. I've wanted to know them, understand them, feel them."[19]

Clinton's empathy was not feigned—its targets found it magnetic, absorbing, an essential element of his charisma. But he also used it as a tool. Underneath the empathy lurked a hard edge of ambition and self-absorption. His Rhodes Scholar classmate, John Issacson, later said: "People would say he was a great listener, and he was in a way, but you were on Bill's topics when you were with Bill. Not that he didn't have a lot of topics, but you were working in Bill's territory. Big territory, but his territory. He was capable of keeping it that way. I was frustrated and awed by it. I was aware of it as a source of power. He was smart and morally earnest, and also a bullshitter who told stories."[20]

Like so many other future presidents, Clinton projected a preternatural certainty about his own abilities and his future success. It was the kind of thing that undoubtedly set teeth on edge. He told a coworker in the Duffy campaign: "As soon as I get out of school, I'm moving back to Arkansas. I love Arkansas. I'm going back there to live. I'm gonna run for office there. And someday I'm gonna be governor. And then one day I'll be callin' ya, Billie, and tellin' ya I'm running for president and I need your help."[21]

Some of this was undoubtedly bravado, papering over deep insecurity. One of his close friends and gubernatorial aides, Betsey Wright, commented: "There's a terrible insecurity there! It's huge! And that in some ways defines Bill Clinton, counter to his intellect—which is the other way that defines Bill Clinton!"[22] But that insecurity drove him. Though depressed after electoral defeats in college and again after his reelection bid for governor in 1980, he had the emotional resilience to learn from them. In 1982 he became the first defeated Arkansas governor to regain the office—remaking his (and Hillary Clinton's) image in the process.

Clinton's success in Arkansas politics was remarkable, but also deceptive. Little Rock was a small world. Once he got the hang of it, Clinton dominated it with one hand tied behind his back. Harris writes: "In Arkansas, he had governed by instinct and spontaneity.... Of all the illusions he carried to the presidency, the greatest might have been this failure to appreciate the distance between the statehouse and the White House."[23] Jimmy Carter, another Democratic governor, drew the same treacherous analogy to politics in Atlanta. Like Carter, Clinton was ill-prepared for the presidency—he had never managed a task so big. He did not know the Congress, the Washington bureaucracy, or the national press. He was suspicious of the Washington establishment, an attitude that Hillary shared and cultivated. They saw themselves—and ran their campaign—as outsiders who could conquer Washington and clean up, as Harris puts it, "a capital cluttered by special interests, cynics and hacks." Bill and Hillary knew that the dark, entrenched powers had to be defeated before they could win their progressive reforms.[24]

But they were playing in a different league and their own success and brilliance blinded them. Donna Shalala, Clinton's long-serving secretary of Health and Human Services, would later say: "Bill and Hillary came from Arkansas where they were always used to being the smartest people in the room.... So they naturally assumed they were the smartest people in the room in Washington, too. Anyone who had any different idea than they had was dismissed as part of the system, and part of the problem."[25]

There was also a distinctly rebellious streak. Clinton had seen the other side of Hot Springs and he liked to play the bad boy.

During college, he spent one summer driving Senator William Fulbright (D-AR), for whom he was working, around Arkansas. He fought with Fulbright so obstinately that Fulbright eventually kicked him out of the car. He procrastinated too, tempting the fates.[26] While teaching constitutional law at the University of Arkansas Law School, his first job out of Yale, he wrote most of the final exam at the front of the room while his students labored over the first question. His affinity for chaos had a distinct advantage—it put him in the vortex, and left him in control. Only Clinton, it seemed, was smart enough to clean up the messes he was constantly creating.

Indeed, Bill Clinton had an almost unprecedented ability to live with contradiction: to cultivate it, profit from it, and enjoy it. Bobbing and weaving were skills he had learned early. He was insecure but brash, empathetic but narcissistic, brilliant but intellectually facile. He cherished success but courted disaster. Even in policymaking, he was drawn to contradiction and complexity. He was a southern Democrat—which, by the 1980s, was fast becoming an oxymoron. He looked for a third way in politics that shunned both big government and unfettered markets.[27] Jimmy Carter had started down this path, fighting (unsuccessfully) the liberal Democratic establishment. Clinton, an infinitely more talented politician, took it the next step. He was active in the Democratic Leadership Council (DLC), an organization designed to restore the Democratic Party's fortunes by pushing it toward centrist policies that southerners might live with.[28] He was genuinely skeptical of taxes and regulation, but not of government, which he felt should be both smaller and more activist; public policies, he thought, should be different, new, and unprecedented. This infatuation with combining seemingly contradictory political ideas into some dazzling new package would powerfully shape Clinton's health policy agenda.[29]

### SIX BUSHELS OF FRESH PEACHES

Why did Clinton headline health care policy? He didn't have to, and he would later come to regret it. As we shall see, one reason was calculated—he saw controlling health care spending as key to achieving his economic agenda. But there are also telltale hints in his background that suggest a special affinity for medicine and health.

To start with, his mother, like Jimmy Carter's, was a nurse. This introduced him early in childhood to the health care system of his time and place, and his reaction was much less ambivalent than Carter's. Clinton recalls:

> I loved going to the hospital to visit her, meeting the nurses and doctors, watching them care for people. I got to watch an actual operation once, when I was in junior high.... I was fascinated by the work surgeons do and thought I might like to do it myself one day. Mother took a lot of interest in her patients, whether they could pay or not. In the days before Medicare and Medicaid, there were a lot who couldn't. I remember one poor, proud man coming to our door one day to settle his account. He was a fruit picker who paid Mother with six bushels of fresh peaches. We ate those peaches for a long time.[30]

Illness would also play an important part in his life. He was, of course, surrounded by substance abuse and its penumbra of mental illness and violence. But that probably did not register as a health problem for a southern male of that era, even one as smart as the young Clinton. There was no escaping, however, the repeated physical illnesses of some of his closest relatives. His grandmother, whom he called "Mammaw," was struck first when Clinton was about nine years old. "Mammaw's stroke was a major one, and in the aftermath she was racked by hysterical screaming. Unforgivably, to calm her down, her doctor prescribed morphine, lots of it.... Her behavior became even more irrational ... and in desperation Mother reluctantly committed her to the state's mental hospital ... it was bedlam.... Her problem gave me my first exposure to the kind of mental-health system that served most of America back then."[31]

His grandfather suffered from lung disease, and later his stepfather, Roger, contracted mouth and throat cancer, for which alcohol abuse is a major risk factor. The bills for his father's medical treatments started coming due about when Clinton left Hot Springs for college at Georgetown. He feared that the family wouldn't be able to pay his college costs and rejoiced when he got a job as a clerk for Fulbright: "I had worried about how they could afford Daddy's medical treatments on top of the costs of Georgetown. Though I never told anyone at the time, I was afraid I'd have to leave Georgetown and come home, where college was so much less expensive. Now, out of the blue, I had the chance to stay on at Georgetown and work for the Foreign Relations Committee."[32]

The cancer defied local doctors, and in 1967, Roger Clinton went to Duke Medical Center in Durham, North Carolina for advanced treatment. Clinton drove down to visit: "Every weekend I would drive the 266 miles from Georgetown to see him, leaving Friday afternoon, returning late Sunday night.... It was one of the most exhausting but important times of my young life.... On those weekends, Daddy talked to me in a way he never had before."[33]

Treatment failed, and later that year, Bill Clinton returned home for his stepfather's final moments. "Daddy's last days brought a classic country deathwatch into our house. Family and friends streamed in and out to offer their sympathy.... It was raining the day of the funeral. Often, when I was a boy, Daddy would stare out the window into a storm and say, 'Don't bury me in the rain.'"[34]

Virginia Clinton had survived two husbands. She would outlive one more. After Roger's death, she married Jeff Dewire, a diabetic who died in his sleep in 1974. Diabetes is a powerful risk factor for heart disease, which often causes sudden death. Clinton would have other exposures to diabetes: "It subsequently killed my 1974 campaign chairman, George Shelton. It afflicts two children of my friend and former chief of staff Erskine Bowles.... That's a big reason why, as President, I supported stem cell research and a diabetes self care program."[35]

Bill Clinton knew first-hand both the personal and financial effects that illness could have on families. The effect may have been greater because his mother was so often the indirect victim—losing her own mother and two husbands to disease while Clinton was still young. She was the one constant in his life, a strong woman struggling with abuse, professional and family obligations, death, and loss. Later, another strong woman's passion for health care issues would sharpen Bill Clinton's affinity for the daunting challenge of health care reform.

Nor was the substance of health care policy foreign to the future president. He had taken up health issues at several points along his political journey. During an unsuccessful run for Congress in 1974, he supported national health insurance. In his first term as governor in 1978, he tried to tackle the poor quality of and limited access to care in rural Arkansas. He fought off local physicians, won federal funds, and opened four rural clinics staffed primarily by nurse practitioners.[36] In a notable preview of things to come, he appointed Hillary to chair a rural health advisory committee. All this introduced him to the political perils of health care reform. Arkansas physicians lined up with his enemies, called for his resignation, and helped to defeat him in his first reelection bid.

During that first gubernatorial term, he also got a glimpse at the electricity the issue could generate. In December 1978 the Democratic Party convened a midterm convention in Memphis, Tennessee. Ted Kennedy (D-MA) and Jimmy Carter had been stomping about the Democratic ring, testing each other like sumo wrestlers. A Kennedy primary challenge to Carter was in the air. The main issue was Kennedy's frustration over Carter's health care policy, and the featured event of the convention was a health care panel, on which Kennedy would debate Secretary of HEW Joe Califano, representing the Carter administration. To moderate, the party turned to the newly elected Democratic governor from Arkansas. Clinton drew lessons from the masters: "Califano was articulate in his defense of the President's more incremental approach to health-care reform, but Kennedy won the crowd with an emotional plea for ordinary Americans to have the same coverage that his wealth provided for his son, Teddy, when he got cancer." Clinton added the inevitable bottom line—"I enjoyed the national exposure."[37] There were memorable lessons: health care could be a big-time issue, and bold policy trumped wonky incrementalism.

Speaking of Clinton's attraction to health care, Rockefeller would later observe: "Health care expressed not only his youth, but expressed his success—he cut the infant mortality rate in half in Arkansas—and expressed his love of people. It's basic. It combines everything."[38]

When Bill Clinton bulled his way onto the national stage during the 1991 primary season, not many voters would fathom the complicated mix of talent and weakness that he brought with him. He was brilliant, politically gifted, charming, supremely confident, charismatic. He was also undisciplined, insecure, impulsive, narcissistic, untrustworthy, and self-destructive. He could inspire a hall full of skeptical union members into a standing ovation one moment and then go on television to bob and weave around a tawdry sexual dalliance in the next. He liked playing with fire. And few issues burned as hot—or spoke to the many sides of Bill Clinton—as health care reform.

HEALTH CARE REFORM

When Clinton began his run for the White House, health care issues were firmly on the national agenda. Even George H. W. Bush had groped for a plan after underdog Harris Wofford—promising health care for all—won the special 1991 Senate election in Pennsylvania. Predictably, the Democratic primary became a kind of echo chamber, amplifying the venerable liberal call to spread health care coverage to the uninsured. But not every party member signed up for the crusade. Senator Jay Rockefeller, for one, advised candidate Clinton that the issue of coverage was overplayed and lacked political punch. The public, he thought, was more concerned about the rising costs that directly touched middle-class Americans.[39]

### The 1992 Campaign

But in the heat of a primary, the pressures on Democrats to have a health plan covering all Americans were virtually irresistible. Clinton committed right from the start—in the Little Rock speech announcing his bid for the presidency.[40] But he did not detail a plan, and his rivals were soon pushing him to get specific. Senator Robert Kerrey (D-NE) proposed a single-payer plan. Paul Tsongas, a former Massachusetts senator (ill with lymphoma himself), touted a new formulation that emphasized "managed competition" as a way to make the health system more efficient.

On January 19, 1992, in a New Hampshire primary debate, Clinton spoke again of his commitment to universal health coverage and expressed support for a so-called "pay-or-play" approach to financing expanded coverage. This would require that employers either play (provide insurance to their workers) or pay (contribute to a national fund that would purchase insurance for workers when their companies did not.) Clinton had thrown the position together hastily with the advice of a domestic aide and Hillary Clinton, but it had a long political provenance and was on the shelf, ready to go. Its roots dated back to Richard Nixon's Comprehensive Health Insurance Plan, which would have required all employers to insure their employees. Pay-or-play was a variation on the employer responsibility theme. It enjoyed the support of the congressional Democratic leadership and had been endorsed by a highly visible 1990 congressional policy committee, the Pepper–Rockefeller Commission.[41]

However, for months Clinton resisted the pressure to flesh out the details.[42] This may have reflected political wisdom: though good primary politics, a very specific health care proposal leaves candidates open to attack during elections. Clinton's political advisors routinely counseled him to stay as general as he could. The same political team had guided Wofford into the Senate without ever getting bogged down in the specifics of the promised health plan.[43]

But Clinton's delay also seems to have reflected division, both within the campaign and in his own mind. And, of course, there was Clinton's inveterate tendency to procrastinate in making difficult decisions. One group of advisors, representing the Democratic mainstream, supported pay-or-play as a way of financing universal coverage; they were willing to pay the hard political price—raise taxes or regulate health care prices—to generate the necessary funds. A second group, however, pushed for an alternative to this traditional liberal, protax, proregulatory approach. They pushed for managed competition, an idea that dated back to 1976, when Joseph Califano had tasked a Stanford University economist named Alain Enthoven to develop a private-sector approach to health system reform.[44]

Managed competition would work, according to its advocates, by promoting competition among health care plans (the Kaiser Permanent Plan was the archetype). Consumers, choosing among multiple health plans, would drive costs down without the political pain of raising taxes or forcing employers to pay or play (which economists condemned as a hidden tax on business). To be sure, the competition had to be regulated—or managed—to prevent abuses; for example, the contending health plans had to be stopped from cherrypicking healthy patients. But, properly governed, managed competition might make health care affordable so that more businesses would offer it; the government could cover the remaining uninsured using the savings that managed competition generated for Medicare and Medicaid. At the end of the managed competition road, some advocates perceived a kind of health care nirvana—universal coverage paid for not by taxes or regulation, but rather by the magic of the markets. Competition, wisely overseen by impartial officials, would flush wasteful dollars right out of the health care system, solving the age-old cost problem and making it simple to cover everyone.

Within the Clinton camp, the managed competition group included Ira Magaziner, a former Rhodes Scholar classmate of Clinton and a Rhode Island business consultant. Assisting Magaziner was a brilliant young medical student named Atul Gawande, who had worked on a managed competition proposal for another southern Democratic Congressman, James Cooper (D-TN).

After Clinton secured the nomination, President Bush began attacking his vaguely defined commitment to the pay-or-play approach as a tax increase and began hectoring him as just another big-government, tax-and-spend liberal. The last thing this New Democrat wanted was to be tarred with the traditional big-government brush. He needed to deflect the fire; he needed a new approach.

In August 1992, Gawande and Magaziner organized a series of meetings with outside advisors, representing both traditional Democratic stalwarts and the new managed competition crowd. Recognizing the political vulnerabilities associated with pay-or-play, as well as the preferred access Magaziner and Gawande enjoyed to Clinton, the Washington group retreated and embraced what Hacker would call a "new liberal synthesis" ideally designed to appeal to Clinton's affinity for innovative policies that harnessed seemingly conservative methods to win progressive goals. Ira Magaziner, Atul Gawande, and Paul Starr, a Pulitzer Prize–winning Princeton sociologist who had recently cofounded the liberal *American Prospect* magazine, refined the concept of managed competition. Their health plan would organize a new regime of competing managed care organizations. The competition would be orchestrated and controlled by the federal government to assure that it was fair and that the desired savings were achieved. To assure universal coverage, the plan advocated an employer mandate—all businesses would have to insure their employees. The implicit tax of pay-or-play disappeared, but insurance for all—the liberal mantra—remained.[45]

For Clinton, avoiding new taxes was absolutely critical. Based on interviews with multiple Clinton aides, political scientists Lawrence Jacobs and Robert Shapiro contend that Clinton saw health reform first and foremost as a way to control health costs, reduce the federal deficit, and spur economic growth. The humanitarian and political benefits were a welcome dividend. Any proposal that increased spending on health care—even to cover the uninsured—was a nonstarter, and increasing taxes to cover those costs was just salt on the wound. Clinton, they argue, would never have gone down the health reform road had he known what he subsequently learned—that there was no painless way to finance universal coverage.[46]

Gawande and Magaziner presented the new vision to Bill Clinton in East Lansing, Michigan, on September 22, 1992. They brought along skeptics of managed competition, including Judy Feder, a Georgetown political scientist who had written the Pepper–Rockefeller pay-or-play report. The Democratic health policy elite appeared to have coalesced around a dramatic, innovative approach to health care reform. Clinton bought it.

On September 24, at the headquarters of the pharmaceutical giant Merck and Co., Clinton unveiled his plan. At his side were Harris

Wofford, the Pennsylvania champion of universal coverage, and Jay Rockefeller, cochair of the Pepper–Rockefeller commission—more apparent evidence of party solidarity behind Clinton's New Democratic health care plan. Clinton continued to glide over possibly controversial details, such as precisely what requirements the government might place on competing managed care organizations, and exactly how the predicted savings would be accomplished. Secretly, advocates of the pay-or-play approach within the Clinton camp doubted that such savings were possible in the short run. They believed, the federal government would have to raise new monies to cover the uninsured. But the lure of a bold "third way," Clinton's skepticism of traditional liberal nostrums, and Magaziner's access to Clinton doomed efforts of the "Washington" clique to make this case to Clinton.[47]

The new position made for perfect campaign optics. Managed competition was new, vague, and almost impervious to effective Republican attack. It sounded market-oriented and regulatory at the same time. It promised conservatives savings and liberals universal coverage. In the October debates with Bush, it left the Republican spluttering. And it would provide president Clinton with an apparent mandate to do something dramatic about health care. Precisely what, however, was still not clear.

### The Transition

Bill Clinton won with only 43 percent of the vote, a shaky base for what he hoped would be a dramatic, reform-oriented presidency.[48] Where health care was concerned, his management of the crucial transition period—from election to inauguration—only further undermined the administration's weak foundations.

During the campaign, Clinton had promised a health care plan in one hundred days—the FDR legacy was haunting still another American president. Clinton's team recognized that this was a formidable challenge—one that left them both excited and anxious. To take it on, Clinton's advisors commissioned a transition task force to prepare a health care proposal for the new administration. Atul Gawande and Judy Feder led the group,[49] and tensions between new and traditional Democrats, between managed competition and tax-or-regulate immediately reemerged.[50]

Absorbed with staffing his Cabinet, Clinton and his inner circle of aides offered virtually no guidance to the team. The transition team aimed to produce a 150–200-page document, halfway between legislation and a set of principles, and fleshed out options for unveiling it at either fifty or one hundred days. They knew speed was essential.

In early January, however, Feder and her staff learned from Magaziner that he had been working on health care for Clinton's economic transition group. Other rumors circulated that Magaziner had organized his own shadow health care transition team, although he flatly denied this. Hearing that an economic policy meeting scheduled for January 10 in Little Rock would be dealing with health care budget issues, Feder— still isolated from the Little Rock inner circle—lobbied fiercely to be included so that the health care group could present its own findings. She finally secured an opportunity to brief the president-elect on how his health care plan was evolving.

The January 10 meeting convened in the dining room of the governor's mansion, where about thirty top advisors squeezed in around the table and along the walls. All the key economic advisors to the president attended—Robert Rubin, Lawrence Summers, Robert Reich—and Hillary Clinton. Vice President–elect Gore and Secretary of HHS– designate Donna Shalala were also there. The transition health team included Feder; Gawande; Ken Thorpe, a young health economist; and Stuart Altman, who had featured so prominently in Richard Nixon and Wilbur Mill's near miss at health reform in 1973–74. The health team had been told to present their plan from a budgetary perspective— focusing on its economic effect. Thorpe, the group's economic modeler, did most of the talking. They had concluded, he said, that the savings from managed competition would not cover the costs of insuring uncovered Americans, at least for the foreseeable future. Thorpe, Feder, and Altman were all skeptics of the managed care approach (Washington rumors had, for a time, charged that Feder was trying to nudge the administration toward regulating payment rates—the classic old Democratic approach). Now, the team delivered their bad news. Even if it was successful, it would take years for competing managed care organizations to fundamentally change the efficiency of health care delivery. Meantime, as much as $100 billion in new revenues would be needed to cover the uninsured and all the benefits promised as part of the campaign's health platform. The transition group provided a range of cost-control options that might cut into that number, including price controls and managed competition.

Clinton was not happy. These, he said, were the biggest numbers he had ever seen. One of Rubin's aides volunteered that there were innovative approaches (presumably managed competition) to reduce the new expenditures. Hillary Clinton and Stuart Altman had a brief exchange in which Altman, citing his long experience in policy development, stated emphatically that radical revision of the insurance system, of the type contemplated by managed competition advocates, was politically impossible. Magaziner pointedly disagreed. If other nations provided universal insurance at far less expense, then America could do it too.[51]

At this point, Clinton adjourned the meeting. He had heard enough. This was traditional, backward-looking, stuck-in-the-mud, liberal Democratic thinking. This was what he had been elected to purge from Washington. There had to be a better way. "She [Feder] got crushed. They were furious at her," Jay Rockefeller, a Feder confidant, later told Johnson and Broder.[52] The two reporters concluded: "[I]nstead of heeding the message, he [Clinton] sent the messenger home in disgrace."[53]

After the meeting, the transition group waited more than an hour in an airport van for Rubin, who was to accompany them back to Washington. He had stayed behind to confer with Clinton. When he joined them, Rubin, no fan of Magaziner, unhappily announced a new presidential decision. Henceforth, Magaziner was running health policy development. Feder would ultimately be banished from the inner circle of advisors, and later secured a job on the periphery of policy-making working for Donna Shalala. Having sided with the Feder group, Gawande, too, was now on the outs, and returned to medical school after a brief stint working for Shalala at HHS. Altman returned to Brandeis University. A group with deep health policy experience on both sides of the political aisle was sent packing while the consultant who promised his buddy a brand new health policy mousetrap was in charge.

Still the one hundred–day deadline loomed. After dismissing the transition team, Clinton had no detailed health care plan to present to the nation—or to submit to Congress. In 1965, LBJ had had the King–Anderson proposal ready to go on Inauguration Day. It became H.R. 1 and S. 1. It needed work—LBJ knew that—but to him, the details didn't matter; he had been hectoring Wilbur Mills (D-AR) to work them out for over a year and had dispatched Wilbur Cohen to help him. Now, Clinton needed a health care proposal fast, and to this brilliant, intellectually restless, former Rhodes Scholar, the details did matter—a lot. In a decision that would haunt his legacy, his wife's political career, the fortunes of the Democratic party, and the history of health reform, he turned to Ira Magaziner and Hillary Clinton to jump-start health care reform. Magaziner would be Mr. Inside—running the day-to-day policy development. Hillary would be Madame Outside—making the case to the public.

The choice of Magaziner reflected Clinton's friendship with the abrasive, eccentric former Rhodes Scholar, as well as Magaziner's assurances that he could develop a radically new solution. Like Clinton, Magaziner had an instinctive affinity for dramatic, convoluted, holistic policy proposals. As Johnson and Broder put it: "Boldness and complexity were hallmarks of his work."[54] Magaziner had been a business consultant and had no links to the Washington establishment—two other attributes that undoubtedly appealed to the New Democrat heading to the White House. Of course, when it came to managing the most complex political issue on the president's agenda, lack of Washington experience would have its downsides.

We cannot see through the mists of the Clintons' relationship and explain exactly why Bill chose Hillary to codirect the reform effort. The decision was unprecedented—no first lady had ever assumed such a substantive role. But times were changing. Hillary Clinton had made it clear that she was not going to bake cookies in the White House's overstaffed kitchen. And she was brilliant, articulate, shrewd, hard-driving, and much better organized than her husband. She had run similar task forces in Little Rock, including one on health care. Time would also prove that she cared passionately about universal coverage—indeed, the very intensity of her commitment to vulnerable, uninsured Americans could make her appear uncompromising. Clinton could count on her, as he could on few others, to protect his own interests. Rumors also insinuated that Bill had promised Hillary some major leadership role to make up for the accusations of infidelity that nearly swamped his campaign. In his memoirs, Clinton only restates conventional wisdom: "I decided Hillary should lead the health-care effort because she cared and knew a lot about the issue, she had time to do the right job, and I thought she would be able to be an honest broker among all the competing interests.... I knew the whole enterprise was risky: Harry Truman's attempt to provide universal coverage had nearly destroyed his presidency, and Nixon and Carter never even got their bills out of committee."[55]

By turning to Magaziner and his wife, Clinton was also continuing a trend to centralize control of health care policy in the White House. Their power came only from their relationship with the president. Because it was important, Clinton wanted health care policy development under his thumb. Delegating to Feder and company—the Washington establishment—had failed. Turning to Magaziner and Hillary was one way he could keep health care from becoming infected with tired Beltway thinking.[56] The designated secretary of Health and Human Services, Donna Shalala, had little health policy background (she had been president of the University of Wisconsin), and that made it even easier to dismiss HHS as a player in health policy development.

On January 25, Clinton announced that Magaziner and the first lady would lead a new task force to shape his health care proposal. Ultimately its many subgroups would encompass over 600 health care experts, congressional staff, and stakeholder representatives. The task force strategy seems to have had multiple precedents. Hacker traces its roots to the president-elect's Little Rock experience and to Lyndon Johnson's administration. Between 1965 and 1968, Johnson had relied on small, short-lived groups of policy analysts—very different from what the Clinton process would become—drawn from within and outside the Washington establishment, to develop new policy initiatives. Under Johnson's guidance (and with shrewd help from his chief domestic advisor, Joseph Califano), the device had worked well—quickly producing bold ideas that the two men could move into play.[57]

Magaziner himself had also convened huge advisory groups for other projects he had performed as a consultant, often with disastrous results. "The Greenhouse Compact," his effort to produce a Rhode Island economic strategy, had been supported by most of the state's political establishment but proved politically tone-deaf and was routed by the voters (almost 4–1). Jacobs and Shapiro believe that the new task force had still another purpose: to legitimize a proposal that would actually be developed by a tight insulated core of Clinton loyalists with little attention to outside experts or political advisors. In this view, the entire process was an elaborate kabuki, designed to give outside groups the appearance of access and of deliberation while Magaziner, a few aides, and President and Mrs. Clinton made all the decisions.[58]

In any case, two individuals with no Washington experience and no official governmental roles designed an unwieldy and untested process—with its sprawling advisory group and tight inner circle—to develop an unwieldy and untested health system proposal all under daunting time pressures. Clinton did not have a well-developed internal White House organization to provide any counterweight to the task force. He didn't like hierarchy, and his new chief of staff, childhood friend Mack McClarty, would prove pleasant but ineffective. There was, as yet, no domestic policy council of the type that vetted Richard Nixon's or Jimmy Carter's health care proposals. Indeed, Carol Rasco, a former Clinton gubernatorial aide who would become the staff director of the Domestic Policy Council once it was up and running, played very little role in health reform.

Clinton himself later concluded that he had made some important mistakes during his transition. "Looking back, I think the major short-comings of the transition were two: I spent so much time selecting the cabinet that I hardly spent any time on the White House staff; and I gave almost no thought to how to keep the public's focus on my most important priorities, rather than on competing stories that, at the least, would divert public attention from the big issues." The big competing story exploded around an offhanded suggestion that the military would permit gay men and women to serve; the president-elect spent more time handling the fallout from that than he did organizing his signature health policy.[59]

As a result, health policy came flying out of the transition like a brake-less truck careening down a mountain trail. And because the president's wife and one of his longtime friends were in charge, it became personal: even the president's most trusted and senior aides, including Cabinet secretaries, hesitated to challenge Hillary, Ira, and their minions. But the ride was exciting, and Clinton was at the wheel which was the way he liked it.

## Kicking the Health Care Can down the Road

Lyndon Johnson had also liked being in control, but he had been a much more disciplined driver than the young man from Arkansas. In the early days of Clinton's administration, the President's aversion to careful process, his distractability, his tardiness, and his fascination with the details of policy became the stuff of Washington gossip and con-cern.[60] Clinton's door was always open. No one directed Oval Office traffic. Meetings became policy seminars in which the president and his staff indulged in endless discussions about the latest issue to land on the president's desk. Experienced Beltway insiders began to liken the White House to a kids' soccer game, where aides swirled around whatever policy ball was in play at the moment, casting discipline, team play, planning, and strategy to the winds.[61]

By early February, however, Clinton's economic advisors seemed to have settled in at the vital center of the White House policy scrum. In the complex contest between progressive and conservative groups that had always roiled the Clinton camp, voices of caution—in the form of Secretary of the Treasury Lloyd Bentsen and National Economic Council Chairman Robert Rubin—prevailed.[62] They convinced Clinton that deficit reduction should be his first priority. The rationale: it would result in lower interest rates and a burst of economic growth. After all, Clinton had been elected in no small part because of the economic slowdown that had plagued the latter part of the Bush administration ("It's the economy, stupid!").[63] What's more, the economic team felt that Clinton's health care goal was sheer folly: too expensive, too ambitious, too reckless. It could balloon the deficit and stoke inflation.[64] Once again, health reformers ran headlong into economic advisors—a great debate that has marked every administration back to Truman and that become especially vivid after the Nixon administration and the creation of OMB.

Magaziner and Hillary protested. Congressional advisors, including Senate Majority Leader George Mitchell (D-ME) and House Majority Leader Richard Gephart (D-MO), had counseled them that for health reform to succeed, it needed to be done quickly, and it needed the president's unwavering, undistracted support.[65] Waiting until the fall or beyond would enable the opposition to mobilize (get those dead cats off the porch!). Clinton, however, felt pinned by his economic aides. Bentsen, in particular, brought political heft to the economists' pitch.[66] The former Texas senator was tall, gray-haired, patrician, handsome, rich and conservative. He had been chair of the Senate Finance Committee (the standard liberal jibe had it that Clinton chose him as secretary to remove the inevitable reform roadblock from Finance), and he knew the Senate better than any of the green Clinton team (except, perhaps, Vice President Al Gore). Bentsen had made a national name for himself during the 1988 vice presidential debate, when he had shot down Senator Dan Quayle's attempt to seize the mantle of John F. Kennedy: "Senator, I served with Jack Kennedy, I knew Jack Kennedy, Jack Kennedy was a friend of mine. Senator, you are no Jack Kennedy!"[67]

On February 17, Clinton spoke to a joint session of Congress and served notice that he would make balancing the federal budget his first goal. Included in his budget proposal, to the chagrin of his health policy team, was a substantial reduction in Medicare and Medicaid spending.[68] This money would go back to the treasury instead of into the pot that had been intended to fund expanded benefits for the uninsured. Clinton notes laconically in his memoirs: "In the second week of February, we decided to kick the health care can down the road and complete the rest of the economic plan."[69]

Clinton and his health care team still held out hope, however, that a legislative gimmick might enable them to move health care reform despite—or maybe because of—the focus on the budget. A key element of the congressional budget process is the passage of a resolution, called budget reconciliation, that lays out the Congress's fiscal goals for the coming year. The Congress has to pass such a bill annually, and it cannot be filibustered—it needs only fifty-one votes to pass the Senate, whereas breaking a filibuster requires sixty. Senate rules also limit the length of debate on the measure. Bill, Hillary, and Ira, together with Senate and House advisors, resolved to attach a health care reform proposal to the budget reconciliation legislation in 1993 as a way to outflank congressional opponents. With fifty-six Democrats in the Senate, a simple majority would win health care reform. Perhaps Clinton could get it all—deficit reduction and a new health care system.

There was only one problem. Senator Robert Byrd (D-WV), one of the longest-serving members of the Senate, chairman of its powerful Appropriations Committee, and the self-appointed guardian of that chamber's hallowed prerogatives and processes, objected. It was not a proper use of the reconciliation process; it was an abuse of the Senate rules. A bill as momentous as health care reform should be considered on its own merits, not snuck under cover of reconciliation. Despite pressure from all quarters—including intensive lobbying by the president—Byrd would not budge.[70] There was also the minor detail, of course, that Clinton did not have a bill to attach to reconciliation, and would not have one for months to come. Jacobs and Shapiro speculate that some of Byrd's obstinacy may have arisen from Clinton's own economic team, who were whispering in the senator's ear that the health plan was a disaster.[71] The reconciliation strategy died, and with it any hope of getting health care reform enacted in the first one hundred days—or perhaps ever.

Looking back, Clinton later commented that he should have changed strategy at this point. Having delayed consideration of health care and lost the reconciliation opportunity, he should have curtailed his ambitions. "This is entirely my mistake," he told Johnson and Broder in 1995, "no one else's. I probably made a mistake in not then going for a multiyear strategy, and not trying to say we've got to do it in 'ninety-four.... I set the Congress up for failure.... What we should have said is 'This might take three years.'"[72]

In fact, subsequent events suggest Clinton would probably have enjoyed little more success had he kicked health care even further down the road. But he didn't know that at the time, and neither he nor his team accepted defeat. More miles, much sweat, and many tears, lay ahead before the Clintons abandoned health care reform.

### Squeezing a Bill through the Tollgates

From February to August, when Bill Clinton's budget bill finally squeaked through the Congress, he and his closest aides focused almost exclusively on their economic plan. Ira Magaziner and Hillary Clinton agonized over the delay.[73]

Meanwhile, their task force became a legendary example of complex, disorderly, and chaotic policy development. Hundreds of policy experts inside and outside government labored in its byzantine corridors, all of which led to Ira Magaziner and a few close aides who worked day and night for months. No aspect of the health care system escaped their attention. They were recreating it from the ground up. The system's size and complexity seemed to justify an inordinately complex solution. Ira and Hillary occasionally briefed the president.[74] The intricacy of their developing proposal did not seem to worry him. He seemed instead to relish it. They were creating something genuinely new. Criticized in retrospect for the elaborate process and proposal, Clintonites point out that at the time, they were advised by congressional barons, including Dick Gephardt and Ways and Means Chair Daniel Rostenkowski (D-IL), not to send the Hill an outline or a set of principles. The Congress needed a detailed bill. The administration listened and obliged. Of course, no one on the health team had the experience to question Hill leaders about why they wanted such detail when committees rewrote virtually anything the Executive Branch sent them. One wonders whether a president with Lyndon Johnson's savvy would have taken this insistence on detailed language at face value—especially if it would result in critical delays. He certainly made it clear to Wilbur Mills that he wanted Congress, not the White House, to draft Medicare.

In March 1993, Hillary Clinton's father suffered a serious stroke. She returned to Little Rock and stayed with him for three weeks until he passed away. By several accounts, this loss had a deep effect on Hillary Clinton and—as a result—on the task force process. In her absence, progress slowed. "When Hillary's father died," commented Senator Rockefeller, "the whole thing came to a halt. There was nobody to step in ... it's very hard for her to advance her project except by her own work."[75]

When she returned, Hillary Clinton seemed for a time less engaged and available to staff—further delaying the progress of health care reform. Emotionally, however, the experience strengthened her commitment. "I came back even more convinced that this was not only the economically and politically smart thing for us to take on, but that it was the right thing to do.... So I think my father's experience really reinforced what this was truly about: that it wasn't some policy-wonk abstract discussion."[76]

Despite Hillary's strengthened commitment, the White House dissolved the health care task force in May 1993. By now, even Clinton recognized that the process was dysfunctional. Mimicking Magaziner's private-sector motif, it had become a sprawling warren of feverish policy deliberation divided into eight "cluster teams" and thirty-four "working groups."[77] These dissected particular issues, great and small, and presented their findings in grueling conferences—called "tollgate" meetings—to Magaziner and a few close aides. For reasons known only to Magaziner, these gatherings began on Friday mornings and ran late into the night and through the weekend. Topics were often highly academic, aimed at understanding the underpinnings of complex health policy phenomena. Tollgate meetings would generate unanswered questions that would in turn generate new reports and more tollgate meetings. Ultimately, Magaziner and a few close aides would take the reports and make key decisions—again, in conferences that lasted through the night. Some experienced hill staffers, came to the conclusion that the task force was really about educating Magaziner, Mrs. Clinton, and their inner circle about the basics of writing national health insurance legislation. As one important insider put it, "It was a tremendous spinning of wheels and relatively little opportunity for reflection."[78]

Looking back, even critics had to admit that the process generated fascinating ideas and new insights. But it did not create legislative language, and it sprang constant leaks that distracted the press and the president from their focus on passing their budget plan. One of the task force's last acts was emblematic of its problems and the culture of the early Clinton White House. On May 20, 1993, Clinton, the first lady, Vice President Gore, Mrs. Gore, and fifty top Clinton administration officials gathered in the Roosevelt Room of the White House (was Franklin turning in his grave?) for an Oxford-style debate on one aspect of health reform: how comprehensive should the initial benefit package be? Magaziner organized two teams to joust over the issues. It was all substance. Newcomers relished the focus on pure policy rather than political tactics. This, thought the Clinton team, was what responsible government should be.[78]

Washington old-timers, on the other hand, were flabbergasted at the naïveté and waste—was this a good use of hundreds of person-hours of the most senior officials in Washington? Clinton loved the intellectual gymnastics and showed impressive command of the material. Then reality crashed in on the enthusiastic debaters. Sarcastic details of the meeting—dubbed "Oxford on the Potomac"—were splashed across the pages of the *Washington Post* and the *New York Times*. Embarrassed, the White House indefinitely postponed the three additional debates it had scheduled and imposed a blanket of secrecy over health care discussions.[79]

With the end of the task force and the imposition of secrecy, health care went into hibernation for months. But Clinton had not forgotten it. The health care issue's pull on him clearly went beyond his budgetary agenda; we don't know whether it came from his own passion for the issue, his personal commitments to Hillary and Ira, his political calculations, or the simple inertia of a process already in motion. Likely, it was a mix of all four.

Days after the budget plan passed Congress, the president convened meetings with advisors. He was scheduled to reveal his health care plan in a speech before a joint session of Congress on September 22, 1993—just six weeks away. It was time to make the critical decisions that he had long postponed.[80] Once again, health care advocates confronted economic advisors. Analysts from the Council of Economic Advisers, OMB, and the treasury felt that the estimated savings from managed competition remained unrealistic. The president needed to raise taxes or cut back the benefits of the proposed program, perhaps covering catastrophic illnesses only. Mrs. Clinton and Mr. Magaziner had modified their proposal to include tougher cost controls, including governmentally mandated limits on the amounts that premiums charged by managed care companies could increase each year. This, they felt, provided ironclad guarantees that costs would be controlled (the Congressional Budget Office would later agree). But the economists were not buying it.

By now, however, Clinton was disaffected with his economists.[81] They had not anticipated the bruising budget battle that he had just been through. So far, his administration had bled itself dry fighting an excruciating political struggle that only a Republican could love—cutting federal programs and raising taxes in the name of budgetary discipline. The expansive side of Clinton wanted to do something big and generous for voters, something that would make middle-class Americans grateful to Democrats for generations to come. After months of task force debates, leaks, delay and drift, he embraced, again, the new liberal synthesis that had so appealed to him when he announced it on September 24, 1992. He would propose universal coverage, managed competition, and a new system to control costs and regulate managed care organizations. As political scientist Theda Skocpol points out, much of the plan's complexity originated in its efforts to keep costs under control, which originated in turn from Clinton's unwavering commitment not to raise taxes to cover the expenses of covering the uninsured.[82] Ironically, in trying to lighten the touch of government, Clinton and his team gave birth to a public relations monstrosity that opponents would successfully ridicule as big government gone wild.

Under Magaziner's guidance, a new team of policy experts worked feverishly over the next weeks to turn their proposal into legislative language. Typically, the bill was not ready by September 22, nor was Bill Clinton prepared for his speech about it. Clinton was redrafting his remarks until minutes before he appeared in the well of the House, where 535 legislators and a national television audience awaited him. The result was a classic example of Bill Clinton's unique ability to tempt the fates and win. Clinton's aides did not have time to put his just-in-time speech on the teleprompter before the president clambered up the podium to face the American people. For seven harrowing minutes, the leader of the Free World watched the wrong speech scroll before him as he spoke.

No one noticed. Roger Blythe's son was a natural. By all accounts, it was one of his great performances. In those seven minutes, he told his audience: "If Americans are to have the courage to change in a difficult time, we must first be secure in our most basic needs. Tonight I want to talk to you about the most critical thing we can do to build that security. This health care system of ours is badly broken, and it is time to fix it.... At long last, after decades of false starts, we must make this our most urgent priority, giving every American health security, health care that can never be taken away, health care that is always there. That is what we must do tonight."

Recalling FDR, Clinton placed his health reform in the proudest traditions of the Democratic Party and its long fight to stand up for middle-class America.

> It's hard to believe that there was once a time ... when retirement was nearly synonymous with poverty ... and older Americans died in the street. That's unthinkable today, because over a half a century ago Americans had the courage ... to create a Social Security System that ensures that no Americans will be forgotten in their later years. Forty years from now, our grandchildren will also find it unthinkable that there was a time in this country when hardworking families lost their homes, their savings, their businesses, lost everything simply because their children got sick or because they had to change jobs.[83]

All those hours and hours immersed in the details of health reform paid off in a president who could talk confidently and spontaneously about the topic and capture the imagination of the country in the process. The reaction to the speech was enormously favorable. Bill Clinton, through force of intellect, personality, and a silver tongue, had put reforming the American health care system back on the political agenda despite months of missteps and diversions. He had created a mess. Then he had cleaned it up. Public support for health reform soared in opinion polls. The transformation was launched. Or so it seemed—briefly. In fact, health care's moment had already passed. First of all, there was the reform proposal itself: not yet ready. The accumulating effects of delay, mismanagement, distraction, and inexperience began to take their toll. Unlike the reformers, the opposition was ready and loaded with slashing advertisements. In LBJ's words, their letters opposing the plan were not only written, but delivered. In the 1990s, the letters came in the form of highly professional grassroots organizing and media campaigns fueled by millions of special-interest dollars. Leading the effort were the Health Insurance Association of America (HIAA) and the National Federation of Independent Business (NFIB). The former saw red over the total reformation of the insurance business that the new Clinton plan would have required, which included regulation of premiums. The NFIB attacked the employer mandate. Together with a coalition of like-minded interest groups, HIAA and NFIB had begun organizing to beat the Clinton plan in May 1993—four months before Clinton's speech.[84] The HIAA had launched a now legendary ad campaign that featured an attractive, articulate couple—Harry and Louise—sitting at a kitchen table. Exuding middle American appeal and earnestness, they expressed confusion and doubt about the complex Clinton plan—"they choose, we lose," the couple concluded, playing to the public's fear of government involvement in health care. The ad only had to run a few times in one market—Washington. But it looped endlessly as the media filled the vacuum created by Clinton's delays.[85] For its part, the NFIB began a nationwide campaign to mobilize its small business constituents throughout congressional districts of America. The small business lobby allied itself with the hot, savvy, rising Republican conservatives in the House.

Congressional Republicans had time to think about their response to the Clinton health care initiative. Originally, they had been divided between conservatives, such as Newt Gingrich (R-GA), who saw beating Clinton's reform as part of a strategy for retaking the House from the Democrats; and moderates, including Senator John Chafee (R-RI), who wanted to find a compromise plan. Senate Majority Leader Robert Dole (R-KS) was planning his own run for the presidency against Clinton. He sat on the fence, at first signing on to the Chafee bill and hinting he would work with the administration. Dole and the Republicans did not want to be blamed for beating a still-popular health initiative. But they also feared the political gains that would accrue to the Democrats if the Clintons succeeded. Dole worked quietly to sink Clinton's health reform as soon as the outside interest group campaign began to take its toll on public support for the program. Senator Chafee himself described the progress of the Republican alternative: Dole, he said, went from calling it "my plan" (when Clinton's reform seemed inevitable) to "the Chafee–Dole plan" (as reform teetered) to "that god damn plan of Chafee's" (as Republicans united against it).[86]

As the health plan began a free fall in the polls, the Clintons decided to take the health care reform issue to the American people, but they failed to pull off their campaign. Things started well. The first lady made a triumphant tour of congressional health committees during the week after the speech. She dazzled Democrats and cowed Republicans with her poise and command of the issues. The president and his wife were planning a national tour to promote health reform, but events intruded.

On October 3, 1993, a U.S. military mission to capture a Somali warlord in Mogadishu went badly astray, leading to multiple U.S. casualties and a public relations disaster for the administration. Then a crisis burst out in Haiti and the administration dispatched American forces. Next Bill Clinton worked on getting the North American Free Trade Agreement (NAFTA) through Congress. NAFTA pinned congressional Democrats between their Third Way president and their base, including the unions and the environmental community. The bill squeaked through both chambers with more Republican votes than Democratic (House Democrats voted nay 156–102). The result dispirited the party activists and opened a rift with organized labor—one of the few reliable supporters of health reform. This was a breach that health reform could ill afford. The White House needed labor's organizing clout in local districts and its money to buy counterads to the HIAA. And it needed enthusiasm from the liberal grassroots that had fought the administration hard on NAFTA. Clinton had spent his dwindling political capital on another Republican issue—a free-trade bill negotiated by the Bush administration.

Trying to rekindle the old magic, Clinton gave another health care speech to Congress on October 27, 1993, trying to focus renewed public attention on the legislation. The nominal reason for the talk was to announce the final bill, but it *still* wasn't ready. The talk garnered little attention. Finally, on November 20, a year after his election, Clinton finally sent legislative language to the Hill—three days after the final, bruising NAFTA vote.

Other problems were taking their toll as well. Johnson had predicted that his own public standing would erode with every minute he was in the Oval Office. The Clintons were experiencing this in spades (and they started with a 43 percent election compared to LBJ's 61 percent). Clinton seemed to make one public relations blunder after another—some real, others exaggerated, but all of them damaging. He blundered into the firestorm over gays in the military without any thought about how to manage (much less win) the controversial issue. The White House fired the staff of its travel office, causing a negative buzz in the press. The press had a field day with a story that the president had delayed air traffic in Los Angeles for hours while he received an expensive haircut from a celebrity stylist (the story of the delays were later shown to be false, but the fancy haircut was real).[87]

And then there was Whitewater. In December 1993, the press reported accusations that when Clinton was governor, he and Hillary had tried to protect a well-connected bank officer and Democratic fundraiser from regulatory scrutiny in the aftermath of the failure of his savings and loan. An old story that right-wing journals had been hawking for months, it broke into the mainstream media while Clinton was recovering from his tough first year in office and was trying to focus—after the budget, NAFTA, Somalia, and Haiti—on health reform. Whitewater became a media obsession, spurred on by conservative talk shows, conservative money, Hillary Clinton's reluctance to make her personal papers public, Bill's penchant for flying near the flame, and the administration's decision to appoint a special prosecutor to investigate.

As much as any other of Clinton's missteps and afflictions, Whitewater undermined his effort to pass health reform. It eroded trust in the president, and trust was critical to advocating for health care change. Harold Ickes, a Clinton political advisor hired to help with health reform, saw this instantly: "Our research shows this is very, very personal. People don't give—to use the vernacular—a fuck about the national interest when they think about health reform. They want to know: How is this going to affect me, my children, my parents? ... That's why trust in the Clintons is going to be a critical element in carrying the day."[88]

The polls reflected all the troubles. They dropped below 50 percent after four months (in May 1993) and bounced around in the 40 percent range for the rest of the year. After rising back into the 50 percent range at the start of the second year (right after the proposal was finally submitted), they drifted down through the winter and spring (as Congress debated health reform) until the Clintons were dipping into the danger zone below 40 percent (by August 1994, as reform collapsed).[89]

There was still one more basic problem. Clinton had not organized a pro–health reform movement that remotely competed with the swelling, well-funded opposition. He faced a number of obstacles. His NAFTA battle and his Medicare and Medicaid cuts had blunted the enthusiasm of liberal Democrats, as well as, perhaps, the two most important potential supporters of health reform: labor and the American Association of Retired Persons. The Clintons had hoped that some large businesses would stand with them—after all, companies that offered generous health benefits were at a distinct disadvantage in a global economy—but in the end, they, too, backed away. Without organized backing, it was exceedingly difficult to combat the insurance and small business lobbies—or, more important, to intimidate some Republicans in the Senate (they needed at least four to get to sixty) and to entice conservative Democrats in the House to support the bill.[90]

More ominously, the Clintons seemed unable to focus on and execute the politics of health reform. In December 1993, when the administration had finally delivered its legislation to Congress—too late for action before the Christmas recess—Jay Rockefeller told Johnson and Broder: "I am in a state of rage, befuddled, all the rest of it. I'm furious right now at the White House.... There's still no organization on health care. There's nothing out there."[91] Skocpol added, "Ira Magaziner and Hillary Rodham Clinton coordinated extensive resources to devise the technical details that went into the Clinton Health Security proposal. But no comparable organizational effort was made on the *political* side, because for many months there was a remarkable vacuum of top-level White House leadership for the politics of health care reform."[92]

Clinton had hired Harold Ickes in November 1993 (already late) to fill this leadership vacuum, but his arrival had been delayed because of Ickes's indecision over whether he had the Washington experience, and the control over Magaziner, to do the job.[93] Magaziner had acquired the reputation of a Rasputin-like figure, with a seemingly unbreakable lock on Clinton's health care decisions. Would Ickes be able to work with him? Would Magaziner be willing to report to him?

When Ickes finally arrived in January 1994, he was immediately diverted to working on the Whitewater controversy. It was as though, captivated by the intellectual challenge of remaking the health care system, Clinton's policy seminar had failed to schedule the final and most crucial session—the session on how presidents lead a reluctant Congress and skittish nation to enact sweeping changes in its largest industry. In 1962, at the dawn of the modern media age, Kennedy's aides had debated whether to pursue an outside strategy on major health reform. Thirty years later, the issue was no longer in doubt. Presidents who did not have an outside strategy—and a damned good one—would be wiped out by the chorus of interests yelling nay.[94]

## Denouement

In January 1994, Congress cranked up its legislative machinery for a new session that would run until the November election. By tradition, each congressional session starts with the president's State of the Union address. Trying once again to invigorate health reform, Clinton made it the centerpiece of his address. The tall, still-young-looking president, his hair graying but not yet snow-white, said he was open to ideas other than his own, was willing to talk, but then he held up the presidential pen and made a startling pledge: "I have no special brief for any specific approach, even in our own bill, except this: If you send me legislation that does not guarantee every American private health insurance that can never be taken away, you will force me to take this pen, veto the legislation, and we'll come right back here and start all over again."[95]

Clinton's advisors had divided over whether to include this language, but Hillary had strongly favored it, and other proponents thought it would give heart to beleaguered supporters of reform. Moreover, Clinton had earned a reputation as a waffler, and members of Congress had become wary about sticking their necks out for a position that he might negotiate away at any moment (in Washington parlance, this was known as being BTU'd after the House Democrats reluctantly voted for a politically risky energy tax, based on British Thermal Units, only to have the White House jettison the tax when the Senate balked). The veto pen looked like a promise to hold firm for the great liberal reform.[96]

Harris believes that Clinton himself had doubts—liberals would say he was waffling—about inserting the veto threat, but that Hillary Clinton's influence was decisive. The exchange reflected the complex dynamic in their marriage. "Hillary Clinton thought the veto threat was a good idea, and [White House advisor David] Gergen was struck that Bill Clinton seemed entirely deferential to her on this and seemingly every question. This was just weeks after the *American Spectator*'s embarrassing exposé of yet another sexual scandal and just days after Clinton acquiesced to demands for a special counsel on Whitewater. 'Watching him in that time,' Gergen recalled, 'I think it put him in a situation where on health care he never challenged it in a way he ordinarily would have.'"[97]

Despite throaty liberal approval from the Democrat-controlled Congress, the president eventually came to see his veto threat as a blunder. He was now committed to covering everyone—there could be no compromise without political embarrassment. He had lost the room to maneuver.[98]

On the other side, Republicans were already at the barricades. Sensing blood in the water, their opposition to the Clinton plan was hardening.

Senate Minority Leader Dole delivered a withering Republican rebuttal to Clinton's speech that featured a putative diagram of the Clinton plan sprouting a thicket of boxes and arrows. Like Doc Bowen mocking the conservatives' voucher plan in the Reagan Cabinet—line, line, line, line—Dole drew a diagram of the Clinton chaos. The message? This was big-government craziness run amok.

But Clinton even had problems with the Democrats. The flamboyant, unpredictable Senator Daniel Patrick Moynihan (D-NY) didn't see what all the health care fuss was about. The former Harvard professor and Nixon advisor thought welfare redesign was much more urgent. The problem for the Clintons was that Moynihan was chairman of the Senate Finance Committee, through which their health care legislation had to pass. Despite many personal conversations, neither Bill nor Hillary would ever change Moynihan's views. Senate Finance never reported out a health care reform bill, although the less influential Senate Committee on Health, Education, Labor and Pensions, chaired by Senator Edward Kennedy, did.

In the House, two key committees, both chaired by proponents of health reform, were also deeply divided. Representative John Dingell Jr. (D-MI), son of the legendary Congressman John Dingell (of Murray–Dingell–Wagner fame) had stepped into office when his father died and now, thirty-nine years later, wanted desperately to honor his father's legacy by enacting national health insurance. The chairman of the critical House Commerce Committee, Dingell worked tirelessly to gather enough Democrats to overcome solid Republican opposition, but Representative Cooper, who was running for Senate, as well as other moderate-to-conservative democrats, were leery of the employer mandate and of the regulatory aspects of the Clinton bill. Cooper, with Republican cosponsors, had introduced his own legislation, which he characterized as "Clinton lite." Lacking an employer mandate, the Cooper bill would not cover everyone, but it had a number of Clinton-style managed competition provisions. The White House was not interested in compromise; nor were traditional Democratic liberals. Dingell failed.

Dan Rostenkowski, the powerful chair of the House Ways and Means Committee and a Clinton ally, had resigned in the midst of scandal in May 1994. Health reform lost a critical supporter. His replacement, Sam Gibbons (D-FL) was also strongly behind the Clinton plan, but he didn't have Rostenkowski's heft. He managed after much wrangling and compromise, to eke out a 20–18 vote in favor of a version of the Clinton bill. But the proreform forces did not have the votes to get it through the full House. Speaker Tom Foley (D-OR) concluded that "... the basic problem, which the Clintons did not want to acknowledge, was that there was no consensus to support a plan as ambitious as they offered—not in the country, not in the Democratic Party, not in the House."[99] Foley imagined a lack of national consensus in the country. Other observers focused on the inevitable buzz of hostile interests, or the smart tactics of the Republicans, or the broken spirit of the Democrats. But a political scientist from any other system in the world would be flabbergasted by something that Foley took for granted: the infernal complexity of the American legislative process itself. After all the agony of the tollgates, the Oxford debates, and the long weekends drafting reform language, the plan finally went to Congress, where the House Ways and Means, House Commerce, Senate Finance, and the Senate Committee on Health, Education, Labor and Pensions (we won't even go into the matter of subcommittees) each tossed aside the carefully drawn provisions and debated, marked up and reported or defeated a different version of the bill. Only an extraordinarily talented leader can win big reforms out of machinery so fiendishly (or, from those who prefer inaction from their legislature, brilliantly) devised to frustrate.

Over the summer, Majority Leader George Mitchell concluded that the Senate would not pass a universal coverage plan either. He wanted to develop a proposal that would get to 95 percent coverage of Americans, as well as drop the employer mandate that so angered small business. He hoped to draw in some moderates from the other side of the aisle: John Chafee (R-RI), David Durenberger (R-MN), and John Danforth (R-MO). The White House agreed to let him explore this possibility. As Mitchell was trying to negotiate a compromise, Clinton spoke to the National Governors Association in Boston on July 19, where he responded to a question by hinting that he was open to compromise: "There may be some other way to do this [besides an employer mandate]," he said. Noting that only 98 percent of Americans were covered by Social Security, he implied that getting to 95 percent coverage might be good enough at first.[100] As soon as the president's remarks hit the wires, his phone buzzed. At least as Harris tells the story, the president was overruled: "[T]he White House operator was calling, with Hillary Clinton on hold. She was in a rage, according to a White House aide who listened to the call. 'What the fuck are you doing up there?' Clinton tried to explain that what he had said was not quite the way it was being reported. She cut him off. 'You get back here right away.' When he returned to the White House, Clinton immediately went up to the residence. The next day, he retracted his remarks to the governors, professing that he was still committed to universal coverage."[101] Just this once, Mrs. Clinton wanted the president to stick to his guns.

On July 22, Clinton called Magaziner at home in Rhode Island to say that he thought health reform was dead. They had one last arrow in their quiver: a national bus tour led by Hillary Clinton, the Health Security Express, that would weave its way in late July from Portland, Oregon to Washington, trying to arouse the American people in support of health reform. Instead of enthusiasm, Hillary drove into the tenacious efforts to demonize her and her husband: there were protests and heckling, some of it personal, much of it enraged. If health care ever had a moment, it was clearly gone.[102]

Mitchell had fifty-six Democratic votes for reform in the Senate—four short of cloture on the Republican filibuster. By now, midterms loomed three months ahead, and every move would be filtered through partisan calculations. Mitchell decided to let health care reform die without a vote. At the end, White House aide Chris Jennings met with Mitchell, desperately seeking some way to make it possible to move forward. Jennings recalled: "I kept on saying 'Could we compromise here, or could we do this?' ... And he looked into my eyes ... almost like a father looks toward their son and ... said, 'You know, Chris, it's dead. It's dead.... We did everything we could, but it's over.'"[103]

The Republicans were elated—and nimbly avoided any blame for the defeat. Senator Robert Packwood (R-OR), ranking minority member of the Senate Finance Committee, commented memorably: "We've killed health care reform. Now we've got to make sure our fingerprints are not on it."[104]

For Bill Clinton, of course, the Republican fingerprints were indelible. His election had brought the Democrats back after twelve years out of executive power. But after two tumultuous years, the Republicans were poised to win the biggest midterm sweep—of House, Senate, governors' mansions, and state legislatures—in sixty years. The Republicans would take the House for the first time in thirty-eight years and then hang on to it in the next election for the first time since 1928. Clinton concluded wanly: "Though I felt for months that we were beaten, I was still disappointed, and I felt bad that Hillary and Ira Magaziner were taking the rap for the failure. It was unfair.... The plan was the best Hillary and Ira could do, given the charge from me: universal coverage without a tax increase; and it wasn't they who had derailed health care reform—Senator Dole's decision to kill any meaningful compromise had done that."[105]

In retrospect, he wished he had done welfare first—like Jimmy Carter. "We might not have lost either house if, as soon as it became clear that Senator Dole would filibuster any meaningful health reform[,] I had announced a delay in health care until we reached a bipartisan consensus, and had taken up and passed welfare reform instead. That would have been popular with alienated middle-class Americans who voted in droves for Republicans."[106]

Clinton's own bottom line was something he later did most successfully: steal the other side's thunder (welfare reform). Down the road, perhaps he could have come back for a bipartisan try at a smaller sort of health reform (perhaps something like the State Children's Health Insurance Program [SCHIP] that a Republican Congress would pass in 1997). His health plan, Clinton seems to have concluded, was doomed from the outset because of the opposition of one man. He had made a tactical political error in not realizing this sooner, and this had cost his party the Congress, which seemed, in retrospect, to have troubled him a good deal more than the outcome of the health debate.

There is no shame in losing health reform—Clinton got much deeper into the Congressional process than, say, Harry Truman. But there is a stunning difference in the epilogue. Truman never abandoned his ideal. He kept roasting its opponents long after his reform was dead and buried. Truman left office a deeply unpopular president, but his reform survived him thanks to the boundless energy of his defense. It is no coincidence that LBJ decided to honor Harry Truman when he signed Medicare into law.

Contrast Clinton. His reflections are all about strategy and blame. He felt bad for Hilary and Ira. But where was the memory, now, of those "hardworking families [who] lost their homes, their savings, their businesses, lost everything simply because their children got sick or because they had to change jobs"? The fiery faith of September was burned out by August. The opposition killed the plan, wiped their fingerprints off the corpse, and took uncontested control of the postmortem; the Republican spin about Clinton's clumsy health reform entirely won the day, even as large swaths of the private sector were pursuing some parts (managed care, competition) without others (regulations for fairness, universal coverage).

## Lessons of Clinton Health Reform

The Clinton administration leaves us another long list of presidential don'ts. Many of the lessons simply reinforce the conclusions we drew from Lyndon Johnson's success—and Jimmy Carter's failure. The Clintons violated most of the Johnson precepts, and their party paid the price. But, of course, each administration—and each historical moment—is unique. Each effort offers its own variations on the great themes of success and failure. We can find nine lessons—many familiar, some new—in the Clinton failure.

*Speed.* The Clintons came to office with something rare: an electoral mandate for health reform coupled with solid majorities in both chambers of Congress. But neither the president nor his advisors had any idea how swiftly mandates evaporate. After two big health care elections—Wofford and Clinton—they became "overconfident about the momentum of reform," as presidential health advisor Paul Starr put it. "We misjudged the health care politics of 1993 as a change in the climate when it was only a change in the weather."[107] They should have heeded LBJ: "Every day ... I have less power left."

The Clintons understood this intellectually—their allies in Congress made sure that they did—but the hyperactive and distractable president fought his bruising battles for a balanced budget and NAFTA while his political power drained away. Clinton's own idea of coming back to a bipartisan health bill three years later sounds like wishful thinking. As the opposition surged, routed the Democrats in Congress, and undercut the president's authority, he was not likely to win anything major—not on his terms.

*The Transition.* The importance of speed highlights the vital role of presidential transitions. Successful health care reform may have been doomed the moment Clinton sent Feder, Gawande, and the transition task force packing on January 10, 1993. If he was serious about health reform, Clinton needed a proposal soon after taking the oath of office. Instead, he started health care all over again in January 1993. As the president himself admitted, he had failed to understand the vital role of the ten weeks between election and inauguration. He failed to focus on key issues, as well as on who was staffing them or what they were preparing for him. He permitted a deep division within the staff (Washington realists versus Third Wayers) to rage for two months before he angrily intervened.

*Organization.* Too tight an organization can squelch creativity—precisely what Dick Darmon did to President Bush and Ike did for himself. Clinton, like Carter before him, made the opposite mistake: too much chaos, too little organization to back up the president. He needed an effective chief of staff and a domestic policy process. He had neither until months after he took office. A good organization could have made choices between competing health care camps—or alerted the president that he needed to intervene.

*The Danger of Policy Hubris.* Another lesson reflects Jimmy Carter's experience: Incoming presidents—especially those with no Washington experience—arrive with a profound contempt for the people and ideas that preceded them. Carter and Clinton shared that bias. Carter slapped down powerful potential allies (such as Tip O'Neil and Dan Rostenkowski) and instead spent hours poring over health care minutia, scribbling marginal notes about bureaucratic entities (PSROs?) that only a policy wonk could love. Clinton went even further than his predecessor from Georgia: he wanted Magaziner to give him something new, something awesomely clever and innovative, a proposal that blew away the old truism that new revenues were needed to cover the uninsured. Even if it had been practical, this policy breakthrough would have demanded months of deliberation and vetting. Clinton relished the challenge, wallowed in the detail, delayed the product, and paid dearly for his mismanagement. To be sure, the president can develop new ideas in the Oval Office—Richard Nixon and George H. W. Bush both did so. But remaking the political agenda is an entirely different project from delivering on a campaign promise, cashing in on a mandate, and winning reform.

*The Seductions of Technique.* As Jacob Hacker summed it up, the Clinton strategy was driven almost entirely by policy considerations: each time someone raised a problem, the specialists hammered out a technical adjustment. But technical adjustments are no answer to political attacks.[108] Ira Magaziner did not design a robust plan well geared for the political scrum of Washington politics. He was the wrong person for that job. After Senator Byrd squashed the budget reconciliation strategy, Clinton was left with the wrong team, the wrong strategy, and still no bill (he might not have been able to take advantage of the budget reconciliation strategy even if Senator Byrd had winked it through). There is no technical fix—no better algorithm or more scientifically verifiable modality—that can answer the partisan blasts of Washington politics. Americans rally around big reforms that inspire them; complex programs invite caricature.

*It Takes a Movement.* Roosevelt, Kennedy, and Johnson all understood something fundamental about the president's role: there's nothing to match the bully pulpit, especially in a new media age. Kennedy went public for Medicare and kept at it, setting the agenda for his successor. In contrast, Clinton and his team—like Carter before him—focused on policy development. Clinton had the gifts, as his first address to Congress vividly demonstrated. But he never subordinated the policy process to his persuasive powers (the proposal still was not ready). Clinton never mobilized his allies. On the contrary, he alienated his own troops—liberals, labor, environmentalists, the AARP—by taking on causes they did not share. When he finally launched his health care battle, he led a dispirited and mutinous army against opponents who were locked, loaded and ready.

*The Inside Game.* Clinton and his team also lacked any deep knowledge of the Congress and how to work with it. This is another occupational hazard for presidents who ride into Washington as outsiders and reformers. Hillary and Bill understood the importance of Congress. They listened closely to what senior congressional leaders— Mitchell, Gephardt, Rostenkowski, Dingell—told them. They worked hard to bring around the irascible Moynihan. They did what they were told in developing and introducing a detailed proposal that later became an embarrassment. But they were minor-leaguers playing in the majors. And Congress is an extraordinarily difficult institution to manage.

In contrast, LBJ was as likely to give as to get advice from the congressional barons of his time. They respected him and feared him. They wondered what he had up his sleeve. Ronald Reagan managed to intimidate Congress with his personal popularity, a lopsided electoral victory, and a rising conservative movement (which terrified Democrats in conservative districts) lined up strong behind him. Even Richard Nixon found a way to work with Congressional leaders, hooking Wilbur Mills and Ted Kennedy through savvy staff members and a desire to accomplish something. Clinton had neither the experience nor the wisdom to work out a way. He became much more nimble later in his presidency, but by then, it was too late for health reform.

*The Limits of History.* Comparing Clinton to prior presidents can mislead. Times change. The LBJ era of old bulls chairing congressional committees was long gone by the 1990s. Raw partisan politics—more ferocious than anything in recent memory—gusted up with the brash new Republican leadership keen to end their party's long (thirty-eight years in the House) sojourn in the political wilderness.

The presidency was also different, in part because of the increased authority of economic institutions. By the time Clinton took office, OMB was a force to be reckoned with. Equally important, the Congressional Budget Office had a stranglehold over forecasting the costs of proposed legislation. Concern about how CBO would score the Clinton plan helped drive the White House to add regulatory features to convince the agency that the proposal would not need new taxes. This made the plan more complicated—and vulnerable. In a simpler era, before these agencies existed, it was easier for presidents, such as Kennedy or Johnson, to manipulate, ignore, or overrule their economists. Clinton, too, ultimately had to override his economists' advice when he introduced health reform, but his decision came much later, after he felt their views were not serving his political needs. Even then, he felt compelled to propose a bill that was budget-neutral by some economic calculations. The new governmental machinery made it—and continues to make it—harder than ever to complete that crucial requirement for health care reform: hush the economists.

*Harry Truman's Final Lesson.* Clinton took enormous risks for health care reform. His bold choices and his management of their consequences reflected a unique blend of attributes: empathy, childhood memories, the strong women around him who cared deeply about health care, charisma, intelligence, inexperience, hubris, self-indulgence, and political recklessness. All played a role in pushing him toward embracing health care, endorsing the plan he did, delivering it late, and deciding to jettison the issue after it went down.

One question that looms over the Clinton health care experience is how things might have been different if (Truman-like) he had stuck to his principles after his effort lost. Might he have left a different legacy? For more than a decade after George Mitchell threw in the towel in September 1994, health care reform disappeared from public discourse. The Democrats lost their signature issue. And, perhaps not coincidentally, they lost their grip on power in every branch and level of government. In that period, the Republicans consolidated their own control on the national level for the first time since 1928. The political wreckage signals one final rule that every health care reformer ought to bear in mind: *learn to handle defeat skillfully.*

# CHAPTER 11

# George W. Bush

*Bring It On—Reforming Medicare*

George W. Bush was a child of privilege, but not always a privileged child. Grandson of a senator, son of a president, descendant of financiers, oilmen, and industrialists—he never lacked for money or opportunity. Compared to many presidential stories—FDR's polio, Ike's D-Day gut-check, Nixon's poverty, Clinton's child abuse—W.'s path to the presidency looked, in the words of another Texas president, like "a dose of salt going through a widow woman."[1]

But it wasn't quite that easy, and if it had been, George W. Bush might have been a different kind of health care president. Under the placid surface of a sheltered youth, cold currents buffeted this heir to a political dynasty. They made him both tougher and more compassionate, more iconoclastic and more alert to the domestic issues that his father shunned.[2]

By the end of his eight years, the Bush legacy looked bleak: a catastrophic foreign policy, a plunging economy, a collapsing financial system, allegations of torture, violations of civil liberties, lost majorities in Congress, and approval ratings in the tank. But these end-times portents do not tell the whole story of Bush's presidency—certainly not the entire health care story. When the spirit and the politics moved him, Bush could set health care goals, pursue them relentlessly, give and get in the legislative process, and emerge with a program he was proud of. This is the story of the Medicare Modernization Act of 2003, which provided prescription drug coverage for the elderly.

The Medicare Modernization Act was not the only important health care event of the second Bush presidency, but it is the most significant. It was by far the biggest expansion of Medicare (after catastrophic repeal) since its passage thirty-eight years earlier. And Bush made it possible through his leadership. Why did he commit his political capital to this classic Democratic (Johnsonian, no less) mother of all entitlement programs? Politics and ideology were important—he was eager to rethink the program. But George Bush also seemed to have an affinity for health care issues, and a commitment to social safety net programs that complicates the standard picture of this conservative president. Even the editorial page of the *New York Times*—never a soft touch for this man—felt compelled to note that "President Bush can also lay claim to some signal achievements in health care—achievements that we urge President-elect Barack Obama to continue and develop further." Health care had an unexpected claim on George W. Bush's heart. The search for why begins with his seemingly privileged past.

## GEORGE W. BUSH

George W. Bush's biography is full of unacknowledged pain, paradox, and complexity. The least introspective of men, W. would dismiss this idea as psychobabble, titillating to the East Coast intellectuals he detested.[3] But the story is compelling and helps explain why this conservative pushed a huge investment in a Great Society health care program.

### We're Both Clowns

W. was a child of New England, born in Yale's shadow while his war-hero dad completed his undergraduate studies. But by the time George W. was a toddler, the Bush family had moved to where the oil was—Odessa and then Midland, Texas. Midland was where George W. would always feel most at home, but, paradoxically, his education, his father's career, and his family roots would force him to ping-pong between the cool, piney hills of the New England and the hot, dusty flats of Texas.

George W. grew up in a typical 1950s family. George H. W. Bush was seldom home.[4] Traveling the Southwest to sell oil equipment and hatch drilling deals, he was the absent breadwinner who dropped in to entertain and be entertained by his growing family. Barbara was the pillar of the household: strong, tart, and verbal—the family's disciplinarian, scheduler, driver, nurse, and cook.

Outgoing and active, little George was the leader of a band of children who roamed his Midland neighborhood. The families were all young, and children were sprouting like wildflowers. In 1949, Robin Bush arrived; then John Ellis (Jeb) Bush in 1953.[5] About the time Jeb was born, George H. W. Bush launched a new oil drilling venture, the Zapata Petroleum Corporation, that would soon make his family rich.

Then Robin's leukemia tore through the family. W.'s father continued his hectic business travels—nothing new about that. But now little George's mother disappeared as well, along with his younger sister. Both were absent for months at a time as Robin received experimental treatment in New York City. Six-year-old George W. and newborn Jeb were left in the care of neighbors and visiting family.

And W. never knew why. Nobody ever told him how sick his sister was. She seemed well enough when she came home.[6] After all, she only rejoined the family when her disease remitted. After Robin's quick, unceremonious funeral in Greenwich, George H. W. Bush and Barbara returned to manage their fractured home. Minutaglio recounts the scene and its aftermath:

> It was the middle of a school day, and George W. was struggling down a covered walkway at the small school, weighted down by a Victrola that he and his friend Bill Sallee had been ordered to carry to the principal's office. He turned to watch his parents' car as its wheels crunched over the gravel parking lot and pulled up close to the school.... George W. stared expectantly at the car, assuming, hoping that Robin was there.... He sprinted ahead to his teacher and blurted, "My mom, dad, and sister are home. Can I go see them?"[7]

George was full of childhood questions about the missing Robin. Was she buried standing up or lying down? If she was upright, when the earth rotated, would she end up standing on her head? He had nightmares. Barbara became depressed and withdrawn. Like so many young children confronted by disorienting family trauma, little George—his father often gone—felt compelled to play caretaker. One day, Barbara heard W. tell a playmate at the front door: "I can't come over to play because I have to play with my mother. She's lonely."[8]

Later, Barbara regretted that she and her husband didn't prepare George W. for Robin's loss. "He felt cheated," she later said, "I do think that the death of Robin had a big effect on George. I think it's very, very difficult for a young child to see his parents suffering. And so I think he tried to be lighthearted. I also lost my sister, and I think that is another thing that George and I have in common. You know, we're both clowns. I think kids who lose a sibling often try and find ways to, you know, make things easier in the family."[9]

Nine years later, starting Andover, George Bush's first English assignment at the forbidding New England prep school was to write about a profound emotional experience. Like Richard Nixon, he wrote about losing a sibling. But the result was not the catharsis that Richard Nixon may have experienced with his saccharine but literate tribute to a brother dead of tuberculosis. Displaying what some believe is the dyslexia underlying Bush's frequent malapropisms, he mangled the essay and got a failing grade and a cruel teacher comment: "Disgraceful. See me immediately."[10]

The young Bush's role as caretaker did not end with Robin's death. W.'s grade school and junior high years were long, isolated ones for his mother. She had two more boys: Neil in 1955 and Marvin in 1956. "This was a period, for me, of long days and short years," she recalled, "of diapers and runny noses, earaches, more Little League games than you could believe possible, tonsils, and those unscheduled races to the hospital emergency room, Sunday school and church, of hours of urging homework, short chubby arms around your neck and sticky kisses; and experiencing those bumpy moments—not many, but a few—of feeling that I'd never, ever be able to have fun again, and coping with the feeling that George Bush, in his excitement of starting a small company and traveling around the world, was having a lot of fun."[11] Barbara Bush had episodes of depression, but getting help was not an option in this transplanted, upper-crust New England household.[12] When Barbara had a miscarriage shortly before W. went to Andover, he was the one to drive her to the hospital and comfort her during the aftermath. Picking her up the next day, he asked her earnestly: "Don't you think we ought to talk about this before you have more children?"[13]

Thus did George W. Bush, however unconsciously, struggle to fill his father's shoes as a source of emotional and even physical support to his mother.[14] But there were other, equally salient ways in which his father's example—both present and absent—became burden and inspiration. Quite simply, his father—in school, sports, military service, politics, family, and life—set the standards to which all his children were held—and held themselves. And none took the role model more seriously than the firstborn son. George W. would follow in his father's path for years—with dread, with joy, and later with rebellion and anger.

That rebellious streak would open space for health policy on W.'s Oval Office desk.[15]

## Commissioner of Stickball

Being a Bush was tough for George W. Where his father was school-smart, athletic, and focused, modern psychologists might describe George W. Bush as learning-disabled—perhaps even hyperactive. He did poorly in school. He wasn't a good athlete, but he was kinetic, even frenetic. He had skills, but not the kind that traditional educational institutions valued.

His mediocre grades undoubtedly caused anxiety, self-doubt, and resentment toward Andover, Yale, and all the New England institutions they came to symbolize. As Weissberg puts it, "He had to cope with being treated as dumb, without even being a jock."[16] After that failing grade in his first English assignment, he worried desperately that he was going to get tossed out of Andover and shipped back to Midland in disgrace.[17] Today school counselors and developmental psychologists would have been all over young George. He would get tutoring in personalized learning techniques. His tests would be untimed. Therapists would bolster his self-esteem by assuring him (correctly) that dyslexia and hyperactivity are biological problems that have nothing to do with native intelligence or ability, and that they can be overcome. He might even get dosed with stimulants to help him settle in and concentrate during those long, dark, cold New England winters.

But these supports were a long way off in the early 1960s, and George W. had to find a different way to be a Bush. Developing a toughness that would later shape his presidency, he used the abilities he possessed. He was outgoing, verbal, friendly, humorous, and fun-loving. He had a good memory, especially for names, and he had already begun watching how his father, by then cultivating a political career in the Houston area, could find success in relationships with crowds. At Andover, he became a cheerleader—another way to be part of the action. He led from the outside: ironically, mockingly. His father had been captain of the Yale baseball team. W. organized a para-athletic program—a stickball league—of which he became "commissioner." At Yale, too, he was a different sort of leader. He didn't just join a fraternity, he was its president. He was a hellraiser and prank-ster: hard-drinking, partying, cool and sardonic, continually testing the limits. He got himself arrested twice during college: once in New Haven for lifting a Christmas wreath from a downtown store, another time in Princeton as part of a melee following a Princeton–Yale football game.[18] He covered his insecurity with brash overconfidence and impulsiveness.[19]

Clearly, George W. Bush was not buying his father's route to success—the tight-lipped, understated, conventional, New England path that relied on a combination of innate talent and golden connections. But despite W.'s overt rebellion, he could not escape the Bush legacy entirely. He confided repeatedly to friends in quiet moments how much he admired the elder Bush.[20] He was his father's political sidekick, sharing GHW's rocky path to and from the Oval Office. Politics brought him close to a father who had been absent in earlier years. In the process, W. internalized the Bush family's political ambitions but rebelled pointedly against the elder Bush's methods, styles, and policies.

W. was never an official member of this father's entourage. He usually had something else going: a string of failed businesses after graduating from Harvard Business School, service in the Texas National Guard (along with the sons of many other famous Texans) during the Vietnam War, an unsuccessful 1978 run for Congress, and then the presidency of the Texas Rangers baseball team during his father's tenure in the Oval Office. He struggled with and overcame a drinking problem. He took a famous (and perhaps mythical) walk at Kennebunkport with Billy Graham and embraced Jesus Christ.[21]

But every time his father ran for office, W. was there. During the White House years—from the 1988 victory to the 1992 defeat—W. played high protector and enforcer: vetting staff for loyalty during the 1988 presidential transition and bringing the boom down on aides (such as Chief of Staff John Sununu) who threatened the family interests. He was a trusted surrogate, organizer, retail politician, and his father's connection to the evangelical right. He developed, said Republican political operative Mary Matalin, an exquisite command of political tactics. He was, she opined, a "political campaign terrorist.... He's much more of a stiletto as opposed to an ax murderer. He comes into a room, you know he's there." He showed his toughness. Said John Ellis, his cousin: "That's what people don't understand about him. They don't understand how fucking tough he is."[22] Perhaps outgrowing and sublimating his childhood hyperactivity, he became intensely focused and disciplined—using exercise to calm his kineticism.

However, he remained a rebel. A Yankee to the core, George H. W. Bush had failed to connect with Sunbelt voters: the cowboy hat and boots never seemed to fit, the barbecue seemed to stick in his craw. In contrast, W. relished and celebrated his Texas roots and ostentatiously scorned the establishment in all its incarnations: the Washington parties, the state dinners, the scribblers and TV pundits. Rather be in Crawford.

## How to Sell a Position to a Bush

His father was always uncomfortable with evangelical religion—not proper, too emotional. W. gave easy voice to his born-again convictions. Southerners and evangelicals saw him as one of their own. Convinced that his father's decision to reverse himself on taxes helped cost him reelection, George W. became an unbending, inflexible tax-cutter. Where the father was slow, methodical, even ponderous in decision-making, the impulsive son would be the decider—quick on the trigger, going from the gut. His father was famously (in his own rebellion against Ronald Reagan) a detail man, at least on matters that interested him. GW would stick to the big picture—those nagging details, difficult to master in any case, could be delegated.

And, perhaps most important for our story, W. rebelled against his father's policy preferences. The elder Bush had loved foreign policy and disdained domestic matters. In the end, domestic policy scuttled his presidency. His reaction to the 1991 recession had been inept, and his tepid conversion to health care reform had been half-hearted and unpersuasive. The younger Bush learned the lesson: he would put domestic issues at the top of his agenda.[23]

George W. Bush's concern for domestic policy issues, however, may have reflected more than a turn against his father. There was, also, a subtle, unspoken embrace of a deeper Bush family legacy. Amidst the cynicism and tactical maneuvering of modern politics, the Bushes shared a tradition of service. This began with the rigid, upright Prescott; flowed down to his loyal son George H. W.; and passed, somehow, to the hyperactive George W. After young George was elected governor of Texas in 1994, Karl Rove, his controversial strategist, found a hidden do-gooder, willing to use government for social purposes, lurking underneath W.'s tough, wisecracking, conservative shell.[24] Early in his first term, Bush made education his signature initiative and proposed a value-added tax to fund better education for Texans. Rove protested.

Raising taxes had gotten his father into big trouble. But Bush thought it was the right thing to do and took it to the legislature—where it lost. As Weissberg notes: "Thereafter, Rove understood that the way to sell a position to Bush was the same way you sold one to his father, by arguing it was the right thing to do, and framing any political advantages around the ethical choice."[25]

Calculation and instinct came together in another political choice: W.'s embrace of "compassionate conservative."[26] The slogan solved some important problems for Bush during his presidential run. It softened the impression that he was a captive of right wing "wackos" and evangelicals.[27] It showed independent voters that this relatively unknown Texan could feel the suffering of the disadvantaged. In the post–Cold War, post-Clinton, pre-9/11 era, a winning Republican platform needed more than national security, tax cuts, and moral values—it needed something for the Americans who were being left behind in the vertiginous global economy.

But Bush's compassionate conservatism was more than a glib election-year pose. As the Medicare story will make clear, something about it grabbed him. George W. Bush wanted to help. The methods would have to be right, but he was anxious to try. Perhaps personal experience fed the impulse: early loss; a mother struggling with grief, stress, and depression; his own fear of failure in a distant boarding school. We may never know the roots of Bush's compassion—especially in a man so scornful of introspection. But they appear to be an essential part of this privileged, insecure, energetic, talented, disabled man always struggling with the legacy of his formidable family.

## THE MEDICARE MODERNIZATION ACT

Like most major legislation, the Medicare Modernization Act (MMA) had deep political roots. LBJ's signature on Medicare was hardly dry before HEW officials, including Joe Califano, began pushing for drug benefits. Johnson—who had squelched the effort to add them to the original bill in the Senate—continued to balk at the projected costs (even he had his limits).[28] The Nixon and Carter administrations wrestled with the issue; when the Reagan administration expanded Medicare coverage to pay for catastrophic costs, the Democrats jumped on the plan and added prescription drug coverage—"lighting up the proposal like a Christmas tree." Medicare drug coverage disappeared with the collapse of Catastrophic Coverage Act and sank again as part of the Clinton health reform plan.

Then, toward the end of the 1990s the tectonic plates began shifting and the health policy terrain changed again.[29] First, the federal budget surplus was growing (it would rise from $70 billion in 1998 to $236 billion in 2000)—the payoff from those tough fiscal decisions in 1993 and 1997 when the Clinton administration pushed through deficit reduction packages. This was the first balanced budget since 1969 and the first multi-year surplus since 1949. For the first time in a half-century, the government had money to spend. A second factor was the resurgent right in American politics, which fueled Republican aspirations to shake up Medicare by increasing the private sector's role in its management. Still a third influence was the changing nature of medical practice: Drugs were now hugely important. By the end of the 1990s, a crop of new, seemingly miraculous agents—lowering cholesterol and blood pressure, preventing heart attacks and strokes, stopping cancer in its tracks—offered hope to Medicare beneficiaries, and, at the same time, terrible frustration as drug prices soared out of reach. Unhappy seniors, in turn, caused hypertension in Congress.

Not surprisingly, the Democrats pounced first. Eying the 2000 election and the presidential bid of Vice President Al Gore, Bill Clinton used his 1999 State of the Union address to call for a Medicare prescription drug benefit (dubbed Part D) with a New Democrat twist: The new program would permit beneficiaries to purchase drug coverage from private health care plans. The government would subsidize premiums for those with lower incomes (up to 150 percent of poverty level). The drug plan would cost $650–700 billion over ten years. But no problem—the federal budget surplus now projected out to $4.4 trillion over that period. This was the liberal definition of paradise.[30]

Wary congressional Republicans, also eyeing the looming election, pledged to work on a bipartisan drug package.[31] As if to confirm the fundamental change in the national politics of Medicare drug coverage, the pharmaceutical industry announced in January 2000 that it was dropping its longstanding opposition to a Medicare drug benefit, provided it was administered through the private sector. In April, the Republicans introduced their own drug prescription plan.

### The 2000 Presidential Campaign

The Democrats pounded the prescription drug issue right from the start of the primaries. Bush was slow to embrace it, but by May 2000 he jumped on the bandwagon: "Our nation must reform Medicare, and, in doing so, ensure that prescription drugs are affordable and available for every senior who needs them. As with Social Security, Medicare reform must be guided by clear tenets.... When I am president, I will lead Republicans and Democrats to reform and strengthen Medicare and set it on firm financial ground. And I make this pledge to seniors: Every senior will have access to prescription drug benefits."[32] Medicare reform came first—in the Republican lexicon, this meant injecting private insurance companies into the government program; drug coverage, however, would be part of the package. Bush remained vague about what precisely he would do. Gore, in typical contrast, trumpeted a number: $339 billion over ten years.

Throughout the summer and fall, the Democrats pressed their advantage on the issue, which was polling well among the elderly—no small matter in battleground states such as Florida. On August 29, 2000, Gore challenged Bush to "put up or shut up" on Medicare drugs and then launched a series of ads condemning the drug industry and Republican reluctance to help the elderly with drug costs.[33] In September 2000, Bush finally put up: his plan combined conservative commitment to Medicare reform with a dash of compassion. Bush would transform Medicare into a program of competing private insurance plans that would (presumably) offer drug benefits to all enrollees. In the short term, however, he would offer $12 billion a year in matching grants to states to support state-run programs to subsidize drug expenses for low-income elderly Americans.

During the first Bush–Gore debate on October 4, 2000, moderator Jim Lehrer opened with the Medicare drug issue. The candidates sparred over whether the Bush plan would cover all the elderly or just the poor.[34] Bush accused the Democrats of failing to to enact a drug benefit during their eight years in power. Elect him, he promised, and he would get it done. By the end of the debate, Bush had made passing the Medicare drug benefit a test of presidential mettle.

### Out of the Box

George W. Bush, the first MBA president, would not be remembered for his management skills ("Brownie, you're doin' a heck of a job!"),[35] but his transition got him off to a quick start on the Medicare drug issue. According to Scott McClellan, Bush's former press secretary, Bush put his close friend Clay Johnson in charge of transition planning more than a year before he was elected.[36]

On January 29, 2001, ten days after his inauguration, Bush released a proposal that reflected his campaign positions: grants to the states to assist poor elderly Americans with the costs of their drugs. A comprehensive Medicare reform package would follow later. *New York Times* correspondent Robert Pear noted acidly: "Mr. Bush's debut in the health policy arena could scarcely have been more different from the approach of his predecessor. Bill Clinton recruited more than 500 experts to advise him and his wife, Hillary, and after nine months of work ... he sent Congress a 240,000 word plan.... By contrast, President Bush, on his 10th day in office, with fewer than a half-dozen health policy experts, issued a 2100 word sketch of his ideas for Medicare drug benefits."[37]

Republicans and Democrats promptly rejected the Bush proposal. Charles Grassley (R-IA), about to become Republican chair of the Senate Finance Committee (until the defection of Senator James Jeffords [R-VT] four months later, tossed control back to the Democrats), noted that the president's plan had little chance of enactment because it didn't help all the elderly, but he thanked the president for keeping the heat on. And Bush's spokesman, Ari Fleischer, as much as conceded that the plan's chances were slim, saying that it was "not inconsistent or incompatible that this becomes part of the longer, broader Medicare reform."[38] Bush was already telegraphing a style that he would follow on Medicare drugs and related issues: set ambitious goals, stir the pot, stay flexible, see what happens.

For most of the spring, Bush focused his energy on his top priority: tax cuts. He got them by late May and in the summer returned to Medicare and demonstrated another strategy that would mark his Medicare reforms. He laid out principles—a framework—for what he wanted from the Congress, but he avoided detailed legislation. The simple framework, announced July 10, 2001, had two key tenets:

- All seniors should have the option of a subsidized prescription drug benefit as part of a modernized Medicare.
- Medicare should provide better health insurance options, like those available to all Federal employees.

The message: the new administration would support Medicare as an entitlement and drug coverage as a benefit, but it wanted to reform— the administration always called it modernizing—the program along conservative lines. It should be reorganized to resemble the Federal

Employees Health Benefit Program, in which the federal government solicited bids from insurance companies, made the resulting options available to employees (in this case, the elderly) and let the employees (Medicare eligibles) pick a plan, for which government covered part of the premium. There would be no guarantee of drug coverage, but beneficiaries could purchase it by picking a plan that included it. Of course, these plans would cost more, and the elderly would have to pay extra for more generous coverage. The poor would get help with the costs. The Republicans would take the old big government entitlement—as they saw it—and bring it into the twenty-first century of market competition, beneficiary cost-consciousness, improved efficiency, and cost containment.

Democrats saw an assault on a cherished principle: the social insurance idea that all beneficiaries were treated the same, that all beneficiaries went into the same national insurance pool. Ted Kennedy (D-MA) made it clear that at least in the Senate, Bush's modernization was a nonstarter. He told the *New York Times:* "It's going to become increasingly apparent through the summer that 'Medicare reform' is not going to take place. But there will be a real attempt to pass a good, effective prescription drug program."[39] But through the summer, Bush continued to pair the notion of drug coverage with a broader revamping of Medicare to make it more like private health care markets. He seemed to relish the boldness of his proposal and the controversy it would engender.

Bush liked being the game-changer, the risk-taker, the leader who disrupted established thinking and challenged political assumptions. Fans on Capitol Hill, such as Congresswoman Nancy Johnson (R-CT), who chaired the health subcommittee of House Ways and Means, saw Bush as a creative health care force. "I have served under Reagan, Bush 1, Clinton and Bush 2," Johnson would later say, "and in my mind there has never been the kind of dynamic, out of the box, creative thinking about health care."[40] Where Johnson saw boldness and creative disruption, of course, Democrats saw recklessness and ideological obsession. In their view, markets were hell on social justice, they were engines of inequality, they were making a mess of the American health care system. They would fight this brand of modernization. George W. Bush pushed back. He traveled to Truman High School in Independence, Missouri (hallowed Democratic ground) on August 21, 2001, and made his typical pitch. He started out on the politics, warning opponents that he would not be intimidated:

Medicare is—they usually call it, in the political lexicon, "Mediscare." See, when you talk about Medicare, then somebody takes your words and tries to twist it and frighten people who rely upon Medicare. That's an old tactic, an old political tactic. That doesn't deter me, however, from talking about making sure the system works.

Then he went on to talk substance:

Medicare is an incredibly important program. It's a promise the Nation made to our seniors, and we've got to make sure it works.... Now, I've asked Congress to—both Republicans and Democrats—to think about how to do the following things: Make sure prescription drugs is [*sic*] available for seniors; make sure seniors who like their current Medicare system can stay in it, the way it is; but make sure seniors have got a variety of options from which to choose. I said, "Why don't you all look at your own health care plan?" It's not a bad place to start. If the Senators and Congressmen have got a variety of options from which to choose, if their own health care plan trusts them to design a program that meets their needs, why shouldn't we do the same thing for our seniors? Why shouldn't we say, "Let's give seniors choices."[41]

President Bush's framework made little progress. First, Democrats had wrested control of the Senate at the start of the summer, and they were not going to step aside for what they saw as a Republican assault on Medicare. Second, even Republicans were reluctant to reform Medicare when elderly were mostly happy with the program and were not calling for competition and choice; what they really wanted was prescription drug coverage. Finally, the terrorist attack on 9/11 wiped the administration's domestic agenda right out of mind.[42]

The 2002 State of the Union address focused on terrorism—famously (and controversially) describing an "axis of evil" that threatened the homeland. President Bush barely mentioned the Medicare program, although his budget included $190 billion for an expanded Medicare drug benefit. Congressional Republicans, however, could not ignore the issue. Facing the 2002 midterms, GOP congressmen were anxious to show their continued concern for the elderly, and the Republican House moved aggressively on Medicare prescription drug coverage in the spring and summer. The Republicans tossed the Medicare modernization agenda overboard and fashioned a prescription drug entitlement that would be made available through competing private plans. House Democrats proposed their own initiative, which differed from the Republicans mostly in the generosity of the package: $800 billion from the Democrats, compared with the GOP's $310 billion.[43] The

Republican bill narrowly prevailed in the House but ran into the Democrat-controlled Senate. Senate liberals opposed the idea—a benefit run by competing private plans—and opted, instead, for a prescription drug benefit offered as part of the traditional Medicare program, just like physician and hospital services. They also upped the House benefit to nearly $600 billion. With the Democrats holding a precarious 51–49 majority, neither party could round up the 60 votes necessary for cloture, and prescription drug coverage died on July 31. The White House largely sat on the sidelines during this debate.[44]

President Bush was still riding high in the polls (up to 70 percent approval through much of the summer), and he kept pressing his Medicare reform as he stumped for congressional Republicans. During a July 25 appearance on behalf of Senator Elizabeth Dole (R-NC), he repeated his pitch: "We need a Medicare plan that is modern. You know, Medicare is a great idea, except that it's antiquated. It was made for another time. It's time to reform Medicare so seniors have got prescription drugs and more options from which they can choose. It is time the Federal Government trusts the American people."[45]

In the summer, the administration initiated a comprehensive review of the Medicare program under the guidance of Tom Scully, administrator of the Center for Medicare and Medicaid Services (which administers the program) and Mark McClellan, chief White House health policy advisor. Eventually, Douglas Badger, special assistant to the president, replaced McClellan who went off to run the Food and Drug Administration. The White House policy bureaucracy included an interesting twist: responsibility for Medicare was in the hands, not of the domestic policy council, but of the National Economic Council. This meant that whatever emerged would, willy-nilly, have the backing of the administration's number-crunchers.

The review heavily involved the president and his senior staff. Through the fall, White House staff produced detailed memoranda on Medicare prescription drug policy issues and then met for a series of about ten hour-long policy discussions with the president; Vice President Cheney; Andy Card, the White House Chief of staff; Karl Rove; Cabinet secretaries, and others. By all accounts, the president was a dominant presence in these meetings: he came well prepared, he spoke without notes, he asked probing questions.

This image of a highly engaged, detail-oriented president Bush is startling. It is different from almost every other account of the president's management style, even in areas as vital as the economy and Iraq.[46] Why did George W. Bush—the well-known delegator—apparently dive into the weeds of Medicare prescription drug coverage?

A number of factors may have been at work. First, Bush himself had made the passage of a drug benefit an acid test of presidential effectiveness. His mind was turning toward November 2004; failing to produce a Medicare drug bill would leave him exposed to Democratic attacks.

Second, in November 2002, the Republicans retook the Senate (51–49), so that for the first time since 1955, they controlled the presidency and both houses of Congress. This raised hopes that the president might actually achieve his Medicare reform agenda. Of course Republican dominance also increased the pressure on the president to deliver his campaign promises.

But to manage the politics, the president did not need to be as involved as he seems to have become in the particulars of Medicare policy. This suggests that something else was at work. Perhaps it was his continuing rebellion against his father's example. The first Bush had ignored the details of health policy. The older Bush never read the briefing books, showed up late, and filibustered the health experts with talk of other things; his son tackled the books, focused on the subject, and almost made a fetish of punctuality during the sixty-minute sessions.

Perhaps Medicare policy resonated with his self-image as both caring (expand benefits) and tough (make Medicare more efficient, introduce market discipline). Or perhaps he liked the bold risk—a frontal assault on a program dubbed the third rail of American politics. In a sense, as more than one participant suggested to us, his bust of the old paradigm approach marked his thinking on Medicare, the Middle East, and other areas. "He's a systems thinker," Congresswoman Nancy Johnson told us.

Whatever the impetus, the president showed a rare level of personal involvement in the passage of an expanded Medicare drug program in the fall and winter of 2002–3.

Several critical decisions emerged from the policy review. The administration increased its commitment for drug coverage from $190 billion to $400 billion over ten years. This brought the White House into line with congressional Republicans, who had put this figure in their own budget reconciliation bill. Conservatives and economists in the administration grumbled, but the president made it clear that he wanted a bill, and $400 billion (not a penny more) was the price he was willing to pay.

Second, the administration softened its approach toward Medicare reform. Instead of directly restructuring all Medicare around competing private plans, it took a less direct route and tried to get Medicare beneficiaries to *choose* private health plans by dangling the prescription drug carrot before them. Medicare would offer drug benefits only under private plans; beneficiaries would choose whether to stay in the traditional program or switch for the new benefit.

## Home Stretch

In January 2003, the president released the broad outlines of his Medicare proposal in a State of the Union address. The speech focused on the looming war with Iraq. Nevertheless President Bush devoted several minutes to Medicare drug coverage. He then took to the road to sell the program, which received a mixed reception. Congressional Republicans applauded the administration's commitment to a more realistic funding level but were nervous about denying drug benefits to elderly Americans enrolled in traditional Medicare.[47] The Republican leadership warned the White House against the approach.

Over the next four weeks, the president made two additional decisions. He would introduce a framework for a prescription drug benefit, not a full bill. Though the language was ready and vetted, and the details available, Hill Republicans counseled against setting the specifics in stone. With the Clinton example still looming large, Bush decided he would leave the Congress as much running room as possible in designing the new benefit.[48]

Secondly, the administration backed off its signature innovation: it would no longer insist that drug benefits be available only to enrollees in private plans. Participants in traditional Medicare would get some drug coverage, but drug benefits under private plans would be more generous. This was a concession—still not sufficient, it would turn out—to congressional anxieties about offending the nearly 90 percent of elderly who preferred traditional Medicare.

The administration released its blueprint on March 3, and the legislative battle began. There were many favorable signs. The administration had managed its role well. It had gotten its proposal into play early—two months—into the new Republican-dominated congressional session; it had sketched out the principles and delegated the critical details to

Congress. And it had stayed flexible, backing off the full reform plan, at the advice of Congressional leaders. All were lessons learned from Clinton errors.

The politics seemed favorable. The elderly were, of course, a crucial voting block. The formidable AARP—clearly trying to accommodate what looked like a Republican era—had made it clear in discussions with Karl Rove that it would support a benefit at the $400 billion level, although it was holding out for some additional concessions that would be negotiated with legislators. Other big interest groups were on board: the pharmaceutical and insurance industries.[49] Congressional Republicans had forged alliances with some key Democrats, notably Senators Edward Kennedy (D-MA), Max Baucus (D-MT), and John Breaux (D-LA). We have watched Kennedy play a role in almost every chapter of the book. By now, he no longer had to negotiate with labor (as he had during the Nixon administration) or anyone else to forge a compromise across the aisle. His support guaranteed liberal votes. Senators Baucus and Breaux brought along more moderate and conservative members of the party. Furthermore, Senate Majority Leader Bill Frist (R-TN) was a respected physician and health policy expert who was firmly committed to passing the prescription drug benefit.

But the politics were still not easy. The stakes for the next election were huge. If Republicans could claim credit for a big Medicare expansion, they could erode the Democrats' longstanding claim to be the program's champions against Republican knives. GOP success might even snatch Medicare (and, who knew, even the health care issue) away from the Democrats. As a result, some Democrats would be tempted to block the initiative. And for many liberals, any move toward Medicare markets was not modernization (as the Republicans saw it) but an erosion of the universal, social insurance principle that they still believed in deeply—even while it was being routed at almost every policy turn. They would not give up their Medicare without a fight.

The administration and congressional leaders faced ideological faultlines crisscrossing both parties. Conservative Republicans opposed this enormous open-ended entitlement—just the sort of thing they usually dubbed big government and railed against. At the same time, they were attracted to the idea of introducing private plans into Medicare to administer the drug benefit. And, more generally, they cheered the first step toward turning the program over to private plans. Many Democrats found the idea of private plans abhorrent but had long wanted to add a drug benefit. In fact, many wanted to spend more than $400 billion on it.

Congressional leaders and administration officials formed a team to lobby members and monitor the program's progress. Secretary of Health and Human Services Tommy Thompson played a major role. So did the Director of CMS Tom Scully. Both would prove effective—at least in the eyes of many Republican colleagues—in the legislative negotiations over the next months. While some Democrats demurred, both earned the respect of GOP leaders on the Hill. One Republican participant, who asked to remain anonymous, described the group's legislative teamwork as "seamless." For their part, Democratic staff grudgingly acknowledged the political effectiveness of the administration but saw it as either uninterested or unprepared to contribute on substantive legislative issues.

In June 2003, President Bush made another tactical retreat. He backed away from the position that the drug benefit for private health plan enrollees should be more generous than for traditional Medicare. In this, he was acceding to the strong views of Republican allies on Capitol Hill.[50] To keep pressure on senators, Bush convened a bipartisan group of supporters at the White House on June 18 to give them a pep talk about passing the bill.[51]

Eventually, the center held. Parallel Medicare bills—containing both expanded drug benefits and many other changes in the program, large and small—passed both houses. But—again the infernal machinery of American government—passage was by no means assured. When the House and Senate met in conference to reconcile the two measures, the Republican leadership excluded virtually all Democrats from the sessions—except the highly sympathetic Baucus and Breaux. This left the negotiations almost entirely within Republican hands. But the leadership was jolted when the House and Senate negotiating teams, both Republican, could not find common ground. Charles Grassley, the quirky, plainspoken chair of Senate Finance, and Bill Thomas (R-CA), the brilliant but mercurial and condescending chair of House Ways and Means, nearly came to blows in extended intemperate sessions that lasted from July through early November of 2003. By all accounts, Thomas played a dominant role in crafting the substance of the legislation, but he also kept the conference in turmoil. He even ejected White House representatives (though he permitted the CMS's Scully to stay for expert backup) and threatened to exclude the two moderate Democrats on the Senate side as well. At one point, a delegation of angry House

Democrats marched on Thomas's office, demanding to be admitted to the conference. Thomas blew them off.

Desperate House and Senate Republican leaders eventually resorted to a virtually unprecedented device. They negotiated at the leadership level, and presented conferees a fait accompli. The explosive Thomas was so infuriated that he charged out of the conference room and headed for the airport to catch a plane home. House leaders had to coax him back to Capitol Hill to finish the negotiations.

One of the issues that froze the conference was the last remnant of Bush's original vision of turning all of Medicare into a privately managed insurance program. The House had included a provision that would have allowed private plans in a number of metropolitan areas to submit bids for Medicare business. Private plans would compete with traditional Medicare in these areas; if the traditional program cost the feds more, the elderly would have to pay more to stay in it. For the conservative House Republicans, this was an essential provision that gave them something—a market challenge to the traditional big government program—in exchange for expanding the Medicare entitlement. For the Democrats, the Republican provision was an assault on essential principle. Grassley, knowing how closely divided the Senate was, had tried to limit the competition demonstration. Thomas had balked. In the final compromise, Thomas won competitive bidding demonstrations for Medicare in four markets starting in 2010.[52]

The AARP played a critical role by endorsing the plan. It had negotiated with Republican leaders—Senator Frist and Representative Denny Hastert (R-IL)—on several key provisions: subsidies to employers to prevent them from dropping drug coverage for retirees and limits on the number of competitive demonstrations. The AARP figured that it would be a long time before it would again have Republican support for a $400 billion Medicare expansion. President Bush had called the CEO of the AARP, James Parkel, to help secure the endorsement, building on months of lobbying by House and Senate Republicans.[53]

The bill emerged from the conference decorated with a slew of other reform provisions designed to inject private-sector innovations into Medicare. These were less controversial and included experiments designed to improve the quality of care, reduce the cost of managing chronic illness, and require reporting of data on quality of care by providers. Although the conference report did not come close to the wholesale restructuring that Bush and his conservative allies had contemplated during the 2000 campaign or even the vision of Part D that they first sent to the Hill, the bill injected a distinctly Republican set of innovations into the Medicare program.

Now the leaders had to win approval of the compromise. House Republicans, angry that the market reforms had been watered down while spending was still at $400 billion, threatened mutiny. During the floor debate on Friday afternoon, November 22, Bush phoned conservative Republicans from Air Force One as he headed back from a trip to England, where he had been a guest of Queen Elizabeth. Karl Rove had already been twisting arms from Buckingham Palace.[54] After landing, the jet-lagged president dialed Republican holdouts until early Saturday morning. Breaking precedent, Secretary of HHS Tommy Thompson went onto the House floor to lobby balky Republican representatives. The House leadership played hardball, allegedly threatening one holdout Republican with retaliation against his son, who was contemplating a run for Congress. Then they broke House rules—and infuriated the Democrats—by letting the voting period drag on and on. The fifteen minutes allowed for voting turned into forty-five, but the bill was going down by four votes; the vote stayed open for over two hours (until 5:50 A.M.) while Republican leaders twisted arms, bent ears, and horse-traded with the reluctant representatives.[55]

Eventually, the conference report squeaked through by a near party-line vote: 220–215. Twenty conservative Republicans voted against it. Hours later, President Bush used his Saturday morning radio address to pressure the Senate to follow the House's lead: "In the nearly 40 years since Medicare was launched, this is the most significant opportunity for any Congress to improve health coverage for our seniors," he told them.[56] The Senate complied. Kennedy had now defected, claiming that the competitive demonstrations (not in the Senate bill) were unacceptable, and a number of liberals fell off with him. But Frist was able to cobble together 61 votes to end debate, and the measure ultimately passed 54–44.

## GEORGE W. BUSH AND HEALTH CARE

When the dust settled, it was clear that the Congress had played the dominant role in writing the MMA. The bill bore little resemblance to the plans Bush had introduced. Nevertheless, the passage of the Medicare Modernization Act of 2003 appeared to be a major victory for George

W. Bush and the Republicans. For Bush, it blocked a potential Democratic attack in the 2004 election. The president went on to win a difficult reelection despite approval ratings that lingered into the mid–40 percent range for much of the spring and summer. The Republicans picked up four Senate seats for decisive control (55–45) in that chamber and picked up another three in the House, where they now had their largest margin in more than fifty years (232–202).

And yet, as many Capitol observers told us, the Republicans as a party never managed to win credit for health care. The issue remains securely in Democratic hands—indeed, public opinion polls in the run up to the next election, the 2006 midterms, showed that voters trusted Democrats over Republicans on health care by a larger margin than on any other issue. The Republicans would lose the House and Senate in 2006 and slipped further into the minority in 2008—a stunning reversal in four years. The Medicare Modernization Act—despite its growing popularity among beneficiaries—seemed to do the GOP little political good. On the contrary, Democrats attacked the program's complicated benefits structure and—getting to the heart of the major question about "modernization"—the difficulty seniors (and their children) were having in negotiating the private-sector offerings.

Still, it is a remarkable story: The conservative Bush administration won the largest expansion in Medicare history and the biggest new health care entitlement in almost four decades (not much thanks to the Democrats who, in the end, largely opposed it). In the process, the George W. Bush health care story confirms and elaborates many of the lessons about presidential leadership and the management of health policy: personal commitment, a variation on the rule of speed, flexibility (an extreme case), handling economists, the possibilities and limits of bipartisanship.

W's exertions contrast dramatically with the growing pile of books that picture a president blithely disinterested in the details. For a hands-off president—the Great Delegator—George Bush was surprisingly involved in the Medicare Modernization Act. Everyone we interviewed described exactly the same behavior: crisp, prepared, knowledgeable, interested, and (always) punctual.

Health care seems to have been different—this was not the Bush MO on many other matters. The health care issue reflected W.'s personal proclivities: It seemed, at least before Congress got involved, to offer an opportunity to be bold and disruptive, to change the whole framework. It also offered a chance to engage a domestic issue that his father had muffed. And perhaps, too, it permitted a return of compassionate conservatism that had evaporated early in the Bush presidential years.

W. offers a corollary to the old rule of speed. His team was prepared with a Medicare plan within weeks of the inauguration. Then tax cut battles, the loss of the Senate, and 9/11 delayed a serious effort. Months before the November 2002 election, however, the administration began a systematic health policy review, and when the election put Republicans back in command of Congress, the administration was ready to go. In a way, the November 2002 election constituted a new start for the Bush presidency. From this perspective, the Medicare review resembled a well-managed transition. And offers a different sort of lesson: the Bush team had a plan ready to go if and when opportunity struck—for, as the Clinton team had learned, the policy opportunity usually passes swiftly. And perhaps the whole notion of moving fast is more important for introducing new programs than expanding old ones—especially Medicare. The elderly are always there, politically potent and ready to throw their weight behind more generous benefits.

The Bush effort, like Clinton's before it, raises the great tactical question: how flexible should the White House be? W. provided general policy direction but avoided getting mired in detailed proposals, which he instead delegated to the Congress. The president was flexible even on his strongly held ideological principles—compromising on the subject of bold Medicare reform. The administration's legislative team reacted nimbly to the politics on the Hill—retreating again (and again) from the essential principle of private competition. George Bush got a bill, but it was far less than he had originally wanted. Did W. prove too flexible? The opposite mistake, perhaps, of Bill Clinton waving his veto pen? Time will tell whether the Medicare Modernization Act starts the program down the Republican road toward increased private sector involvement (as Republicans hoped) or proves to be just another big government entitlement (as they fear).

Put Lyndon Johnson aside, and something quite astonishing emerges from the record. The Republicans have been far more successful at health reform than the Democrats. Nixon got national health insurance through the Ways and Means Committee. Reagan added catastrophic health insurance to Medicare (later repealed). And W. won a prescription drug benefit. Always, it's a variation on the same theme. Republicans get into it because of a president's personal bent, whether for systems reform (competition) or election-year insurance; Democrats go along for benefits they have invariably wanted for some time. W.—like

Nixon—was able to attract Ted Kennedy to his cause and hold him almost till the end. This was critical to outflanking liberal Democrats in the Senate and breaking a likely liberal filibuster.

President Bush managed his own economists and the conservatives around him. He announced unequivocally that he would go with a $400 billion price tag and no more.

Finally, the Bush years demonstrate, more than most, how every administration sits in a great political context. George W. Bush came to office in what appeared to be a powerful conservative era. Democrats were retreating. Even Bill Clinton had declared that the era of big government was over. Conservatives arrived touting an armful of policy blueprints—and in health care, that meant restoring private markets.

President Eisenhower—an establishment Republican—had started the GOP down the path—private mechanisms could solve the public's health problems. But Ike was proposing markets in a social Democratic era. By the Bush era, the Sunbelt GOP could promote a more radical market philosophy that would uproot even Ike's signal innovation (tax cuts for employer health insurance). A new generation of conservatives would try to get the big institutions—employers, government—out of the middle, put individuals in charge of health care insurance choices, and make everyone feel the cost consequences of their market decisions. The elderly should own their health care choices, just like every other member of the ownership society. In 2003, all this seemed within reach to the confident GOP—and even to Democrats such as Baucus and Breaux.

And yet, for all that, not much of the new market paradigm made it into the final bill. The Bush administration would not get to redesign Medicare. Their national demonstrations of market power were reduced to just four settings and would not begin for another seven years—talk about "kicking the can down the road."

It is, of course, too early for any side to render a judgment on the Medicare Modernization Act. But we can put the crucial question—the fate of markets and Medicare: Will future generations see the Bush administration reform as the opening wedge of markets and competition, thanks to the competing plans offering prescription drug benefits, or the demonstrations yet to launch, or other features buried in the bill? If so, the administration will look extraordinarily astute as it flexibly negotiated the plan into place against the opposition of both left and right. Or was this the last best chance, the highwater mark, for a market revolution that is now fast receding in the face of a global economic crisis and perhaps even a new era—of big government? If so, the administration's willingness to negotiate so much away will come to seem like a final health care retreat before savvy Democrats who stood up as the market tide crested—and then began to recede.

In short, the final judgment about Bush administration effort to reshape Medicare rests on such great questions as the future of the market culture, the role of government, and the outcome of elections that we cannot foresee.

Of course, the George W. Bush health care legacy will include a variety of other decisions, such as his veto—in the face of considerable criticism from both parties—of the extension and expansion of the State Child Health Insurance Program in 2008, and his successful advocacy—to cheers from many quarters—of funding to combat AIDs in developing countries.

But one thing is clear. The Medical Modernization Act story will surprise critics of George W. Bush's presidential leadership (though not critics of his conservative ideology). Indeed, the details of an engaged, interested, and flexible president Bush surprised us. For scholars of the health care presidency itself, W. provides an intriguing example of how a president's personal history, ability, disability, and health care experience can mesh with political opportunity to produce a bold and unexpected health care reform.

# Conclusion

*Eight Rules for the Heart of Power*

President Nixon shunned people. He didn't want to meet strangers, and he didn't like to talk to his subordinates. Two tough staff members kept almost everyone at a distance while Nixon sat alone in his hideaway and—fire crackling, air conditioner humming—scratched down his often brilliant plans on pad after pad of yellow paper. Ten years later, President Ronald Reagan dutifully kept a White House diary. The old actor recorded every review, every compliment, every applause line. His gauzy optimism almost never failed him—even rocky performances had morphed into minor hits by the end of the entry. He was the child of an alcoholic, and he acted it: constantly searching for approval, affable to a fault, gregarious like no one in Washington, and just one intimate relationship (Nancy, whom he called mommy). The first conclusion that emerges from seventy-five years of the presidency is a vivid sense of how every president is unique. Each brings his own skills, passions, and pains to the White House; each takes a different approach to the challenge of health care policy.[1]

Each president also operates in a different era, stamped with its own controversies, conditions, and conventional wisdom. We began our story in the depths of the Great Depression, watching Franklin Roosevelt set the tone for an entire generation: "These dark days will be worth all they cost us," he told the nation as he took the oath of office, "if they teach us that our destiny is ... to minister to ... our fellow man." The idea echoed through American politics for decades; it cemented a coalition, inspired Democratic presidents, and shaped the health policies they pursued—until President Reagan put his finger on an entirely different national beat. "Government is not the solution to our problem," said Reagan as he stepped into office almost a half-century after Roosevelt. Now, government was the problem. A new vision—the vibrant, deregulated, health care marketplace—animated a new majority that crested with the control of both executive and legis-lature under George W. Bush.[2]

In the preceding pages, we have explored the unique features of eleven administrations: the biography of the presidents, the ideas they promoted, the institutions they built, and the health policies they pur-sued. Different times, different parties, different men. But despite all the variation, we've watched the nation's health care troubles climb up every president's agenda. Each president had to face up to the issue. And when he did—whether in good times or bad, whether fighting the political tide or cruising with it—each encountered the same stubborn requirements of presidential leadership. In this final chapter, we reflect on eight lessons we have culled from the past to advise future adminis-trations when they face—as they will inevitably face—the problems of the health care system.

## PASSION

Major health care reform is virtually impossible: difficult to understand, swarming with interests, powered by money, and resonating with popu-lar anxiety. The first key to success is a president who cares about it deeply. Only a president with real commitment will invest in such a dangerous and risky venture. It costs time, energy, and political capital. This is no arena for half-hearted efforts.

Of course, the chances of success vary. President Johnson had what seemed like a sure thing (although, as we now know, it took all his leg-islative magic to get what he got). Bill Clinton had a reasonable shot. Harry Truman would have needed a miracle. But across time and place, all successful health care presidents share the same attribute: they care passionately.

Of course, the rule of passion extends to any big issue. The Oval Office is a cacophony of demands and causes. Presidents can normally win only a handful of great changes, and the way to win them is to focus intensely on the prize and push, push, push. This leads directly to our voter's guide for judging candidates: What's the big idea? What's the passion? What does he or she seem to care about most intensely? Focus on the two or three issues that seem lodged in the candidate's gut, because—with all the tumult that surrounds a president—those are the ones most likely to emerge from the Oval Office. And that goes double for health care.

## SPEED

The day after the presidential election, the savvy health policy analyst will slip his or her president-elect a message: "Hurry up—you're almost out of time." The window of opportunity always slams shut quickly. Lee Hamilton, a congressional veteran (and cochair of the 9/11 Commission) once remarked, "[H]ealth care is so difficult because Congress is an incremental body and health care is a non-incremental issue."[3] It does not fit naturally into the pulling and hauling of Washington politics. Once the legislative docket fills up, it is hard to squeeze a big program through. Moreover, each president's power is at its height while the vote count is still warm. As Lyndon Johnson warned his staff after the 1964 landslide, "[E]very day while I'm in office, I'm gonna lose votes." And then, the irresistible lesson about Medicare: "We gotta get this legislation fast."

President Bill Clinton offers a cautionary tale about violating the rule of speed. After his election, national health insurance looked like a winner: even some Republicans began lining up behind health plans (or staking out bargaining positions, as they might more accurately be called). A full year later, when the administration finally submitted its proposal, Clinton's election—and a squeaker at that—was ancient history and Congress was maneuvering for advantage over the upcoming midterms. Clinton's political capital had, inevitably, bled away in bruising battles over the deficit and NAFTA. The reform moment and all its energy had evaporated even before a bill appeared in Congress.

Occasionally, a bolt from the blue upsets the normal calendar: 9/11 offered the Bush administration a grisly sort of elbow room. The shock over the terrorist attack on the Twin Towers—followed by a solid midterm victory that delivered both houses of Congress to the Republicans—offered the president a new beginning. On the domestic front, he adroitly cashed in his renewed political capital on a Medicare prescription drug bill that was designed—here was Bush's passion—to drag Medicare toward the Republican idyll of competition and markets.

W.'s success offers a corollary to the rule of speed: the opportunity may arise unexpectedly. When it does, the chance is not likely to last long. Have a plan ready to go.

Finally, a caveat. It is far easier to modify an existing program—add new benefits to Medicare, expand eligibility for Medicaid—than it is to create one from scratch. Existing programs already have supporters, and they are more difficult to bomb with hot charges of socialism or cool pleas from Harry and Louise. For all that, however, the LBJ rule remains the prime reformer's directive: "You've got to get it during my honeymoon."

## BRING A PLAN WITH YOU

The White House is no place to be scheming up health reform legislation. This corollary to the rule of speed stresses the importance of coming into office with a legislative proposal in hand. FDR made the first one hundred days famous; today, health reformers ought to begin their work one hundred days before that.

And all this makes the transition particularly important as a time to position an agenda. Contemporary campaigns usually have a policy shop in full operation long before any votes are cast. Presidents should use it. The transition needs to begin well before the victory speech, and it needs to be managed with exquisite care. Clinton came to regret that he had lost track of health care during those precious weeks between November and January. He—and his party—paid dearly for his error. Carter made the same mistake. In contrast George W. Bush got started a year before his election. And when that plan went nowhere, he began another health policy review months before the 2002 midterm (the 9/11 midterm) gave him fresh majorities in both chambers.

Of course, the ideas will not always be ripe. New coalitions and different perspectives require time to mature their health care vision. For example, Richard Nixon entered the Oval Office when Washington had been dominated by Democrats for almost four decades. The conservative larder had not been stocked with ideas about health care. He used a talented team to rethink the Great Society approach and transplant national health insurance from the Social Security Administration to employee benefits offices. Ironically, as national politics moved to the right, it would be Democrats who latched onto Nixon administration's health care concoction. Likewise, George H. W. Bush reluctantly gathered a team to develop a more fully market-based health care plan—which he bequeathed to future conservative administrations—such as the one run by his son.

One surprise in our survey is that every administration makes a difference. Even maladroit administrations and failed proposals reshape the national conversation about health care.

Another surprise: the Democrats may own the health care issue—the beloved New Deal's lost reform—but it has been the Republicans who have more often won the big changes. Dwight Eisenhower was too cautious to push through his private sector plans, but by locking in the tax deduction for employee health benefits, he secured the distinctive American health insurance regime. Nixon, for his part, redefined the idea of national health insurance—the patchwork of employers and government that soon became the mainstay of Democratic plans—and even as his administration was going down in scandal, he managed to get a positive vote out of Ways and Means. Presidents Ronald Reagan and George W. Bush managed the largest health care entitlement expansions after LBJ's Medicare. For Republicans, there's always the same agonizing tradeoff: push more competition into the system, address national needs, and inoculate the party for the next election, all in exchange for permitting Democrats to expand their big-government entitlement programs. From Richard Nixon to George W. Bush, Republican presidents weigh the conflicting imperatives while conservatives furiously denounce the deal their own party is making.

Republican proposals pose a tough choice for Democrats that go far beyond the metrics of the next campaign. Yes, there are new benefits and entitlements. But each expansion erodes the social insurance ideal—we're all in this together, the rich and the healthy help the poor and the sick—and expands the marketplace ethos: everyone looks out for themselves.

## HUSH THE ECONOMISTS

The most heretical rule in the historical record: expanding health coverage requires presidents who are able and willing to overrule their economic advisors. Getting health care to large populations is expensive; economists invariably oppose it. The generalization holds across every administration from Harry Truman to George W. Bush: no expansion of health care coverage fit the budget; each drew cautions—and usually outright condemnations—from the economic team. Health reform always faces a phalanx of nays from the Office of Management and Budget, the Council of Economic Advisors, the team at the treasury, and the green-eyeshade circle on the president's staff.

"Those fools had to go to projecting it [Medicare costs] down the road five or six years," growled Lyndon Johnson, who knew full well that accurate cost estimates (and honesty about the expense of the Vietnam War) might have sunk the entire reform. And even Johnson—dispensing blithe metaphors about needing health care like Lady Bird needed coffee and sugar—reined in the Senate in 1965 when members moved to add additional benefits to the Medicare plan he and Wilbur Mills had cooked up. His economists told him a bigger program would create "fiscal drag." The benefits he squashed—catastrophic health insurance, outpatient prescription drug benefits—would themselves be the subject of great reform battles in the decades ahead.

But overruling the economists becomes ever more difficult. One of the great themes we've followed across eleven administrations marks the growth of the economic infrastructure in the Executive Office of the President. The rising technical sophistication in the executive branch is matched by counterparts on the other end of Pennsylvania Avenue—most notably in the Congressional Budget Office. More sophistication brings better analysis and more levers to control government operations. But it also binds the president in a web of technical arguments, arcane rules, and budget limits. The tilt against new entitlements is now built into the machinery of government.

Republican presidents—notably Nixon, Reagan, and George W. Bush—have been quicker to leap ahead with health care entitlements. Reagan overruled almost his entire Cabinet. On the other hand, the Democrats—Jimmy Carter, Bill Clinton, and even Harry Truman—felt a need to prove their cost-cutting chops and were far more hesitant to hush their economists without at least offering them concessions. In any case, the lesson is repeated in every administration. Presidents who seek to expand health coverage need to find the self-confidence to overrule their dismal scientists and plunge ahead. To be sure, system reforms that control costs are essential, but their success can never be certain—and covering the costs of people without insurance invariably involves higher costs. When Clinton officials suggested that they could cover some 35 million uninsured Americans without raising costs in the short run (through all kinds of budget bells and whistles), they lost their credibility. Economists are in the business of broadcasting the risks.

Presidents interested in systematic health reform are in the business of taking risks.

## GO PUBLIC

There is one job that only presidents can do: create popular momentum for reform. Any ambitious policy needs heat from the grassroots—a wave of phone calls, letters, e-mail, text messages, blogs, and, of course, high poll numbers. Popular movements convert the fence-sitters in Washington. No office in American politics—perhaps in the world—has tools for going public and shaking up national opinion like the presidency.

The job begins on the campaign trail. Presidents who want to enact major new health programs bring a clear mandate from the electorate. This requires that they make health care a priority as they run for office—not an item on the long checklist of promises (as with Jimmy Carter) but a vigorous part of the election strategy (Lyndon Johnson and Bill Clinton).

After the election, the campaign continues. We have watched a long, slow history of going public on health care. When some of Franklin Roosevelt's team pleaded with him to add national health insurance to the Social Security Program, he seemed to agree, then took one look at the conservative southern bulls sitting astride the major congressional committees and had second thoughts. He put his finger directly on this lesson when told his team: "The only one who could explain this to the people is me." But FDR never got around to it. Harry Truman campaigned hard on the issue during the 1948 campaign but ducked it after winning reelection. Eisenhower preferred the hidden hand to the bully pulpit. John Kennedy's aides debated whether to take Medicare to the people—insiders preferred a quiet deal cut behind closed doors. His congressional liaison team despised the idea of public spectacles. But Kennedy took the plunge, using the new medium of television.

The media continues to offer contemporary presidents (as well as their critics) ever greater, wider, louder amplification. In the era of twenty-four-hour media cycle and the pulsating blogosphere—thick with spin, instant news analyses, viral videos, and late-night comedy riffs on the politics of the day—going public is a subtle, difficult, and indispensable presidential task. And it increasingly requires a president—and a team—able to handle the continuous revolution in digital media.

Successfully going public requires a clear, often-repeated narrative that places the arcane details of health care reform into a popular conception of human need, the good society, the logic of government, and the role of markets. The debate that we've followed across the generations is so rich in symbols (the cries of socialism, the call to help thy neighbor, the individual's right to choose) because it provokes the deepest questions Americans can ask themselves: How do we respond to suffering? In a land where it is always morning, how do we deal with aging and death?

## MANAGE CONGRESS

The American political system is famous for its sheer, infernal complexity—it is quite possibly the world's most unwieldy democratic apparatus. When Clinton finally lobbed his national health insurance proposal to the Hill, seven different committees and subcommittees asserted jurisdiction; we watched four committees each devise (or bury) a different version of the proposal. The American legislative system offers plenty of back alleys in which to mug health reform. Political scientists have focused a sophisticated eye on the way different presidents have greater or lesser leverage in Congress—the president often has special influence, for example, in districts that he carried by a wider margin than the member of Congress did. But regardless of the advantages and disadvantages that presidents bring to the task, their role is always crucial. The successful president must be nimble at making our convoluted legislative machinery work.[4]

Here, again, Lyndon Johnson was the master. The famous Johnson treatment flattered, cajoled, intimidated, bluffed, blustered, wheedled, and recycled bawdy tales while his big hands plucked the jacket, squeezed the arms, and insinuated themselves around the shoulders. Ronald Reagan was an entirely different kind of politician. Whereas Johnson had spent a lifetime in Congress, Reagan had barely set foot in Washington. On the contrary, he made his political fortune by bashing it. But in his first year—at least—he handled Congress like an old pro. Reagan genuinely enjoyed inviting leaders from both sides of the aisle to the White House living quarters for long bouts of old stories and Irish jokes—I probably told a few too many stories, he confessed in his journal after a long dinner session with the Speaker of the House Tip O'Neil (their wives, Mommy and Millie had heard them all before).[5] Or take George W. Bush. He could not have been more different from Johnson and Reagan, but he took the new Republican Congress (won in the 2002 election) and negotiated the most ambitious expansion in Medicare's history.

Successful presidents deploy talented legislative liaison teams. Again, Johnson and Reagan had crackerjack operations—Johnson gave his chief congressional staffer the pick of anybody in the executive branch. And for presidents who lack the necessary touch to deal with Congress—JFK is a good example—an outstanding legislative team becomes even more important.

Still, no matter how good the liaison, the phone call from the Oval Office remains the most powerful move in Washington. The astute legislative liaison team identifies the crucial fence-sitters who may be open to a presidential nudge. And, thanks to invaluable telephone recordings (kept during the Kennedy, Johnson, and Nixon years) we know that of all the many things a president can say or do, nothing works like deflecting credit back to the hungry legislator. As President Johnson so often told Wilbur Mills (D-AR)—"We will applaud you." Even Richard Nixon, cloistered and paranoid, learned this lesson. "Why don't you make an agreement with [Wilbur] Mills," he cracked to his aides: "[H]e takes credit one week and I take credit the next week." As his guys laughed at the boss's joke, Nixon underscored the crucial lesson: "I am not concerned about ... getting credit."[6]

### FORGET THE PSROS

The president who poses as a policy wonk is heading for trouble. There is a long list of things the presidents do better than anyone else: watch the big picture, manage the experts, negotiate the economists, rouse the public, bring along wavering legislators. Above all, health care change demands presidential leadership: the ability to lay out a vision and a compelling case for moving toward it. But the byzantine technical details should be delegated to aides and legislators. "I'm not trying to go into the details," said Lyndon Johnson again and again. But he'd plunge in and secure the big principle he cared about—broader coverage for more people.

In contrast, Jimmy Carter pored over his paperwork, scribbling sophisticated opinions in the margin: "I'm personally inclined to think," he scrawled on one memo, "we need ... [to] make PSROs work."[7] A president talking about PSROs (physician panels that reviewed expensive Medicare cases) is in trouble, whether he knows it or not. He isn't focusing where he should be: on the big picture, the national debate, or the congressional process. President Carter lost sight of all three.

For his part, Bill Clinton made the same mistake. He mobilized a huge policy process—a spiderweb of experts—and sat at the center, delighting in the complexity and technical wizardry. But the president failed to manage his moving parts. He lost track of time, layered on complexities to appease his economists, and once again let the big political picture elude him. Bill Clinton knew what he needed to do as a political leader. His speeches were often masterful. But in the end the sheer size and complexity of the policy process—the effort to devise a better health care machine with technical magic to meet every objection—crushed his effort to persuade the people and their representatives.

Delegation begins with the chief of staff—one of the most important personnel decision in the life of any administration. It should be the first presidential appointment after Election Day. Indeed, the presumptive chief of staff should probably be on board before that, getting the transition up and running.

This is the man or woman, after all, who manages the unmanageable office: What did the president actually decide in that meeting? Who should get to see the president? When is the next press conference, big public address, or Rose Garden photo op? A lot of presidents, in each party, muffed this choice. Democrats commit the sin of hubris. They like to imagine they can do the job themselves: Carter skipped the office altogether, and Clinton selected an old friend with little experience in politics (much less with Washington politics) and then made his job impossible by opening the Oval Office door to anyone wandering by. In both cases, they were perhaps overreacting to the errors of their Republican predecessors (Richard Nixon and George H. W. Bush), whose administrations ran into grief in part because of imperious White House managers who kept their bosses isolated.

## LEARN HOW TO LOSE

One familiar story running across the modern presidency is the limitations of the office—especially when it comes to winning domestic reform. The president is hemmed in by Congress, his own office, chance events, economic imperatives (and the economists who divine them), experts (speaking their strange dialect studded with acronyms), interest groups, and the limits of time and imagination. Ambitious health reform is always a long shot. The honest health advisor should probably inform the boss: prepare to lose.

As we have seen, losing itself is an art—for it sets up the expectations for the future. Franklin Roosevelt never even joined the fight for health care. But he encouraged the reformers around him, pushed them to develop plans, and always held out the elusive hope of "taking on the fellows in Chicago." Harry Truman inherited the Roosevelt plan and made it his life's great mission. He never had much of a chance. Congress was stacked against him, the American Medical Association was primed and funded, and Harry was never much good at persuading legislators. Truman lost, but in the process of losing, he defined the terms of the debate. He gave the reforming generations that followed him a cause, a plan, and a patron saint to rally around.

In contrast, Bill Clinton walked away from the wreckage speculating about tactics and musing that he should have tried welfare reform instead. Opponents completely controlled the spin—and the history. And national health reform—the Democrats' signature cause—slipped out of political sight for a decade. The scorecards that list a president's batting average with Congress are deeply misleading, at least on this issue. The thing to score is more subtle than how many times you won. The deeper question is how you left the issue.

These eight rules may apply to plenty of other political arenas. But across seventy-five years we have seen them illustrated—by success and (more often) failure—as presidents pursue health reform. At first glance, the most useful lesson might seem to be one we have not mentioned: duck this issue at all costs. Health care is too perilous. Almost no one wins. After all, putting aside the initial enactment of Medicare, the major successes we have described are all expansions of that program. And no surprise: the elderly are unique constituents, and the program is enormously popular. If you are talking about Medicare expansion, you can bend these rules here and there—Doc Bowen got his increased coverage in Ronald Reagan's seventh year; Bush got Medicare Part D in his third.

But presidents do not have the luxury of slipping the issue. Why? Because hurting, sickness, and death are an unavoidable part of the human condition, and our system for coping with these universal sorrows is in critical condition. Most presidents know this in their bones—they get sick, they hurt, they grieve for people they love. And on the campaign trail, the issue wells up in town meetings and debates. Every president enters that first budget meeting and learns how the rising burden of Medicare and Medicaid spending threatens every other aspiration and promise. The issue will continue to vex the president as long as we have so much trouble caring for sick Americans.

When the challenge arises—as it will for the current president, and for the next—our history offers a very rough guide to action. These suggestions are not, of course, foolproof. Every great political change requires more than a checklist drawn from the past. It always takes imagination, heart, brains, skill, cool—and a whole lot of luck.

Each one of the eleven presidents we studied was an extraordinary man (quite to our surprise, we came to admire many things about every one of them). Each brought his own kind of political genius into the Oval Office. Each, of course, also came with weakness and limits. Although some accomplished great changes in American health care, most failed to do so. And, whether as a success or failure, each passed the problem on to the next president. Even great policy victories, when they come, create new dilemmas to be resolved.

In the end, perhaps health care simply stretches indefinitely into the future. It is, after all, the place where politics and interests meet the human condition, the issue that reflects the greatest challenge to any society: how well do we minister to our fellow humans? Seen this way, health care will always challenge the head and the soul of the vulnerable human who sits at the heart of power.

# Notes

ABBREVIATIONS

FDR Library                 Franklin D. Roosevelt Presidential Library: Hyde Park,
                            New York
Truman Library              Harry S. Truman Library: Independence, Missouri
Eisenhower Library          Dwight D. Eisenhower Library: Abilene, Kansas
JFK Library                 John F. Kennedy Library: Boston, Massachusetts
LBJ Library                 Lyndon B. Johnson Library: Austin, Texas
Nixon Library               Nixon Presidential Library and Museum: Yorba Linda,
                            California
Carter Library              Jimmy Carter Library: Atlanta, Georgia
Reagan Library              Ronald Reagan Library: Simi Valley, California
Bush Library                George H. W. Bush Library: College Station, Texas
Presidency Project          The American Presidency Project, UC Santa Barbara

INTRODUCTION

1. See chapter 6 for notes and details. Rose McDermott, *Presidential Leadership*: Illness and Decision Making (New York: Cambridge University Press, 2008), 164–65 [dry eyed].

2. Alexander Hamilton, *Federalist Number 67* and 69.

3. Mortality data from Robert E. Gilbert, *The Mortal Presidency: Illness and Anguish in the White House* (New York: Fordham University Press, 1998), 4–5.

4. See chapter 4 for notes and details.

5. Pat Caddell, memo to "Governor Carter," "Additions to December 10 Working Paper," December 21, 1976, Staff Secretary Presidential Handwriting

File, Box 1, Folder: Caddell, Patrick, 12/76–1/77, Carter Library. For a detailed analysis of the Republican perspective across policy domains, see Jeremy Johnson, "The Republican Welfare State." PhD dissertation ms. (Providence, RI: Brown University, 2009).

6. See Otis Bowen, oral history, "Interview with Otis Bowen MD," Charlottesville, Virginia, taken as part of the Ronald Reagan Oral History Project, page 57, November 8–9, 2001, Miller Center for Public Affairs, Charlottesville, Virginia.

7. Stephen Skowronek, *The Politics Presidents Make* (Cambridge, MA: Harvard University Press, 1993), 362–63.

8. Lyndon B. Johnson, taped telephone conversation with Wilbur Mills, 9:2 A.M., June 9, 1964, "Recordings and Transcripts of Conversations," Citation 3462, LBJ Library. For further notes and details, see chapter 5.

9. See chapter 5 for notes and details.

10. Richard Reeves, President Kennedy: *Profile of Power* (New York: Simon and Schuster, 1993), 100.

11. Hubert Humphrey, audiotape, 11:25 A.M., March 6, 2005, "Recordings and Transcripts of Conversations," Citation 7024–7025, LBJ Library.

12. Lyndon B. Johnson, taped telephone conversation with Edward Kennedy, 11:32 A.M., January 9, 1965, "Recordings and Transcripts of Conversations," Citation 6718, LBJ Library.

13. Joseph Califano, interview with the authors, June 15, 2006.

14. Richard Nixon, RN: *Memoirs of Richard Nixon* (New York: Simon and Schuster, 1990), 352; Joseph Califano, interview with the authors, June 15, 2006.

15. For both data and a fine analysis, see Matthew Dickinson, "The Executive Office of the President: The Paradox of Politicization," in *The Executive Branch*, eds. Joel Aberbach and Mark Peterson (New York: Oxford University Press, 2005), 135–73.

16. John Morton Blum, ed., *From the Morgenthau Diaries: Years of War, 1941–1945* (New York: Houghton Mifflin, 1967), 71–72.

17. Clayton Knowles, "Kennedy Exhorts Public to Support Medicare Bill," *New York Times*, May 21, 1962, 1.

18. Theodore Marmor, *The Politics of Medicare* (New York: Aldine, 2000).

19. Lyndon Johnson, *The Vantage Point* (New York: Holt, Rinehart and Winston, 1971), 215 [bombshell]; 216 [brother]. Richard Harris, who interviewed Cohen, has a more colorful version of this story in *A Sacred Trust* (New York: New American Library, 1966), 189.

20. Johnson, *The Vantage Point*, 216.

21. Wilbur Cohen, oral history, taken by David G. McComb, tape 3, March 2, 1969, LBJ Library.

22. Lyndon B. Johnson, taped conversation with John McCormack, 4:54 P.M., March 23, 1965, "Recordings and Transcripts of Conversations," Citation 7141, LBJ Library.

23. White House Central File, LE/IS1 IS1, LBJ Library [dressed formally]: the full story is recounted by Lawrence F. O'Brien, oral history, taken by Michael L. Gillette, interview XI, July 24, 1986, Internet copy, LBJ Library.

24. Wilbur Mills, oral history, taken by Michael L. Gillette, interview 2, tape 1 of 2, March 25, 1987, LBJ Library.

25. Dwight D. Eisenhower, address at the Alfred E. Smith Memorial Dinner, New York City, October 21, 1954, *Public Papers of the Presidents, Dwight D. Eisenhower, 1953–1961*, Eisenhower Library.

26. See Marie Gottschalk, *The Shadow Welfare State* (Ithaca, NY: Cornell, 2001); Jacob Hacker, *The Divided Welfare State* (New York: Cambridge, 2002).

27. Stuart Altman, interview with the authors, July 23, 2007. Altman served as Deputy Assistant Secretary for Health Planning and Evaluation at HEW in the Nixon administration.

## 1. FRANKLIN DELANO ROOSEVELT

1. Franklin D. Roosevelt, "'I Pledge You—I Pledge Myself to a New Deal for the American People,' Chicago, Illinois, July 2, 1932," in *The Public Papers and Addresses of Franklin D. Roosevelt*, ed. Samuel Rosenman (New York: Random House, 1938), 1:647–48.

2. Franklin D. Roosevelt, *Public Papers and Addresses*, 2:17 [Special Session], 24–29 [bank holiday], 30–45 [press conference], 59–66 [first Fireside Chat], quoted at 64.

3. Stephen Skowronek, *The Politics Presidents Make* (Cambridge, MA: Harvard University Press, 1993), 292 [mass of farmers]; Sidney Milkis, *The President and the Parties* (New York: Oxford, 1993), part 1.

4. Richard Neustadt, *Presidential Power and the Modern Presidents: The Politics of Leadership from Roosevelt to Reagan* (New York: Free Press, 1990), 136.

5. Frances Perkins, *The Roosevelt I Knew* (New York: Viking, 1946); Ross T. McIntire and G. Creel, *White House Physician* (New York: G.P. Putnam's Sons, 1946).

6. For a fine account of the two Roosevelts and their social statuses, see Roy Jenkins, *Franklin Delano Roosevelt* (New York: Henry Holt, 2003) [completed with the assistance of Richard Neustadt], ch. 1.

7. See the description of the illness in Conrad Black, *Franklin Delano Roosevelt: Champion of Freedom* (New York: Public Affairs, 2003), ch. 4.

8. Black, *Franklin Delano Roosevelt*, ch. 4, quoted at 148 [water].

9. McIntire and Creel, *White House Physician*, 33–40.

10. Francis Perkins, *The Roosevelt I Knew* (New York: Viking, 1946), 29–30; James Roosevelt and Sydney Shallet, *Affectionately, FDR: A Son's Story of a Lonely Man* (New York: Harcourt Brace, 1959).

11. Robert Gilbert, *The Mortal Presidency* (New York: Fordham University Press, 1998), ch. 3, FDR quoted on 47.

12. Roosevelt, "Annual Message to the Legislature," January 2, 1929 [keep them well], "Annual Message to the Legislature, January 7, 1931" [special commission], "A Radio Report to the People on the 1931 Session of the Legislature," April 24, 1931 [absolutely declined], *Public Papers and Addresses*, 1:84, 102–3, 558; Black, *Franklin Delano Roosevelt*, 194 [*New York Times*], 215 [governors].

13. Black, *Franklin Delano Roosevelt,* 276.

14. See Michael Nelson, "The Psychological Presidency," in *The Presidency and the Political System,* ed. Michael Nelson (Washington, D.C.: CQ Press, 2006), 170–94.

15. Black, *Franklin Delano Roosevelt,* 340 [associates], 395 [IRS].

16. For a more extensive analysis of the Roosevelt management style, see James Morone, *The Democratic Wish: Popular Participation and the Limits of American Democracy* (New Haven: Yale, 1998), ch. 4.

17. Black, *Franklin Delano Roosevelt,* 354.

18. Neustadt, *Presidential Power and the Modern Presidents,* 115.

19. Arthur Meier Schlesinger, *The Coming of the New Deal, 1933–1935* (New York: Houghton Mifflin, 2003), 528.

20. Black, *Franklin Delano Roosevelt,* 272.

21. Morone, *The Democratic Wish,* 131.

22. Edwin E. Witte, *The Development of the Social Security Act* (Madison: University of Wisconsin Press, 1962), 8.

23. Arthur Altmeyer, *The Formative Years of Social Security* (Madison: University of Wisconsin Press, 1966), 12.

24. Witte, *The Development of the Social Security Act,* 19–21.

25. Altmeyer, *The Formative Years of Social Security,* 14.

26. *The Evolution of Medicare: From Idea to Law* (Washington, D.C.: U.S. Social Security Administration, Office of Research and Statistics, 1969), ch. 2; Peter Corning, *The Evolution of Medicare* (Washington, D.C.: U.S. Social Security Administration, Office of Research and Statistics, 1969), ch. 2, www.ssa .gov/history/corningchap2.html; Witte, *The Development of the Social Security Act,* 24.

27. Franklin D. Roosevelt, correspondence with Harvey Cushing, multiple dates, *President's Personal File,* Box 1523, FDR Library. Richard Rovit, William T. Couldwell, "No Ordinary Time, No Ordinary Men: The Relationship between Harvey Cushing and Franklin D. Roosevelt, 1928-1939," *Journal of Neurosurgery,* August, 2001, Volume 95, No 2, 1-33, www.thejns.net.org/jns/ issues/v952/full/no950354_r.html, accessed September 29, 2003.

28. Fulton, *Harvey Cushing,* 655; Harvey Cushing, letter to Franklin D. Roosevelt, January 15, 1935, President's Personal File, Box 1523, FDR Library; Richard Rovit, William T. Couldwell, "No Ordinary Time, No Ordinary Men: The Relationship between Harvey Cushing and Franklin D. Roosevelt, 1928-1939," *Journal of Neurosurgery,* August, 2001, Volume 95, No 2, 1-33, www.thejns.net.org/jns/issues/v952/full/no950354_r.html, accessed September 29, 2003. Corning, *The Evolution of Medicare,* ch. 2, p. 8, www.ssa.gov/history/ corningchap2.html.

29. Fulton, *Harvey Cushing,* 650.

30. Witte, *The Development of the Social Security Act,* 30.

31. Witte, *The Development of the Social Security Act,* 174.

32. Corning, *The Evolution of Medicare,* ch. 2, p. 8.

33. Franklin D. Roosevelt, "White House Address to Advisory Council of CES, draft and reading copy, November 14, 1934," Presidency Project, www .presidency.ucsb.edu/ws/index.php?pid=14777.

34. Witte, *The Development of the Social Security Act*, 181.

35. Daniel S. Hirshfield, *The Lost Reform: The Campaign for Compulsory Health Insurance in the United States from 1932–1943* (Cambridge, MA: Harvard University Press, 1970), 44.

36. Corning, *The Evolution of Medicare*, ch. 2, p. 44.

37. Harvey Cushing, letter to Franklin D. Roosevelt, January 6, 1935, Correspondence with Harvey Cushing, President's Personal File, Box 1523, FDR Library.

38. Witte, *The Development of the Social Security Act*, 182.

39. Witte, *The Development of the Social Security Act*, 187.

40. Steven Early, memo to Marvin McIntire, January 21, 1935, President's Personal File, Box 3467, Folder: American Medical Association, FDR Library.

41. Witte, *The Development of the Social Security Act*, 184–85.

42. Perkins, *Roosevelt I Knew*, 299.

43. For a description of the leftist alternatives, see James A. Morone, *Hellfire Nation: The Politics of Sin in American History* (New Haven: Yale University Press, 2003), 356–57.

44. Witte, *The Development of the Social Security Act*, 188.

45. Witte, *The Development of the Social Security Act*, 188; Altmeyer, *The Formative Years of Social Security*, 57.

46. Altmeyer, *The Formative Years of Social Security*, 57.

47. Gerald Morgan, letter to Franklin D. Roosevelt, July 1, 1935, Official File 103, Health, Box 1, FDR Library.

48. Franklin D. Roosevelt, letter to Gerald Morgan, July 26, 1935, Official File 103, Health, Box 1, FDR Library.

49. Corning, *The Evolution of Medicare*, ch. 2, p. 11.

50. Altmeyer, *The Formative Years of Social Security*, 58.

51. Corning, *The Evolution of Medicare*, ch. 2, p. 12.

52. Franklin D. Roosevelt, "Address by the President, Medical Center, Jersey City, New Jersey City, October 2, 1936," Presidency Project, www.presidency.ucsb.edu/ws/index.php?pid=15150.

53. Stephen Early, letter to Ross McIntire, October 7, 1936, President's Personal File, Box 528, Health Matters, FDR Library.

54. Fulton, *Harvey Cushing*, 653.

55. Franklin D. Roosevelt, memo to Francis Perkins, November 13, 1934, Official File 103, Health, Box 1, FDR Library.

56. Francis Perkins, memo to the president, May 2, 1935, Official File 103, Health, Box 1, FDR Library.

57. Francis Perkins, memo to the president, May 2, 1935, Official File 103, Health, Box 1, FDR Library.

58. Franklin D. Roosevelt, memo to Francis Perkins, May 8, 1935, Official File 103, Health, Box 1, FDR Library.

59. Stephen Early, memorandum to Francis Perkins, August 2, 1935, Official File 1731, Interdepartmental Committee for Coordination of Health and Welfare Activities, 1933–1942, FDR Library.

60. Franklin D. Roosevelt, "Presidential Order Creating the Interdepartmental Committee," August 15, 1935, Official File 1731, Interdepartmental Committee for Coordination of Health and Welfare Activities, 1933–1942, FDR Library.

61. Hirshfield, *The Lost Reform,* 71; Corning, *The Evolution of Medicare,* ch. 2, p. 12.

62. Corning, *The Evolution of Medicare,* ch. 2, p. 12.

63. Paul Starr, *The Social Transformation of American Medicine* (New York: Basic Books, 1982), 278–79; Corning, *The Evolution of Medicare,* ch.2, p. 19.

64. Franklin D. Roosevelt, "Letter to the American Medical Association," February 3, 1938, President's Personal File 3467, FDR Library.

65. Altmeyer, *The Formative Years of Social Security,* 94.

66. Corning, *The Evolution of Medicare,* ch. 2, p. 13.

67. M. H. McIntyre, letter to Senator J. Hamilton Lewis, July 2, 1937, President's Personal File, Box 3467, FDR Library; "Nationalized Doctors," *Time,* June 21, 1937.

68. Hamilton Lewis, letter to Franklin D. Roosevelt, August 25, 1937, President's Personal File 3467, FDR Library.

69. Josephine Roche, note to Franklin D. Roosevelt, February 11, 1938, President's Office File 1731, Interdepartmental Committee for Coordination of Federal Health and Welfare Activities, 1933–1942, FDR Library.

70. Hirshfield, *The Lost Reform,* 107–8.

71. Stephen Early, memorandum to Arthur Altmeyer, March 8, 1938, Official File 103, Health, 1938–39, FDR Library.

72. "Try Socialized Medicine, Says Mrs. Roosevelt," *Washington Post,* June 17, 1938, 28.

73. Corning, *The Evolution of Medicare,* ch. 2, p. 13.

74. Josephine Roche, telegram to Franklin D. Roosevelt, July 23, 1938, Official File 1731, Interdepartmental Committee for Coordination of Federal Health and Welfare Activities, 1933–1942, FDR Library.

75. Josephine Roche, telegram to the President, undated, Official File 1731, Interdepartmental Committee for Coordination of Federal Health and Welfare Activities, 1933–1942, FDR Library.

76. Corning, *The Evolution of Medicare,* ch. 2, p. 14.

77. Corning, *The Evolution of Medicare,* ch. 2, p. 14.

78. Corning, *The Evolution of Medicare,* ch. 2, p. 15.

79. Hirshfield, *The Lost Reform,* 115.

80. Technical Committee, memo to Franklin D. Roosevelt, October 12, 1938, Box: Health and Welfare Activities, Interdepartmental Committee to Coordinate, 1935–41, Folder: Memorandum to the President Regarding the National Health Program, 10/12/38, FDR Library.

81. Hirshfield, *The Lost Reform,* 116–17.

82. Technical Committee, memo to Franklin D. Roosevelt, December 15, 1938, Box: Health and Welfare Activities, Interdepartmental Committee to Coordinate, 1935–1941, Folder: Memorandum to the President, 12/15/38, FDR Library.

83. Altmeyer, *The Formative Years of Social Security,* 96; Corning, *The Evolution of Medicare,* ch. 2, 16.

84. Corning, *The Evolution of Medicare,* ch. 2, p. 16.

85. Altmeyer, *The Formative Years of Social Security,* 115.

86. Hirshfield, *The Lost Reform,* 140; Altmeyer, *The Formative Years of Social Security,* 116.

87. Hirshfield, *The Lost Reform,* 156.

88. Hirshfield, *The Lost Reform,* 156.

89. Altmeyer, *The Formative Years of Social Security,* 117.

90. Hirshfield, *The Lost Reform,* 155–57.

91. Franklin D. Roosevelt, letter to Mary Dublin, January 17, 1940, Office File Interdepartmental Committee, 1939–1941, FDR Library.

92. Corning, *The Evolution of Medicare,* ch. 3, p. 1.

93. Perkins, *Roosevelt I Knew,* 283.

94. Corning, *The Evolution of Medicare,* ch. 3, p. 1.

95. Corning, *The Evolution of Medicare,* ch. 2, p. 2; Starr, *The Social Transformation of American Medicine,* 278–79.

96. Richard Harris, *A Sacred Trust* (New York: New American Library, 1966), 27, 28.

97. "Communize U.S. Medicine?" editorial, *New York Daily News,* July 19, 1943, clipping, the Papers of Oscar Ewing, Federal Security Agency Subject File, Box 33, National Health Insurance, Truman Library.

98. John Morton Blum, ed., *From the Morgenthau Diaries: Years of War, 1941–1945* (New York: Houghton Mifflin, 1967), 53.

99. Blum, *From the Morgenthau Diaries,* 71–2.

100. Blum, *From the Morgenthau Diaries,* 72.

101. Corning, *The Evolution of Medicare,* ch. 3, p. 2.

102. Harris, *A Sacred Trust,* 30.

103. Milton Handler, memo to Judge Rosenman, January 28, 1944, Papers of Samuel I. Rosenman, Subject File: Health, Legislative Proposal, Box 1, Truman Library.

104. Milton Handler, memo to Judge Rosenman, January 28, 1944, Papers of Samuel I. Rosenman, Subject File: Health, Legislative Proposal, Box 1, Truman Library.

105. Monte M. Poen, *Harry Truman versus the Medical Lobby* (Columbia: University of Missouri Press, 1979), 17–20.

## 2. HARRY S. TRUMAN

1. Harry Truman, *Where the Buck Stops,* ed. Margaret Truman (New York: Warner Books, 1989), 371–72.

2. Quoted in Harry Truman, *Memoirs* (Garden City, NY: Doubleday, 1955), 1:19.

3. National Affairs: President: "After 52 Weeks, a Surer Man," *Newsweek,* April 15, 1946, 23–27.

4. "The Presidency," *Time,* April 15, 1946, 19–20.

5. "After 52 Weeks, a Surer Man," *Newsweek,* April 15, 1949, 23–27.

6. "The Presidency," *Time,* April 15, 1946, 19–20.

7. Truman, *Memoirs,* 2:23.

8. Harry Truman, *Autobiography,* ed. Robert Ferrell (Columbia: University of Missouri, 2002), 4–5.

9. "Truman Flies to Missouri to See Mother on Birthday," *New York Times,* November 26, 1945, 1.

10. Truman, *Where the Buck Stops,* ch. 9.

11. *Newsweek,* May 26, 1947.

12. Truman, *Autobiography,* 115.

13. Truman, *Memoirs,* 2:225.

14. Truman, *Autobiography,* 43.

15. David McCullough, *Truman* (New York: Simon and Schuster, 1992), 153–60, quoted at 159.

16. Truman, *Autobiography,* 82.

17. Truman, *Autobiography,* 60–63.

18. Ben Turoff, letter to Mr. Harry S. Truman, April 1, 1949, Vertical File 286-A, Truman Library; Harry S. Truman, letter to Ben Turoff, April 12, 1949, 286-A, Truman Library.

19. Truman, *Autobiography,* 82–83.

20. McCullough, *Truman,* 242.

21. Truman, *Autobiography,* 90.

22. McCullough, *Truman,* 309.

23. Truman, *Autobiography,* 8–9.

24. McCullough, *Truman,* 230.

25. McCullough, *Truman,* 263.

26. McCullough, *Truman,* 585.

27. Harry S. Truman, "Address to Health Assembly," May 1, 1948, *The Public Papers of the Presidents of the United States, Harry S. Truman, 1945–1953* (Washington, D.C.: United States Government Printing Office, 1979).

28. "The Presidency," *Time,* September 9, 1946, 22; "The Presidency," *Time,* April 18, 1946, 18.

29. Truman, *Memoirs,* 2 [bourbon], 225 [pace].

30. Oscar Ewing, Western Union telegram to the president, July 28, 1947, Oscar Ewing Papers, Box 33, the President's File, Truman Library; National Affairs: "Mother and Son," *Newsweek,* May 26, 1947; Truman, *Memoirs,* 2:223.

31. D.M. Giangreco and Kathryn Moore, eds., *Dear Harry—Truman's Mailroom* (Mechanicsburg, PA: Stackpole Books, 1999), 12.

32. Giangreco and Moore, *Dear Harry,* 13.

33. Papers of Harry S. Truman—President's Secretary's Files, B File, Folder 12, Truman Library. This quote is from the notes, written in the president's own hand on White House stationary for the dinner. The formal record—which records the address that Truman actually delivered (cited at footnote 27)—is somewhat stiffer and less personal.

34. Harry S. Truman, "Address to Health Assembly," May 1, 1948, *The Public Papers of the Presidents of the United States, Harry S. Truman, 1945–1953* (Washington, D.C.: United States Government Printing Office, 1979); Harry S. Truman, letter to Ben Turoff, April 12, 1949, 286-A, Truman Library.

35. Harry S. Truman, letter to Representative John Kee, July 15, 1952, President's Secretary's Files, 38 B File, Folder 12, Truman Library.

36. Smith McCoy, letter to Harry Truman, July 6, 1950, Vertical File, Health Care Policy, 121-A, Box 3, File 2, Truman Library; John Kee, letter to President Harry Truman, July 31, 1950, Vertical File, Health Care Policy, 121 A, Box 3, File 2, Truman Library; Harry Truman, letter to John Kee, August 9, 1950, Vertical File, Health Care Policy, 121-A, Box 3, File 2, Truman Library; example of "horse and buggy" in "Address at the American Hospital Association Convention, Philadelphia, PA, September 16, 1952," *Public Papers of the Presidents of the United States: Harry S. Truman, January 1, 1952–January 20, 1953* (Washington, D.C.: U.S. Government Printing Office, 1966), 572.

37. Harry S. Truman, "Address at the Dedication of the Norfolk and Bull Shoals Dams, July 2, 1952," in *Public Papers of the Presidents of the U.S.: Harry S. Truman, January 1, 1952 to January 20, 1953* (Washington, D.C.: U.S. Government Printing Office, 1966).

38. McCullough, *Truman*, 469.

39. For example, National Affairs: "Housing," *Time*, November 19, 1945, 24.

40. Harry S. Truman, "Special Message to the Congress Presenting a 21-Point Program for the Reconversion Period, September 6, 1945," *The Public Papers of the Presidents: Harry S. Truman, 1945* (Washington, D.C.: U.S. Government Printing Office, 1965), 263ff.

41. Truman, *Memoirs*, 1:483–85.

42. Truman, *Memoirs*, 1:483. Some historians question this exchange, suggesting that Rosenman must have already known how Truman felt, but that misses Harry's real point: this message was his great New Deal confession, his liberal testimonial. For an alternative reading, see Monte Poen, *Harry S. Truman versus the Medical Lobby* (Columbia: University of Missouri, 1979), 57.

43. William S. White, "Republicans See 1946 Issue Drawn; Truman Plans 'Out-New Deal The New Deal' Says Martin," *New York Times*, September 8, 1945 [nonsense]; Donald R. McCoy, *The Presidency of Harry S. Truman* (Lawrence: University of Kansas Press, 1984), 48; McCullough, *Truman*, 468 [quoting Martin]; Truman, *Memoirs*, 1:483 [Snyder].

44. Milton Handler, memo to Judge Rosenman, January 28, 1944, Papers of Samuel I. Rosenman, Subject File: Health, Legislative Proposal, Box 1, Truman Library.

45. Sam Rosenman, memo to the president, May 12, 1945, Papers of Samuel Rosenman, Box 105, Truman Library; "Press Conference, June 1, 1945," Presidency Project, www.presidency.ucsb.edu/ws/index.php?pid=12222.

46. Second draft: [Message] "To the Congress of the United States"; Third draft: "[Message] To The Congress of the United States," Samuel I. Rosenman Papers, Box 105, National Health Insurance File, Truman Library.

47. Harry S. Truman, "Special Message to the Congress Recommending a Comprehensive Health Program, November 19, 1945," Presidency Project, www .presidency.ucsb.edu/ws/index.php?pid=12288&st=Comprehensive+health+ program&st1=.

48. Felix Belair, "Truman Asks Law to Force Insuring of Nation's Health," *New York Times*, November 20, 1945, 1.

49. Philip Funigiello, *Chronic Politics: Health Care Security From FDR to George W. Bush* (Lawrence: University of Kansas, 2005), 63.

50. Felix Belair Jr. "Truman Asks Law to Force Insuring of Nation's Health," *New York Times*, November 20, 1945, 1, 13 [Wagner quoted at 13].

51. "270,000 Made Idle in Nation's Strikes," *New York Times*, November 20, 1945, 1; "Hospital Maintenance Men Strike; Visitors, Veterans Run Elevators," *New York Times*, November 22, 1945, 1.

52. Harry S. Truman to Mrs. Albert D. Lasker, December 14, 1945, "President Truman's Health Plan" [copy of newspaper advertisement attached to letter], Papers of Harry S. Truman, Official File, 286A, Box 3, File 11, Truman Library.

53. George Coleman, "Emergency Bulletin, National Physicians Committee for the Extension of Medical Service, Nov 23, 1945," Samuel I. Rosenman Papers, National Health Insurance File, Truman Library.

54. National Affairs: President: "After 52 Weeks, a Surer Man," *Newsweek*, April 15, 1946, 23–27.

55. Harry S. Truman, memo to Watson Miller, March 16, 1946, Harry S. Truman Papers, Official File, 286-A, Truman Library.

56. *Newsweek, Periscope*, April 26, 1946, 20.

57. McCoullough, *Truman*, 213.

58. Harry S. Truman, memo to the secretary of labor, March 28, 1946, Papers of Harry S. Truman, Official File, 286-H, Truman Library; Harry S. Truman, memo to federal security administrator, March 19, 1946, Papers of Harry S. Truman, Official File, 286-A, Truman Library.

59. Poen, *Harry Truman versus the Medical Lobby*, 79.

60. Harry S. Truman, letter to General Omar Bradley, April 1, 1946, Papers of Harry S. Truman, Official File, 286-A, Truman Library; General Omar Bradley, letter to Harry S. Truman, April 3, 1946, Papers of Harry S. Truman, Official File, 286-A, Truman Library.

61. James Murray, letter to President Truman, May 14, 1946, Papers of Harry S. Truman, Official File, 286-A, Truman Library.

62. Harry S. Truman, letter to James E. Murray, April 30, 1946, Harry S. Truman Papers, Official File, 286-A, Box 4, File 3, Truman Library.

63. Harry S. Truman, letter to Jim Murray, May 21, 1946, Harry S. Truman Papers, Official File, 286-A, B-File, Box 4, File 3, Truman Library.

64. Wallace Graham, memo, April 9, 1946, the White House, Harry S. Truman Papers, Official File, 286-A, File 4, Folder 2, Truman Library.

65. Truman, *Memoirs*, 1:329.

66. McCoy, *The Presidency of Harry S. Truman*, 164.

67. McCullough, *Truman*, 530.

68. U.S. Senate, "National Health Program, Hearings before the Committee on Education and Labor, 79th Congress, 2nd Session, Part 1, April 2–16, 1946," 47–52; "Civics Lesson," *Time*, April 15, 1946, 20.

69. For a good description, see Poen, *Harry S. Truman versus the Medical Lobby*, 88–92.

70. Richard Harris, *A Sacred Trust* (New York: The New American Library, 1966), 35–36.

71. McCullough, *Truman*, 500–506; Truman, *Memoirs*, 1:500–502 [Morse].

72. James Morone, *The Democratic Wish* (New York: Basic Books, 1990), 258-61.

73. Clark Clifford, memo to President Truman, May 12, 1947, Papers of Clark M. Clifford, Box 12, Folder 7, Truman Library.

74. Interview with President Harry S. Truman, October 5, 1953, Papers of Harry S. Truman, Post Presidential File, Memoirs File, Box 3, page 22, Truman Library.

75. Harry S. Truman, "Special Message to the Congress on Health and Disability Insurance, May 19, 1947," Presidency Project, www.presidency.ucsb .edu/ws/index.php?pid=12892.

76. National Affairs: Special Section: "A Few Party Members, Using Many Lines ... Message from Moscow to Those Who Toil and Tremble ... Pulpit, Press Stage, Screen Offer Sounding Boards ... But Men Who Have Learned the Tricks Expose Their Work ..." *Newsweek*, June 9, 1947, 23–31; Morone, *Hellfire Nation* (New Haven: Yale University Press, 2003), 388–96.

77. J. Edgar Hoover, "How to Fight Communism," *Newsweek*, June 9, 1947, 30–31.

78. "Enemy Within the Gates," *Newsweek*, November 25, 1947. 22.

79. "Left Wing: Reds Gone Hollywood," *Newsweek*, May 26, 1947, 27–28.

80. J. Edgar Hoover, "How to Fight Communism," *Newsweek*, June 9, 1947, 30–31.

81. Representative Forest Harness, "Address before Executive Secretaries of Indiana State Medical Association," February 15, 1948, quoted by Quadagno, *One Nation, Uninsured*, 31–32, and Poen, *Harry S. Truman versus the Medical Lobby*, 103.

82. National Affairs: "Antitoxin," *Time*, June 21, 1948.

83. Truman, *Memoirs*, quoted at 2:284, 2:285, 2:270. Truman and the Democrats did not stay entirely above the Red-hunting.

84. Harry S. Truman, "Annual Message to Congress on the State of the Union, January 7, 1948," Presidency Project, www.presidency.ucsb.edu/ws/ index.php?pid=13005.

85. Oscar Ewing, "The Nation's Health: A Report to the President" (Washington, D.C.: Federal Security Agency, September 1948), 86–87.

86. Oscar Ewing, *The Nation's Health—A Ten Year Program* (Washington, D.C.: Federal Security Agency, 1948), xi.

87. For a good description of the campaign, see McCoullough, *Truman*, 644–46 (Hague quoted at 635).

88. "A Periscope Preview: Election Forecast: 50 Political Experts Predict a GOP Sweep," *Newsweek*, October 11, 1948, 20.

89. The Election: "The Victorious Rebellion of Harry S. Truman," *Newsweek*, October 11, 1948, 5.

90. "Campaign Barbs That Won the Votes," *Newsweek*, November 8, 1948, 4–5.

91. Quoted in Poen, *Harry S. Truman versus the Medical Lobby*, 130.

92. Harry S. Truman, "Address at the Keil Auditorium," St. Louis, Missouri, pages 20–21, October 30, 1948, 1948 Election Campaign, Campaign Documents, Truman Library, www.trumanlibrary.org/whistlestop/study_collections/ 1948campaign/large/docs/index.php#October.

93. The Election: "The Victorious Rebellion of Harry S. Truman," *Newsweek*, November 8, 1948, 4.

94. Harry S. Truman, "Inaugural Address, January 20, 1949," Presidency Project, www.presidency.ucsb.edu/ws/index.php?pid=13282.

95. Harry S. Truman, "State of the Union Address, January 5, 1949," Presidency Project, www.presidency.ucsb.edu/ws/index.php?pid=13293.

96. Harry S. Truman, "Address at the Jefferson-Jackson Day dinner," the Statler Hotel, Washington, D.C., 10:40 P.M., February 24, 1949, *Public Papers of the Presidents: Harry S. Truman, 1949* (Washington, D.C.: Government Printing Office, 1964), 145–49.

97. Harry S. Truman, "State of the Union Address, January 5, 1949," Presidency Project, www.presidency.ucsb.edu/ws/index.php?pid=13293.

98. Harry S. Truman, press conference, March 24, 1949, questions 19 and 33, press conference, April 21, 1949, question 17, *Public Papers of the Presidents: Harry S. Truman, 1949* (Washington, D.C.: Government Printing Office, 1964), 183, 184, 224.

99. Harry S. Truman, press conference, May 12, 1949, question 6, press conference, May 26, 1949, question 12, *Public Papers of the Presidents: Harry S. Truman, 1949* (Washington, D.C.: Government Printing Office, 1964). 247, 269.

100. Poen, *Harry Truman versus the Medical Lobby,* 159ff.

101. Harry Truman, "Special Message to the Congress on the National Health Care Needs, April 22, 1949," *Public Papers of the Presidents: Harry S. Truman, 1949* (Washington, D.C.: Government Printing Office, 1964), 226–230.

102. "The Moon and Sixpence," *Time,* May 2, 1949, 18–19.

103. "Washington Trends," *Newsweek,* May 2, 1949, 14.

104. John Morris, "Truman Submits Health Care Plan on Enforced Basis," *New York Times,* April 22, 1949, 1.

105. Graveyard metaphor from Mark Peterson, "The Congressional Graveyard for Health Care Reform," in *Healthy, Wealthy and Fair,* eds. James Morone and Lawrence Jacobs (New York: Oxford University Press, 1995), 205–33.

106. For the classic description of this battle, see Harris, *A Sacred Trust,* ch. 8.

107. Harris, *A Sacred Trust,* 44–45.

108. The Truman Library archives simply bulge with this material: folder after folder and box after box of letters—often form letters—denouncing national health insurance. For some excellent examples, see 286-A, Box 7, File 12, Truman Library.

109. "The Voluntary Way is the American Way," no date, the Papers of Oscar Ewing, Federal Security Agency Subject File, Box 33, National Health Insurance File, Truman Library; clipping, labeled *Chicago Herald American,* no date, the Papers of Oscar Ewing, Federal Security Agency Subject File, Box 33, National Health Insurance File, Truman Library.

110. Report of Committee on Federal Legislation, the New York State Bar Association, The Papers of Oscar Ewing, Box 35, National Health Insurance, Truman Library.

111. Lawrence Huntoon, MD, PhD, "Universal Health Coverage—Call It Socialized Medicine," *Medical Sentinel* 5, no. 4 (2000): 134–36.

112. Representative John Dingell, letter to Harry S. Truman, October 12, 1950, President's Secretary's Files, Box 14, File 6, Truman Library; Harry S. Truman, letter to Representative John Dingell, October 20, 1950, President's Secretary's Files, Box 14, File 6, Truman Library.

113. For quotation and analysis, see Morone, *Hellfire Nation*, 392–96.

114. "Politics: All Eyes on November," *Newsweek*, August 14, 1950, 32.

115. Harry S. Truman, letter to Sheridan Downey, September 24, 1945, Harry S. Truman Papers, Box 105, Truman Library.

116. "The Man Doctors Hate," *The Saturday Evening Post*, July 8, 1950; Oscar Ewing, oral history, Chapel Hill, NC, taken by J. R. Fuchs, page 107, May 1, 1969, Truman Library, www.trumanlibrary.org/oralhist/ewing3.htm#transcript; see also Poen, *Harry Truman versus the Medical Lobby*, 163–64.

117. Oscar Ewing, oral history, Chapel Hill, NC, taken by J. R. Fuchs, pages 216–226, May 1, 1969, Truman Library, www.trumanlibrary.org/oralhist/ewing3.htm#transcript.

118. Lyndon B. Johnson, *The Vantage Point* (New York: Holt, Reinhart and Winston, 1971), 219; Lyndon B. Johnson Papers, "Remarks at the Signing in Independence of the Medicare Bill," July 30, 1965, *Public Papers of the Presidents of the United States: Lyndon B. Johnson, 1965* (Washington, D.C.: Government Printing Office, 1966), 2:811–815, entry 394.

## 3. DWIGHT D. EISENHOWER

1. Dwight Eisenhower, *Waging Peace: The White House Years, 1956–1961* (New York: Doubleday, 1965); Sydney Milkis and Michael Nelson, *The American Presidency* (Washington, D.C.: CQ Press, 2003), 299 ["back door"].

2. Dwight Eisenhower, *At Ease: Stories I Tell My Friends* (Garden City, NY: Doubleday, 1967), 69; for a vivid description of Abilene, Kansas, at the time of Ike's childhood, see ch. 5, Fred Greenstein, *The Hidden Hand Presidency: Eisenhower as Leader* (New York: Basic Books, 1982).

3. Stephen Ambrose, *Eisenhower: Soldier and President* (Newtown, CT: American Political Biography Press, 2007), 572.

4. Harry S. Truman, *Memoirs* (Garden City, NY: Doubleday, 1955–56), 2:185–87; Ambrose, *Eisenhower*, 572.

5. Quotations from Milkis and Nelson, *The American Presidency*, 299.

6. The phrase comes from Marie Gottschalk, *The Shadow Welfare State* (Ithaca, NY: Cornell University Press, 2000); see also Christopher Howard, *The Hidden Welfare State* (Princeton, NJ: Princeton University Press, 1999) and, for the most comprehensive treatment, Jacob Hacker, *The Divided Welfare State* (New York: Cambridge University Press, 2002).

7. Letter to Swede Hazlett, quoted in Ambrose, *Eisenhower*, 232.

8. Dwight D. Eisenhower, "The President's News Conference of March 30, 1960," Presidency Project, www.presidency.ucsb.edu/ws/index.php?pid=11734.

9. Eisenhower, *Waging Peace*, 614–15.

10. Dwight D. Eisenhower, "The President's News Conference of December 2, 1959," Presidency Project, www.presidency.ucsb.edu/ws/index.php?pid=11587; on questions about defense policy, see Dwight D. Eisenhower, "The President's

News Conference of January 13, 1960," Presidency Project, www.presidency
.ucsb.edu/ws/index.php?pid=12131.

11. Oveta Culp Hobby, memo to President Eisenhower, November 18, 1954,
Ann Whitman File, Administration Series, Box 9, Folder: Budget, 1955–56 (4),
Eisenhower Library.

12. Arthur S. Flemming, to Dwight D. Eisenhower, January 12, 1961,
Administration Series, Box 15, Folder: Flemming, Arthur S., 1959–61 (1),
Eisenhower Library.

13. Fred Greenstein, *The Presidential Difference* (Princeton, NJ: Princeton
University Press, 2000), 57.

14. Eisenhower, *At Ease,* ch. 10.

15. Eisenhower, *Waging Peace,* 630–38.

16. Greenstein, *The Presidential Difference,* 55.

17. Marion Folsom, oral history, 1968, OH 112 [COHP], Eisenhower
Library; Eisenhower, *Waging Peace,* 630–38.

18. Dwight D. Eisenhower, memo to Secretary Hobby, November 25, 1953,
Ann Whitman File, Administration Series, Box 19, Folder: Hobby, Oveta Culp
(6), Eisenhower Library.

19. For the best-known proponent of the Eisenhower style, see Greenstein,
*Hidden Hand Presidency* (see citation 5); for a skeptical view, see Richard
Neustadt, *Presidential Power and the Modern Presidents* (New York: Free
Press, 1990).

20. Thomas W. Mattingly, "Medical History of DDE, 1911–1987," Box 1,
Folder: General Health (2), Eisenhower Library.

21. Thomas W. Mattingly, "Medical History of DDE, 1911–1987," Box 1,
Folder: General Health (2), Eisenhower Library; Dwight D. Eisenhower,
*Mandate for Change: 1953–1956* (New York: Doubleday, 1963), ch. 22; Jay
Murphy, *What Ails the White House* (Orland Park, KS: Leathers Publishing,
2006), 83–87.

22. See Clarence Lasly, *Eisenhower's Heart Attack* (University of Kansas
Press, 1997).

23. The recipe can be found in all its fatty glory in Eisenhower, *At Ease,* note
2:381–82.

24. Thomas W. Mattingly, "Medical History of DDE, 1911–1987," Box 1,
Folder: General Health (92), Eisenhower Library.

25. Eisenhower, *Waging Peace,* ch. 9 [for symptoms and recovery], which
he titles *A Drastic Personal Test*; more generally, see Thomas W. Mattingly,
"Medical History of DDE, 1911–1987," Box 1, Folder: General Health (92),
Eisenhower Library.

26. Eisenhower, *Waging Peace,* 230.

27. Dwight D. Eisenhower, "Personal and Secret Letter to Vice President
Nixon," February 5, 1958, Ann Whitman File, Administration Series, Box 28,
Folder: Nixon, Richard M., 1958–1961, Eisenhower Library.

28. Dwight D. Eisenhower, press conference with Robert Pierpoint (CBS),
September 28, 1959, "The President's News Conference of September 28,
1959," Presidency Project, www.presidency.ucsb.edu/ws/index.php?pid=11538;
Dwight D. Eisenhower, press conference with William H. W. Knighton

Jr. (*Baltimore Sun*), October 22, 1959, "The President's News Conference of October 22, 1959," Presidency Project, www.presidency.ucsb.edu/ws/index .php?pid=11569; Dwight D. Eisenhower, press conference with Garnett D. Homer (*Washington Star*), November 4, 1959, "The President's News Conference of November 4, 1959," Presidency Project, www.presidency.ucsb.edu/ws/ index.php?pid=11575; Dwight D. Eisenhower, press conference with Marvin L. Arrowsmith (AP), November 4, 1959, "The President's News Conference of November 4, 1959," Presidency Project, www.presidency.ucsb.edu/ws/index .php?pid=11575.

29. See Ike's own description of the Salk vaccine in Eisenhower, *Mandate for Change: 1953–1956* (Garden City, NY: Doubleday, 1963), 494–97. There was an uproar over snafus in mass distribution, leading to calls for Secretary Hobby's resignation. She did resign shortly afterward, with all sides denying that it was over the vaccination issue.

30. Dwight D. Eisenhower, "The President's News Conference of July 6, 1960," Presidency Project, www.presidency.ucsb.edu/ws/index.php?pid=11865.

31. Eisenhower, *Waging Peace*, 586 [inconsolable]; Dr. Arthur S. Flemming, Oral History No. 506, 1978, p. 35, Eisenhower Library [wrecked financially]; Dwight D. Eisenhower, Papers as President of the United States, 1953–1961, DDE Diary Series, Box 45, Folder: Staff Notes, October 1959 (1), Eisenhower Library.

32. Eisenhower, *Mandate for Change*, 51, 53, 54.

33. Dwight D. Eisenhower, "July 14, 1954," in *Campaign Statements of Dwight D. Eisenhower: A Reference Index*, Eisenhower Library; Dwight D. Eisenhower, "President's News Conference of July 4, 1954," Presidency Project, www.presidency.ucsb.edu/ws/index.php?pid=9947 [socialized medicine].

34. Dwight D. Eisenhower, "Los Angeles, October 9, 1952," in *Campaign Statements of Dwight D. Eisenhower: A Reference Index*, Eisenhower Library. It is often argued that Ike denounced socialized medicine in an effort to win over conservatives. However, there is no evidence that he was doing anything more than applying his deeply held principles to health care. Denouncing national health insurance while insisting on helping the needy (without running a deficit) is pure Eisenhower.

35. *Campaign Statements of Dwight D. Eisenhower: A Reference Index*, 139, Eisenhower Library.

36. Dwight D. Eisenhower, "Salt Lake City, October 10, 1952," in *Campaign Statements of Dwight D. Eisenhower: A Reference Index*, Eisenhower Library.

37. Eisenhower, *Mandate for Change*, 134–35.

38. Richard Harris, *A Sacred Trust* (New York: New American Library, 1966), 65.

39. President Dwight D. Eisenhower, letter to Secretary Olveta Culp Hobby, August 20, 1953, Ann Whitman File, Administration Series, Box 17, Folder: Hobby, Oveta Culp (6), Eisenhower Library.

40. Dwight D. Eisenhower, "State of the Union Message, January 7, 1954," Presidency Project, www.presidency.ucsb.edu/ws/index.php?pid=10096.

41. Roswell B. Perkins, Assistant Secretary [probably of HEW], memo to Governor Sherman Adams, Assistant to the President, July 9, 1953, and

accompanying documents, Central File, Official File OF 117-C, Box 599, Folder: 117-C Health Insurance, Eisenhower Library.

42. Harris, *A Sacred Trust,* 65 [Murray]; Hacker, *Divided Welfare State,* 405 [fires]; Jill Quadagno, *One Nation Uninsured: Why the US Has No National Health Insurance* (New York: Oxford University Press, 2005), 45 [first principle].

43. Roswell B. Perkins, Assistant Secretary [probably of HEW], memo to Governor Sherman Adams, Assistant to the President, July 9, 1953, and accompanying documents, Central File, Official File OF 117-C, Box 599, Folder: 117-C Health Insurance, Eisenhower Library (underlining in original).

44. Dwight D. Eisenhower, "Address at the Alfred E. Smith Memorial Dinner, New York City, October 21, 1954," *Public Papers of the Presidents: Dwight D. Eisenhower, 1953–1961,* Eisenhower Library.

45. Quadagno, *One Nation Uninsured,* 46 [stupid]; Dwight D. Eisenhower, "President's News Conference of July 14, 1954," Presidency Project, www .presidency.ucsb.edu/ws/index.php?pid=9947 [lost yesterday].

46. Quoted and discussed in Hacker, *Divided Welfare State,* 239–42.

47. David Blumenthal and James Morone, "The Lessons of Success— Revisiting the Medicare Story," *New England Journal of Medicine* 359, no. 22 (2008): 2384–89.

48. Secretary Oveta Culp Hobby, memo to President Dwight D. Eisenhower, November 18, 1954, Ann Whitman File, Administration Series, Box 9, Folder: Budget, 1955–56 (4), Eisenhower Library.

49. Rowland Hughes, Director of the Bureau of the Budget, memo to President Eisenhower, December 20, 1954, Central File, Official File, Box 598, Folder: Health 1, Eisenhower Library.

50. President Dwight D. Eisenhower, memo to Rowland Hughes, Director of the Bureau of The Budget December 22, 1954, Central File, Official File, Box 598, Folder: Health 1, Eisenhower Library.

51. President Dwight D. Eisenhower, letter to Secretary Oveta Culp Hobby, December 27, 1954, Ann Whitman File, Administration Series, Box 19, Folder: Hobby, Oveta Culp (4), Eisenhower Library.

52. Thomas W. Mattingly, "Medical History of DDE, 1911–1987," Box 1, Folder: General Health (3), Eisenhower Library [grave mistake]; Eisenhower, *Waging Peace,* 226 [crises].

53. Eisenhower, *Waging Peace,* 98, 99.

54. James A. Morone, *The Democratic Wish* (New York: Basic Books, 1993), 202–5.

55. See Eisenhower, *Waging Peace,* 211; David Halberstam, *The Fifties* (New York: Villard Books, 1993), 705.

56. Peter A. Corning, *The History of Medicare,* ch. 4, p. 3, www.ssa.gov/ history/corning.html; Harris, *Sacred Trust,* 68 [tarred].

57. Harris, *Sacred Trust,* 73.

58. President Dwight D. Eisenhower, memo to Cabinet secretaries, April 3, 1956, Morgan, Gerald D., Records 1953–1961, Box 1, Folder: Aging (1), Eisenhower Library.

59. Anne Whitman, note to Maurice Stans, June 10, 1958, Dwight D. Eisenhower, Papers as President, Ann Whitman File, Legislative Meeting Series, Box 3, Folder: Legislative Minutes, 1958 (3) May–June, Eisenhower Library; Harris, *Sacred Trust*, 77.

60. Ann Whitman File, Legislative Meeting Series, Box 3: Legislative Minutes 1958 (4) July–December, Eisenhower Library.

61. Dwight D. Eisenhower, statements to Cabinet, April 12, 1957, Ann Whitman File, Cabinet Series, Box 8, Folder: Cabinet Meeting of April 12, 1957, Eisenhower Library.

62. Dr. Arthur S. Flemming, Oral History No. 506, 1978, Eisenhower Library.

63. Dwight D. Eisenhower, letter to Secretary Arthur Flemming, November 15, 1958, Dwight D. Eisenhower, Papers as President of the United States, 1953–1961, Box 37, Folder: DDE Dictation, November 1958, Eisenhower Library (underlining in original).

64. Halberstam, *The Fifties*, 701.

65. Harris, *Sacred Trust*, 86–7.

66. Ann Whitman File, Legislative Meeting Series, Box 3, Folder: Legislative Minutes 1958 (4) July–Dec, Eisenhower Library.

67. Harris, *Sacred Trust*, 89; Corning, *The History of Medicare*, ch. 4, p. 7.

68. Dwight D. Eisenhower, "Address to the American Medical Association Annual Meeting, June 9, 1959," *Public Papers of the Presidents: Dwight D. Eisenhower, 1953–1961*, Eisenhower Library.

69. Corning, *The History of Medicare*, ch. 4, p. 7.

70. Dwight D. Eisenhower, memo for the files, October 16, 1959, Ann Whitman File, Administration Series, Box 15, Folder: Flemming, Arthur S. 1959–1961 (2), Eisenhower Library.

71. Dr. Arthur S. Flemming, Oral History No. 506, 1978, Eisenhower Library.

72. Dr. Arthur S. Flemming, Oral History No. 506, 1978, Eisenhower Library.

73. Dr. Arthur S. Flemming, Oral History No. 506, 1978, Eisenhower Library.

74. L. A. Minnich Jr., notes on legislative leadership meeting, February 16, 1960, Ann Whitman File, Legislative Meeting Series, Box 3, Folder: Legislative Leaders, 1960 (1) Jan–Feb, Eisenhower Library. Ann Whitman, Eisenhower's trusted secretary, kept an invaluable and meticulous diary on his schedule and activities.

75. Ann Whitman, diary entry, April 20, 1960, Dwight D. Eisenhower, Papers as President, Ann Whiteman Diary Series, Box 11, Folder: April 1960, Eisenhower Library; Dr. Arthur S. Flemming, Oral History No. 506, 1978, Eisenhower Library [Stans].

76. Ann Whitman, diary entry, February ?, 1960, Ann Whitman File, Legislative Meeting Series, Box 3, Folder: Legislative Leaders, 1960 (1) Jan–Feb, Eisenhower Library.

77. Dwight D. Eisenhower, Papers as President, Ann Whitman Diary Series, Box 11, Folder: April 1960 (1); Dwight D. Eisenhower, Papers as President, Ann Whiteman Diary Series, Box 11, Folder: April 20, 1960, Eisenhower Library.

78. Ann Whitman, diary entry, March 18, 1960, Dwight D. Eisenhower, Papers as President, Ann Whitman Diary Series, Box 11, Folder: March 1960 (2), Eisenhower Library.

79. Ann Whitman, diary entry, March 22, 1960, Dwight D. Eisenhower, Papers as President, Ann Whitman Diary Series, Box 11, Folder: March 1960, Eisenhower Library.

80. Editorial board, "Over 65—An A.B.C. of the Problem," Review of the Week, *New York Times*, April 10, 1960, E6; Harris, *A Sacred Trust*, 103.

81. Ann Whitman Series, Legislative Meeting Series, Box 3, Folder: Legislative Leaders, 1960 (2) March–April, Eisenhower Library (underlining in original).

82. L. A. Minnich Jr., notes on legislative leadership meeting, April 26, 1960 Ann Whitman File, Legislative Meeting Series, Box 3, Folder: Legislative Leaders, 1960 (2) March–April, Eisenhower Library.

83. Ann Whitman, diary entry, April 25, 1960, Dwight D. Eisenhower, Papers as President, Ann Whitman Diary Series, Box 11, Folder: April 1960 (1), Eisenhower Library; L. A. Minnich Jr., notes on legislative leadership meeting, April 26, 1960, Ann Whitman File, Legislative Meeting Series, Box 3, Folder: Legislative Leaders, 1960 (2) March–April, Eisenhower Library.

84. John D. Morris, "Medical Aid: The Pressure on Congress," Review of the Week Editorial, *New York Times*, May 1, 1960, E6; Harris, *A Sacred Trust*, 105.

85. Ike called the failure to reach a disarmament agreement his greatest disappointment. The goals seemed within reach. He knew (thanks, ironically, to the U-2 flights) that the United States would be negotiating from strength despite all the furor over Sputnik and the missile gap. And, despite the vast difference in their personal styles, he and Nikita Khrushchev appeared to have developed a good rapport during Khrushchev's ten-day visit to the United States. See Eisenhower, *Waging Peace*, for his own deep disappointment.

86. Assorted memos to the file, Ann Whitman File, Dwight D. Eisenhower Diary Series, Box 50, Folder: Staff Notes, May 1960 (3), Eisenhower Library.

87. Dwight D. Eisenhower, "Press Conference, March 30, 1960," Presidency Project, www.presidency.ucsb.edu/ws/index.php?pid=11734.

88. Assorted memos to the file, Ann Whitman File, Dwight D. Eisenhower Diary Series, Box 50, Folder: Staff Notes, May 1960 (3), Eisenhower Library.

89. Walter P. Reuther, letter to President Dwight D. Eisenhower, May 6, 1960, Central File, Official File OF 117-C, Box 599, Folder 117-C-7: Health Insurance, Eisenhower Library; Harris, *A Sacred Trust*, 106–7.

90. Harris, *A Sacred Trust*, 116.

91. For a more critical discussion of the hidden hand approach, see Neustadt, *Presidential Power and the Modern Presidents*, ch. 13.

4. JOHN F. KENNEDY

1. John F. Kennedy, *Profiles in Courage* (New York: Harper and Brothers, 1956), 217. As Kennedy acknowledges from the start, most of the book was written by others—most notably Theodore Sorensen—but the conclusion has a darker, mordant quality quite different from the other chapters. On public opinion, see Fred Greenstein, *The Presidential Difference: Leadership Style*

*from FDR to Clinton* (Princeton, NJ: Princeton University Press, 2000), 69. On polls, see Robert Dallek, *An Unfinished Life* (Boston: Little Brown, 2003), 609–702.

2. John F. Kennedy, "Inaugural address, January 20, 1961," Presidency Project, www.presidency.ucsb.edu/ws/index.php?pid=8032.

3. For a description of that press conference—and an analysis of Kennedy System that followed—see Samuel Kernell, *Going Public: New Strategies of Presidential Leadership*, 4th ed. (Washington, D.C.: CQ Press, 2007), 94–96.

4. On the essential Medicare history, see T. R. Marmor, *The Politics of Medicare* (New York: Aldine, 2000); Richard Harris, *A Sacred Trust* (New York: New American Library, 1966); Peter Corning, *The Evolution of Medicare* (Washington, D.C.: U.S. Government Printing Office, 1969); Paul Starr, *The Social Transformation of American Medicine* (New York: Basic Books, 1982).

5. Robert Dallek was the first historian to delve deeply into Kennedy's personal health care story. For the most detailed political science analysis, see Rose McDermott, *Presidential Leadership: Illness and Decision Making* (New York: Cambridge, 2008).

6. Dallek, *An Unfinished Life,* 33–35; McDermott, *Presidential Leadership,* 120.

7. Dallek, *An Unfinished Life,* 73–77. Adrenal extracts became available in 1937; Dallek speculates (on the basis of a handwritten note from Jack to his father) that Kennedy was already taking them.

8. Dallek, *An Unfinished Life,* 79–81, 85, 102.

9. John Hersey wrote a mesmerizing account of the incident after interviewing Kennedy and three of the others: "Survival," *New Yorker,* June 17, 1944, 31–42.

10. Rose McDermott, *Presidential Leadership,* 124.

11. McDermott, *Presidential Leadership,* 134; Dallek, *An Unfinished Life,* 76, 105.

12. McDermott, *Presidential Leadership,* 134–35.

13. McDermott, *Presidential Leadership,* 125. On extreme unction, see Richard Reeves, *President Kennedy: Profile of Power* (New York: Simon and Schuster, 1993), 24.

14. Reeves, *President Kennedy,* 146–47, 243. For a darker analysis of the same story, see Seymour Hersh, *The Dark Side of Camelot* (Boston: Little Brown, 1997), 234–37. Theodore Sorensen tells the story very cryptically in *Counselor: A Life on the Edge of History* (New York: Harpers, 2008), 106.

15. McDermott, *Presidential Leadership,* 144–54.

16. Dallek, *An Unfinished Life,* 581.

17. Richard Whalen, *The Founding Father: The Story of Joseph P. Kennedy* (New York: Signet, 1964).

18. Arthur Schlesinger Jr., *Journals: 1952–2000* (New York, Penguin, 2008), 150 (March 31, 1962).

19. Lawrence F. O'Brien, oral history, taken by Michael L. Gillette, Interview III, pages 50–51, October 30, 1985, Internet copy, LBJ Library.

20. Theodore C. Sorensen, interview with David Blumenthal, March 23, 2006.

21. Lawrence F. O'Brien, oral history, taken by Michael L. Gillette, Interview I, September 18, 1985, Internet copy, LBJ Library [semishock]; Arthur Schlesinger, *A Thousand Days* (Boston: Houghton-Mifflin, 1965), 651; Reeves, *President Kennedy*, 55–57 [ballgame].

22. Ralph A. Dungan, oral history, taken by Larry J. Hackman, p. 41, December 9, 1967, JFK Library.

23. Lawrence F. O'Brien, oral history, taken by Michael L. Gillette, Interview I, page 27, September 18, 1985, Internet copy, LBJ Library.

24. Schlesinger, *A Thousand Days*, 652. Schlesinger, a stalwart of the Eastern intellectual establishment, thought the Kentucky comment bizarre. No one would say so a generation later as the Sunbelt and its mores rose to power.

25. Frederick Dutton, from "Reflections on the New Frontier," transcript of a conversation recorded at the JFK Library among former Kennedy staff in January, 1981, available at the JFK Library; Dallek, *An Unfinished Life*, 306–7 [the transition].

26. Richard Rovere, "Letter from Washington," *New Yorker*, February 4, 1961; James Patterson, *Grand Expectations* (New York: Oxford, 1996), [Stevenson] 459; James Morone, "Representation Without Elections: The American Bureaucracy and Its Publics," in *Representation and Responsibility: Exploring Legislative Ethics*, eds. Daniel Callahan and Bruce Jennings (New York: Plenum Press, 1985).

27. Quoted in Sidney Milkis and Michael Nelson, *The American Presidency* (Washington, D.C.: Congressional Quarterly Press, 2003), 310; Sydney Milkis and Michael Nelson, The American Presidency (Washington, D.C.: CQ Press, 2003), 310.

28. Theodore Lowi, *The Personal President: Power Invested, Promise Unfulfilled* (Ithaca: Cornell University Press, 1985); Richard Rovere, "Letter from Washington," *New Yorker*, February 4, 1961; Samuel Kernell, *Going Public*, 95.

29. Ralph A. Dungan, oral history, p. 96; Dallek, *An Unfinished Life*, 158 [overshadows everything]; Patterson, *Grand Expectations*, 465 [drop domestic]; Richard E. Neustadt, *Presidential Power and the Modern Presidents: The Politics of Leadership from Roosevelt to Reagan* (Free Press, New York, 1990), 110, 170.

30. Reeves, *President Kennedy*, 88–114, 537.

31. McDermott, *Presidential Leadership*, 144–55.

32. John F. Kennedy, "Remarks in the Rudolph Wilde Platz, Berlin, June 26, 1963," Presidency Project, www.presidency.ucsb.edu/ws/index.php?pid=9307.

33. Reeves, *President Kennedy*, 537.

34. Reeves, *President Kennedy*, 100.

35. See James A. Morone, *The Democratic Wish* (New Haven: Yale University Press, 1998), ch. 6.

36. Research Background Files, DNC, Box 240, JFK Library [party platform]; Harris, *A Sacred Trust*, 102 [Detroit rally], 117 [tapes].

37. Wilbur J. Cohen, "Health and Social Security for the American People: A Report to President Elect John F. Kennedy," January 10, 1961, Papers of President John F. Kennedy, Pre-Presidential Papers, Transition Files, Box 1071, JFK

Library; on Wilbur Cohen, see Edward Berkowitz, *Mr. Social Security* (Lawrence: University of Kansas, 1995); for his role on the task force, see 136–37.

38. David E. Bell, memo to Mr. Sorensen, Mr. Feldman, January 24, 1961, Papers of Theodore C. Sorensen, JFK Speech Files 1961–1963, Box 63, Folder: State of the Union Message I, 1/30/61, JFK Library; Budget Bureau memo re HEW proposals 1/24/61–1/25/61, Papers of Theodore C. Sorensen, JFK Speech Files 1961–1963, Box 63, Folder: State of the Union Message I, 1/30/61, Drafts 1/29/61, JFK Library.

39. John F. Kennedy, "Special Message on Health and Hospital Care to the Congress of the United States," Papers of Theodore C. Sorensen, JFK Speech Files, 1961–1963, Box 61, Folder: Health Message to the Congress (2/9/61), JFK Library; Harris, *A Sacred Trust,* 123; Berkowitz, *Mr. Social Security,* 166.

40. Theodore Sorensen, interview with David Blumenthal, Boston, Massachusetts, March 23, 2006; Dallek's *An Unfinished Life* makes the same point on page 328.

41. Lawrence F. O'Brien, oral history, taken by Michael L. Gillette, Interview I, page 24, September 18, 1985, Internet copy, LBJ Library.

42. Lawrence F. O'Brien, oral history, taken by Michael L. Gillette, Interview I, page 25, September 18, 1985, Internet copy, LBJ Library.

43. Lawrence [Larry] F. O'Brien, oral history 1; Irving Bernstein, *Promises Kept: John F. Kennedy's New Frontier* (New York: Oxford University Press, 1991), 282.

44. Lawrence F. O'Brien, oral history, taken by Michael L. Gillette, Interview III, page 53, October 30, 1985, Internet copy, LBJ Library.

45. Larry O'Brien, memo to the President of the United States, March 27, 1961, Papers of Theodore C. Sorensen, Box 57, Folder: Legislative Meetings, 1/24/61–3/28/61, JFK Library.

46. John F. Kennedy, press conference, April 21, 1961, *The Kennedy Presidential Press Conferences* (New York: Earl M. Coleman Enterprises, 1978).

47. John F. Kennedy, press conference, April 21, 1961, *The Kennedy Presidential Press Conferences.*

48. Larry O'Brien, memo to the President of the United States, July 24, 1961, Papers of Theodore C. Sorensen, 6, Box 57, Folder: Legislative Meetings, 7/24/61, JFK Library.

49. Edward F. Woods, "President Said to Think Administration's Record in Congress is Excellent," *St. Louis Post Dispatch,* September 17, 1961, section C, Papers of Theodore C. Sorensen, Box 57, Folder: Legislative Meetings, 9/61, JFK Library.

50. Lou Harris, memo to the president, June 22, 1961, President's Office File, Box 63A: Staff Memos, Folder: Harris, Louis, JFK Library.

51. Lou Harris, memo to the president, June 22, 1961, President's Office File, Box 63A: Staff Memos, Folder: Harris, Louis, JFK Library.

52. Jack Bell, "Kennedy–Congress," Associated Press, September 27, 1961, Papers of Theodore C. Sorensen, Box 57, Folder: Legislative Meetings, 8/16/61–9/29/61, JFK Library.

53. Theodore C. Sorensen, memo to the president, Papers of Theodore C. Sorensen, Box 57: Legislative Program 1962, Folder: President's Copy, JFK Library.

54. Henry Hall Wilson, memo to Richard Donahue, January 5, 1962, Personal Papers of Henry Hall Wilson, Box 4, Folder: Medical Care, 1 of 2, JFK Library.

55. Wilbur Cohen, oral history, taken by David G. McComb, tape A, December 8, 1968, LBJ Library; Lawrence F. O'Brien, oral history, taken by Michael L. Gillette, Interview III, page 32, October 30, 1985, Internet copy, LBJ Library.

56. John F. Kennedy, "State of the Union Address, January 11, 1962," Presidency Project, www.presidency.ucsb.edu/ws/index.php?pid=9082.

57. John F. Kennedy, press conference, January 24, 1961, *The Kennedy Presidential Press Conferences.*

58. Kenneth O'Donnell, letter to Ivan A. Nestigen, Undersecretary of Health, Education, and Welfare, March 15, 1962, Personal Papers of Ivan A. Nestingen: Health Education and Welfare, Box 4, JFK Library.

59. Editorial, *New York Times,* May 21, 1962, 1:8 (see also the related article on 1:4); Harris, *A Sacred Trust,* 146.

60. John F. Kennedy, "Address of the President at the Rally of the Three Generations, Madison Square Garden, May 20, 1962," Papers of Theodore C. Sorensen, JFK Speech Files, Box 68: New York City, 5/18/62–5/20/62, Folder: Medical Care Rally 5/20/62, JFK Library. A recording of the speech is available online at www.presidency.ucsb.edu/ws/index.php?pid=8669.

61. Harris, *A Sacred Trust,* 142.

62. Well described in Harris, *A Sacred Trust,* 145. Senator George McGovern (D-SD) forwarded an advance copy of the rebuttal to Sorensen, but JFK's effort to preempt the criticism seemed half-hearted and unpersuasive. George McGovern, memo to Ted Sorensen, Papers of Theodore C. Sorensen, Box 36: Medicare Care for the Aged, 8/17/61–5/28/61, JFK Library.

63. "Squared Off," *Time,* June 1, 1962, 17–18; "Great Medicare Debate," *Newsweek,* June 4, 1962, 28–34.

64. Donald Janson, "AMA Disputes Kennedy Charge," *New York Times,* May 26, 1962, 1.

65. John F. Kennedy, letter to the AMA, June 4, 1962, President's Office File, Box 51, Folder: 6/1/62–11/62, JFK Library (underlining in original).

66. John F. Kennedy, letter to Dr. Leonard W. Larson, President of the American Medical Association, Papers of Theodore C. Sorensen, Box 36: Medical Care for the Aged 6/2/62–6/13/63, JFK Library.

67. Morris Udall, "Medicare: The Battle of Madison Square Garden, June 1, 1962," in *Education of a Congressman: Newsletters of Morris K. Udall* (Indianapolis: Bobs-Merrill, 1972).

68. Wilbur Cohen, memo to Myer Feldman, January 4, 1962. Personal Papers of Myer Feldman, Box 11, Folder: Health Insurance, 12/60–11/62, JFK Library.

69. Wilbur J. Cohen, memo to Theodore Sorensen, July 6, 1962, Papers of Theodore Sorensen, CS, Box 36: Medical Care for the Aged, 6/2/62–6/13/63, JFK Library.

70. Wilbur J. Cohen, memo to Theodore Sorensen, July 6, 1962, Papers of Theodore Sorensen, CS, Box 36: Medical Care for the Aged, 6/2/62–6/13/63, JFK Library.

71. Claude Desautels, memo to Larry O'Brien, July 2, 1962, Papers of Theodore Sorensen, Box 58, Folder: Legislative Leaders Meetings, 7/2/62–7/10/62, JFK Library.

72. Wilbur J. Cohen, memo to Theodore Sorensen, July 11, 1962, Papers of Theodore Sorensen, Box 36: Medical Care for the Aged, 6/2/62–6/13/63, JFK Library.

73. John F. Kennedy, "The President's News Conference of June 27, 1962," Presidency Project, www.presidency.ucsb.edu/ws/index.php?pid=8735.

74. Larry O'Brien to the President, undated, President's Office File Staff Memos, Box 64, Folder: O'Brien, Lawrence, 2/61–8/62, JFK Library.

75. Theodore Sorensen, memo, July 17, 1962, President's Office File Legislative Files, Box 51, Folder: 7/16–31/62, JFK Library.

76. Clinton Anderson, oral history, taken by John F. Stewart, page 48, April 14, 1967, JFK Library.

77. John F. Kennedy, "Remarks of the President, July 17, 1962," Papers of Theodore C. Sorensen, Box 36: Medical Care for the Aged, 6/2/62–6/13/63, JFK Library.

78. John F. Kennedy, "President's News Conference of July 23, 1962," Presidency Project, www.presidency.ucsb.edu/ws/index.php?pid=8784.

79. Sorensen, interview with the authors, March 23, 2006; Harris, A Sacred Trust, 148 [got over].

80. Edward Berkowitz, Mr. Social Security (Lawrence: University of Kansas, 1995), 183–85.

81. Chuck Odell, memo to Dick Maguire, December 18, 1962, Personal Papers of Ivan A. Nestingen: Health Education and Welfare, Box 4, JFK Library [field manager]; Wilbur J. Cohen, memo to Theodore Sorensen, December 19, 1962, Personal Papers of Meyer Feldman, Box 11, Folder: Health Insurance, 12/62–5/63, JFK Library [confusing].

82. "JFK Library Presidential Recordings: Tax Cut Proposals of 1962–1963, B-3 and B-4: Off the Record Meeting with C. Douglas Dillon, David Bell, Walter Heller, Theodore Sorensen, Gardner Ackley, Elmer Staats, Charles Schultze," audiotape 27, item 1, October 2, 1962, JFK Library; Harris, A Sacred Trust, 153.

83. "JFK Library Presidential Recordings: Tax Cut Proposals of 1962–1963, B-3 and B-4: Off the Record Meeting with C. Douglas Dillon, David Bell, Walter Heller, Theodore Sorensen, Gardner Ackley, Elmer Staats, Charles Schultze," audiotape 27, item 1, October 2, 1962, JFK Library.

84. Theodore Sorensen, memo to the president, Papers of Theodore C. Sorensen, 11/19/62, Legislative Files, 1961–1964, Box 58, Folder: Legislation 1963, 1/13/62–12/22/62, JFK Library.

85. Bernstein, Promises Kept, 258; Harris, A Sacred Trust, 153.

86. John F. Kennedy, memo to Secretary Celebrezze, May 6, 1963, President's Office File, Box 68: Departments and Agencies, Folder: JFK Memos to Departments and Agencies, FAA, Justice, JFK Library.

87. Anthony Celebrezze, oral history, taken by William A. Geoghegan, page 20, 1965, JFK Library.

88. Bernstein, *Promises Kept,* ch. 8.

89. Harris, *A Sacred Trust,* 156–57.

90. Andrew Biemiller, oral history, taken by Sheldon Stern, pages 46–47, May 24, 1979, Washington, D.C., JFK Library; Harris, *A Sacred Trust,* 157.

## 5. LYNDON B. JOHNSON

1. Robert Dallek, *Lyndon B. Johnson: Portrait of a President* (New York: Oxford, 2004), 87 [Humphrey]; Carl B. Albert, oral history, Washington, D.C., taken by Dorothy McSweeney, tape A, April 28, 1969, LBJ Library.

2. On measures of presidential success in Congress, see Andrew Rudalevige, "The Executive Branch and the Legislative Process," in *The Executive Branch,* eds. Joel Aberbach and Mark Peterson (New York: Oxford, 2005), 419–51 (data cited from 431).

The White House tapes constantly show Johnson deferring on the details of legislation while overseeing the politics—although after claiming not to care about details, Johnson often dove into the details. For examples, see Wilbur Mills, telephone audiotape, 9:55 A.M., June 9, 1964, "Recordings and Transcripts of Conversations," Citation 3642, LBJ Library; Lawrence [Larry] F. O'Brien, 3:55 P.M., June 11, 1964, "Recordings and Transcripts of Conversations," Citation 3686, LBJ Library; Robert Byrd, 2:50 P.M., July 15, 1965, "Recordings and Transcripts of Conversations," Citation 8343, LBJ Library.

3. For the classic history of Medicare, see Theodore Marmor, *The Politics of Medicare* (New York: Aldine De Gruyter, 2000).

4. Lyndon Johnson, *The Vantage Point* (New York: Holt, Rinehart and Winston, 1971), 216.

5. Marmor introduced the terms quoted here, *Politics of Medicare,* ch. 3 and 4. On Congressional dynamics, see also Mark Peterson, "The Congressional Graveyard for Health Care Reform," in *Healthy, Wealthy and Fair,* eds. James Morone and Lawrence Jacobs (New York: Oxford, 2005), 205–33; Sven Steinmo and John Watts, "It's the Institutions Stupid! Why Comprehensive National Health Insurance Always Fails in America," *Journal of Health Politics, Policy and Law* 20, no. 2 (1995): 329–72.

6. Wilbur Mills, oral history, taken by Michael L. Gillette, interview 2, tape 1 of 2, March 25, 1987, LBJ Library.

7. Wilbur Mills, oral history, taken by Michael L. Gillette, interview 2, tape 1 of 2, March 25, 1987, LBJ Library.

8. Hubert Humphrey, audiotape, 11:25 A.M., March 6, 2005, "Recordings and Transcripts of Conversations," Citation 7024–7025, LBJ Library.

9. "President Lyndon Johnson, Special Message to Congress: The American Promise," March 15, 1965, LBJ Library, www.lbjlib.utexas.edu/johnson/archives.hom/speeches.hom/650315.asp.

10. Myer Feldman, telephone audiotape, 11:15 A.M., September 3, 1964, "Recordings and Transcripts of Conversations," Citation 5444, LBJ Library.

11. Joseph Califano, interview with the authors, June 15, 2006.

12. Robert Dallek, *Lone Star Rising* (New York: Oxford University Press, 1991), 56; Doris Kearns Goodwin, *Lyndon Johnson and the American Dream,* rev. ed. (New York: St. Martin's Griffin, 1991), 19–34.

13. Kearns Goodwin, *Lyndon Johnson and the American Dream,* 65–66.

14. Johnson, *The Vantage Point,* 104; Dallek, *Lyndon B. Johnson,* 29.

15. Dallek, *Lyndon B. Johnson,* 29 [petted]; Kearns Goodwin, *Lyndon Johnson and the American Dream,* 90–91.

16. Wilbur Cohen, oral history, taken by David G. McComb, March 2, 1969, LBJ Library.

17. James Gaither, oral history, taken by Dorothy Pierce, tape 3, November 10, 1969, LBJ Library.

18. Philip R. Lee, oral history, taken by David G. McComb, tape 1, January 18, 1969, LBJ Library.

19. Dallek, *Lyndon B. Johnson,* 92.

20. Robert Caro, *Master of the Senate* (New York: Vintage, 2002, 617–20.

21. Caro, *Master of the Senate,* 621–23.

22. Caro, *Master of the Senate,* 621–24.

23. Dallek, *Lyndon B. Johnson,* 92–93 [blood pressure]; Caro, *Master of the Senate,* 625 [50–50].

24. Philip R. Lee, oral history, taken by David G. McComb, tape 1, January 18, 1969, LBJ Library.

25. Dallek, *Lyndon B. Johnson,* 82.

26. Carl Albert, oral history, taken by Dorothy Pierce McSweeney, interview IV, tape 1 of 1, August 13, 1969, LBJ Library.

27. Senator Clinton Anderson, oral history, taken by T.H. Barker, page 15, May 20, 1969, LBJ Library; Dallek, *Lyndon B. Johnson,* 82 [on Harlow].

28. James Gaither, oral history, taken by Dorothy Pierce, tape 3, November 10, 1969, LBJ Library.

29. Wilbur Cohen, oral history, Silver Spring, MD, taken by David G. McComb, Tape 3, page 8, March 2, 1969, LBJ Library; Dallek, *Lyndon B. Johnson,* 73 [Humphrey].

30. Kearns Goodwin, *Lyndon Johnson and the American Dream,* 186.

31. Carl Albert, oral history, taken by Dorothy Pierce McSweeney, tape C, interview III, tape 1 of 1, July 9, 1969, LBJ Library.

32. Wilbur Cohen, oral history, taken by David G. McComb, tape 3, March 2, 1969, Silver Spring MD, LBJ Library.

33. Wilbur Cohen, oral history, Silver Spring, MD, taken by David G. McComb, tape 3, March 2, 1969, LBJ Library.

34. Joseph A. Califano Jr., *The Triumph and Tragedy of Lyndon Johnson* (Bryan: Texas A&M University Press, 2000), 82–83 [tutorial]; Kearns Goodwin, *Johnson and the American Dream,* 226.

35. Lawrence [Larry] F. O'Brien, oral history, taken by Michael L. Gillette, interview X, June 25, 1986, Internet copy, LBJ Library.

36. Lawrence [Larry]F. O'Brien, oral history, taken by Michael L. Gillette, interview XI, page 29, July 24, 1986, Internet copy, LBJ Library.

37. Wilbur Cohen, oral history, taken by David G. McComb, tape 3, March 2, 1969, LBJ Library.

38. Hubert Humphrey, audiotape, 11:25 A.M., March 6, 1965, "Recordings and Transcripts of Conversations," Citation 7024–7025, LBJ Library.

39. Lawrence [Larry] F. O'Brien, oral history, taken by Michael L. Gillette, interview XI, July 24, 1986, Internet copy, LBJ Library.

40. Arthur M. Schlesinger Jr., *Journals: 1952–2000* (New York: Penguin, 2008), 231 [August 29, 1964].

41. Califano, *Triumph and Tragedy,* 51–52.

42. Karen Davis, President of the Commonwealth Fund and Former Deputy Assistant Secretary for Planning and Evaluation of the Department of Health Education and Welfare (while Califano was secretary), personal correspondence with the authors, July 21, 2008. Dr. Davis reported that Califano himself had told her the story as a cautionary tale about keeping programs safe from White House meddling. On designing the program, see Califano Jr., *Triumph and Tragedy.*

43. Joseph Califano, interview with the authors, June 15, 2006.

44. Fred Greenstein, *The Presidential Difference* (Princeton, NJ: Princeton University Press, 2000), 87–89.

45. Johnson, quoted in Michael Beschloss, *Taking Charge: the Johnson White House Tapes, 1963–4* (New York: Simon and Schuster, 1997), 370.

46. Califano, *Triumph and Tragedy,* 98; Dallek, *Lyndon B. Johnson,* 328.

47. Wilbur Mills, oral history, taken by Michael L. Gillette, interview 2, tape 1 of 2, March 25, 1987, LBJ Library.

48. Kearns Goodwin, *Lyndon Johnson and the American Dream,* 149; Dallek, *Lone Star Rising,* 147–57.

49. Lyndon B. Johnson, "Commencement Address, the University of Michigan, May 22, 1964, Ann Arbor, Michigan," Presidency Project, www.presidency.ucsb.edu/ws/index.php?pid=26262.

50. Wilbur Mills, oral history, taken by Joe B. Frantz, interview 1, tape 1 of 1, November 2, 1971, LBJ Library; Wilbur Cohen, telephone audiotape, March 21, 1964, "Recordings and Transcripts of Conversations," Citation 2612, LBJ Library.

51. Lawrence [Larry] O'Brien, memo to the President, "Medical Insurance," January 27, 1964, Office Files of Mike Manatos, Box 9 (1 of 2), LBJ Library.

52. Wilbur Mills, telephone audiotape, 9:55 A.M., June 9, 1964, "Recordings and Transcripts of Conversations," Citation 3642, LBJ Library.

53. Lawrence [Larry] F. O'Brien, audiotape, 3:55 P.M., June 11, 1964, "Recordings and Transcripts of Conversations," Citation 3686, LBJ Library. Johnson had called O'Brien off the floor of the House and, when Mills walked by, had him put the congressman on the phone.

54. Lawrence Jacobs, *The Health of Nations* (Ithaca, NY: Cornell, 1993), 192–93.

55. Lawrence [Larry] F. O'Brien, audiotape, 3:55 P.M., June 11, 1964, "Recordings and Transcripts of Conversations," Citation 3686, LBJ Library.

56. Earle Clements, audiotape, 4:18 P.M., June 11, 1964, "Recordings and Transcripts of Conversations," Citation 3690, LBJ Library.

57. George Smathers, audiotape, 11:00 A.M., August 1, 1964, "Recordings and Transcripts of Conversations," Citation 4604, LBJ Library.

58. Lawrence [Larry] F. O'Brien, audiotape, 11:05 A.M., August 14, 1964, LBJ Library.

59. Elmer Staats, memo to the President, August 29, 1964, Ex LE/IS1, White House Central File, Box 75, LBJ Library.

60. Mike Mansfield, audiotape, 10:58 A.M., September 2, 1964, "Recordings and Transcripts of Conversations," Citation 5416, LBJ Library; Carl Hayden, audiotape, 11:15 A.M., September 2, 1964, "Recordings and Transcripts of Conversations," Citation 5419, LBJ Library.

61. Richard Harris, A Sacred Trust (New York: New American Library, 1966), 165.

62. Meyer Feldman, audiotape, 11:14 A.M., September 3, 1964, "Recordings and Transcripts of Conversations," Citation 5444, LBJ Library.

63. Alex Rose, audiotape, 5:32 P.M., September 2, 1964, "Recordings and Transcripts of Conversations," Citation 5429, LBJ Library [got enough votes]; Myer Feldman, audiotape, 11:14 A.M., September 3, 1964, "Recordings and Transcripts of Conversations," Citation 5444, LBJ Library [twisted arms]; Bill Moyers, memo to President Johnson, September 2, 1964, White House Central File, LE, Box 75, LE/IS1 February 21, 1964–September 10, 1964, LBJ Library.

64. Carl Albert, audiotape, 11:20 A.M., September 3, 1964, "Recordings and Transcripts of Conversations," Citation 5445, LBJ Library.

65. Carl Albert, audiotape, 6:06 P.M., September 3, 1964, "Recordings and Transcripts of Conversations," Citation 5469–5470, LBJ Library.

66. Carl Albert, audiotape, 6:06 P.M., September 3, 1964, "Recordings and Transcripts of Conversations," Citation 5469–5470, LBJ Library.

67. George Smathers, audiotape, 5:20 P.M., September 24, 1964, "Recordings and Transcripts of Conversations," Citation 5673, LBJ Library; Russell Long, 5:30 P.M., September 24, 1964, "Recordings and Transcripts of Conversations," Citation 5677, LBJ Library.

68. Harris, A Sacred Trust, 171–72; Marmor, Politics of Medicare, 42–43.

69. Harris, A Sacred Trust, 172–77; Marmor, Politics of Medicare, 43–45.

70. Hale Boggs, audiotape, 9:59 P.M., November 4, 1964, "Recordings and Transcripts of Conversations," Citation 6182, LBJ Library.

71. Carl Albert, audiotape, 12:20 P.M., November 9, 1964, "Recordings and Transcripts of Conversations," Citation 6307, LBJ Library.

72. Russell Long, audiotape, 8:25 P.M., November 18, 1964, "Recordings and Transcripts of Conversations," Citation 6403, LBJ Library.

73. Secretary Anthony J. Celebrezze, memo to the President, November 25, 1964, Ex LE/IS 1, White House Central File, Box 75, LBJ Library.

74. Myer Feldman, memo to the President, December 8, 1964, Ex LE/IS1, White House Central File, Box 75, LBJ Library.

75. Lawrence [Larry] F. O'Brien, oral history, taken by Michael L. Gillette, interview X, page 19, June 25, 1986, Internet copy, LBJ Library.

76. Lyndon Baines Johnson, "The State of the Union Message, Monday, January 4, 1965," Presidency Project, www.presidency.ucsb.edu/ws/index.php?pid=26907.

77. Harris, *A Sacred Trust*, 186–90.

78. Wilbur Mills, oral history, taken by Michael L. Gillette, interview 2, tape 1 of 2, March 25, 1987, LBJ Library.

79. Wilbur Cohen, audiotape, 5:00 P.M., March 23, 1965, "Recordings and Transcripts of Conversations," Citation 7142, LBJ Library.

80. John McCormack, audiotape, 4:54 P.M., March 23, 1965, "Recordings and Transcripts of Conversations," Citation 7141, LBJ Library.

81. Lawrence [Larry] F. O'Brien, oral history, taken by Michael L. Gillette, interview XI, July 24, 1986, Internet copy, LBJ Library.

82. Lawrence [Larry] F. O'Brien, oral history, taken by Michael L. Gillette, interview XI, July 24, 1986, Internet copy, LBJ Library.

83. John McCormack, audiotape, 4:54 P.M., March 23, 1965, "Recordings and Transcripts of Conversations," Citation 7141, LBJ Library.

84. Edward Kennedy, audiotape, 11:32 A.M., January 9, 1965, "Recordings and Transcripts of Conversations," Citation 6718, LBJ Library.

85. Francis Bator, "No Good Choices: LBJ and the Vietnam/Great Society Connection," occasional paper, American Academy of Arts and Sciences, 2007, www.amacad.org/publications/nogoodChoices.aspx.

86. Hubert Humphrey, audiotape, 11:25 A.M., March 6, 2005, "Recordings and Transcripts of Conversations," Citation 7024–7025, LBJ Library.

87. Lawrence [Larry] F. O'Brien, oral history, taken by Michael L. Gillette, interview XI, pages 24–25, July 24, 1986, Internet copy, LBJ Library; Mike Manatos, memo to Lawrence [Larry] F. O'Brien, April 14, 1965, EX IS 1, "Accident-Hospital-Medical-Health," White House Central File, Box 1, LBJ Library.

88. Gardner Ackley, memo to the President, March 11, 1965, Ex LE/IS1, White House Central File, Box 75, LBJ Library.

89. Jack Valenti, memo to the President, April 22, 1965, EX LE/IS1, White House Central File, Box 75, LBJ Library. Valenti was a legendary aide—he was in the Kennedy motorcade in Dallas and on the plane as LBJ was sworn in. He was famously and ferociously loyal: if Johnson dropped an atom bomb on a city, went one jibe, Valenti would write it up as urban renewal. See Jack Valenti, *This Time, This Place: My Life in War, the White House and Hollywood* (New York: Crown, 2008).

90. William Moyers, memo to the President, April 26, 1965, EX LE/IS1, White House Central File, Box 75, LBJ Library.

91. Robert Byrd, audiotape, 2:50 P.M., July 15, 1965, "Recordings and Transcripts of Conversations," Citation 8343, LBJ Library.

92. Johnson, *The Vantage Point*, 218.

93. For a superb discussion, see Jill Quadagno, *One Nation Uninsured: Why the US Has No National Health Insurance* (New York: Oxford, 2005), 83–93.

94. David Barton Smith, *Health Care Divided: Race and Healing a Nation* (Ann Arbor: University of Michigan Press, 1999), 115–16.

95. Quoted in Quadagno, *One Nation Uninsured*, 87.

96. Anthony Celebrezze, letter to Senator Byrd, and attachments, April 27, 1965, EX LE/IS1, White House Central File, Box 75, LBJ Library (emphasis added).

97. Douglass Cater, memo to the President, "Memos to the President, May 1966," Office Files of Douglass Cater, Box 14, LBJ Library.

98. Quadagno, *One Nation Uninsured,* 87–89.

99. F. Peter Libassi, memo to Joseph Califano, Douglass Cater and Nicholas de B. Katzenbach, May 6, 1966, EX IS 1, White House Central File, Box 1, LBJ Library.

100. Farris Bryant, memo to the President, May 23, 1966, Ex FG 165, White House Central File, Box 239, LBJ Library.

101. Smith, *Health Care Divided,* 137.

102. Harris, *Sacred Trust,* 215.

103. The meeting is described by Lyndon Johnson in his *Vantage Point,* 218 [his daddy's illness]; Joseph Califano, *Triumph and Tragedy,* 50–51 [Vietnam]; and Harris, *A Sacred Trust* [standing up, the physician's reactions], 215–16.

104. Douglass Cater, memo to the President, August 26, 1965, Ex LE/IS 1, White House Central File, Box 75, LBJ Library.

105. Ernest B. Howard, MD, memo to F. J. L. Blasingame, MD, AMA Board of Trustees, August 30, 1965, "Medicare History, Executive Sessions, William and Mary, 1965," Personal Papers of Wilbur Cohen, series II, Box 13, LBJ Library.

106. Douglass Cater, memo to the President, September 17, 1965, "Memos to the President, September 1965," Office Files of Douglass Cater, Box 14, LBJ Library.

107. The implementation process is analyzed in Judith Feder, *Medicare: The Politics of Federal Hospital Insurance* (Lexington, MA: D. C. Heath, 1977).

108. Lyndon B. Johnson, letter to John Gardner, April 7, 1966, EX FG 165, White House Central File, Box 239, LBJ Library.

109. Douglass Cater, memo to the President, "Memos to the President, May 1966," Office Files of Douglass Cater, Box 14, LBJ Library.

110. Douglass Cater, memo to the President, "Memos to the President, June 1966," Office Files of Douglass Cater, Box 15, LBJ Library.

111. Joseph Califano, memo to the President, October 1, 1965, Ex IS 1, White House Central File, Box 1, LBJ Library.

6. RICHARD NIXON

1. Richard Reeves, *President Nixon: Alone in the White House* (New York: Simon and Schuster, 2001), 42.

2. Bela Kornitzer, *The Real Nixon: An Intimate Biography* (Skokie, IL: Rand McNally, 1960), 20.

3. Rose McDermott, *Presidential Leadership* (New York: Cambridge University Press, 2007), ch. 6; Vamik Volkan, Norman Itzkowitz, and Andrew Dod, *Richard Nixon: A Psychobiography* (New York: Columbia University Press, 1997), 34.

4. Deborah Strober and Gerald Strober, *The Nixon Presidency: An Oral History of the Era* (Washington, D.C.: Brassey's Inc., 2003), 38.

5. Kornitzer, *The Real Nixon,* 50.

6. Robert Dallek, *Nixon and Kissinger: Partners in Power* (New York: Harper Collins, 2007), 7.

7. Roger Morris, *Richard Milhous Nixon: The Rise of an American Politician* (New York: Henry Holt & Co.: 1991), 83.

8. Kornitzer, *The Real Nixon,* 65.

9. See Jonathan Aitken, *Nixon: A Life* (Washington, D.C.: Regnery Publishing, 1996) for the view that the death inspired Richard to make up for the loss. Hannah Nixon would draw a similar conclusion about the death of Richard's older brother (described below).

10. Kornitzer, *The Real Nixon,* 65–66.

11. William Chafe, *Private Lives/Public Consequences: Personality and Politics in Modern America* (Triliteral: Cumberland, RI, 2006), 268–69; Dallek, *Nixon and Kissinger,* 548 [above all else].

12. Roger Morris, *Richard Milhous Nixon: The Rise of an American Politician* (New York: Henry Holt & Co., 1991), 43.

13. Aitken, *Nixon,* 49–50.

14. R. Schreiber, "Richard Nixon: A Mother's Story," *Good Housekeeping,* June 1960, 212, cited in Stephen Ambrose, *Nixon: The Education of a Politician, 1913–1962* (New York: Simon & Schuster, 1987), 57.

15. President Richard Nixon, audiotape, conversations in the Oval Office, Conversation No. 786-21, 12:49 P.M.-1:09 P.M., September 25, 1972.

16. William M. Blairs, "Psychiatric Aid to Nixon Denied," *New York Times,* November 14, 1968, 34, cited in Aitken, *Nixon,* 196–97; Morris, *Richard Milhous Nixon,* 654; Fawn M. Brodie, *Richard Nixon: The Shaping of His Character* (Cambridge: Harvard University Press, 1983), 331, cited in Ambrose, *Nixon,* 351.

17. Aitken, *Nixon,* 274–79.

18. For the foreign policy effects, see McDermott, *Presidential Leadership,* ch. 6.

19. Fred Greenstein, *Leadership in the Modern Presidency* (Cambridge, MA: Harvard University Press, 1988), 108.

20. William A. Lammers and Michael A. Genovese, *The Presidency and Domestic Policy: Comparing Leadership Styles from FDR to Clinton* (Washington, D.C.: CQ Press, 2000), 220.

21. Richard Reeves, *President Nixon: Alone in the White House* (New York: Simon & Schuster, 2001), 97.

22. Chafe, *Private Lives/Public Consequences,* 261–62.

23. Chafe, *Private Lives/Public Consequences,* 261.

24. John Erlichman, *Witness to Power: The Nixon Years* (New York: Simon & Schuster, 1982), 271.

25. Erlichman, *Witness to Power,* 247.

26. Erlichman, *Witness to Power,* 196.

27. Data and discussion from Matthew Dickinson, "The Executive Office of the President: the Paradox of Politicization," in Joel Aberbach and Mark Peterson, *The Executive Branch* (New York: Oxford University Press, 2005),

150–55; Nixon quote from Lewis Gould, *The Modern American Presidency* (Lawrence: University Press of Kansas, 2004), 150.

28. Richard Nixon, *RN: Memoirs of Richard Nixon* (New York: Simon and Schuster, 1990), 352.

29. Chafe, *Private Lives/Public Consequences*, 262.

30. Kenneth Cole, White House Staff File, Staff Member and Office Files, H.R. Haldeman, Box 125, Folder: HRH Group Meetings, Nixon Library.

31. Lammers and Genovese, *The Presidency and Domestic Policy*, 234.

32. Erlichman, *Witness to Power*, 200–201.

33. Andrew Rudalevige, "The Executive Branch and the Legislative Process," in *The Executive Branch*, eds. Joel Aberbach and Mark Peterson (New York: Oxford, 2005), 431.

34. Reeves, *President Nixon*, 172.

35. Reeves, *President Nixon*, 467.

36. Erlichman, *Witness to Power*, 208.

37. Lammers and Genovese, *The Presidency and Domestic Policy*, 225.

38. Chafe, *Private Lives/Public Consequences*, 260 [Disraeli]; Lammers and Genovese, *The Presidency and Domestic Policy*, 225 [warmed].

39. Richard Nixon, White House Staff Files, Staff Member and Office Files, John D. Erlichman, Box 18, Folder: Erlichman Scrapbook Items, 2/2, Nixon Library.

40. Patrick Buchanan, President's Office Files, President's Handwriting, Box 9, January 1971–March 15, 1971, Nixon Library.

41. President Richard Nixon, audiotape, conversations in the Oval Office, Conversation No. 74-4, 9:50 A.M., September 14, 1971.

42. Richard Nixon, "Address to the Nation on the War in Vietnam, November 3, 1969," Presidency Project, www.presidency.ucsb.edu/ws/index.php?pid=2303.

43. Erlichman, *Witness to Power*, 390.

44. Dallek, *Nixon and Kissinger*, 544–47.

45. Reeves, *President Nixon*, 599.

46. Philip Klinker and Rogers Smith, *The Unsteady March* (Chicago: University of Chicago Press, 1999), 292.

47. Lammers and Genovese, *The Presidency and Domestic Policy*, 231.

48. Stanley Jones, interview with the authors, August 6, 2007.

49. Tom Wicker, "Nixon Endorses New Javits Plan for Care of the Aged," *New York Times*, August 21, 1960 [described in chapter 3].

50. Erlichman, *Witness to Power*, 225.

51. Richard Nixon, March 12, 1969, President's Personal File, Memoranda from the President, 1969–74, Box 1, Richard Nixon Memos, December 1968–December 1969, Folder: March 1969, Nixon Library.

52. No author, "Health Message Chronology," no date, White House Central File, Staff Member and Office Files, John D. Erlichman, Alphabetical Subject Files, Box 19, Folder: unmarked, Nixon Library.

53. No author, "Health Message Chronology," no date, White House Central File, Staff Member and Office Files, John D. Erlichman, Alphabetical Subject Files, Box 19, Folder: unmarked, Nixon Library.

54. Richard D. Lyons, "Administration Seeks Short-Run Gains in Nation's Medical System," *New York Times,* January 12, 1970, 19.

55. No author, "Health Message Chronology," no date, White House Staff Files, Staff Member and Office Files, John D. Erlichman, Alphabetical Subject Files, Box 19, Folder: unmarked, Nixon Library.

56. No author, "Health Message Chronology," no date, White House Staff Files, Staff Member and Office Files, John D. Erlichman, Alphabetical Subject Files, Box 19, Folder: unmarked, Nixon Library; Richard D. Lyons, "US to Seek Rise in Medicare Aid," *New York Times,* March 26, 1970, 1.

57. White House Domestic Council, White House Central File, Subject File Domestic Council, Box 1: July 16–July 31, 1970, Nixon Library.

58. White House Central File, Subject File Domestic Council, Box 2: December 1–December 31, 1970, Nixon Library.

59. White House Central File, Subject File Domestic Council, Box 2: December 1–December 31, 1970, Nixon Library.

60. James Cavanaugh, interview with the authors, August 1, 2007.

61. July 1971.

62. Reeves, *President Nixon,* 297.

63. President R. Nixon, audiotape, conversations in the Oval Office, Conversation No. 454–4, tape 2, February 19, 1971.

64. Louis Harris, "Harris Poll: 80% Fear Health Care Cost Gap," *New York Post,* April 26, 1971; Jill Quadagno, *One Nation Uninsured: Why the US Has No National Health Insurance* (New York: Oxford University Press, 2005), 116 [22 bills].

65. President Richard Nixon, audiotape, conversations in the Oval Office, Conversation No. 60–1, tape 2 of 5, June 8, 1971.

66. President Richard Nixon, audiotape, conversations in the Oval Office, Conversation No. 66–2, tape 3 of 7, July 23, 1971.

67. President Richard Nixon, audiotape, conversations in the Oval Office, Conversation No. 97–2, March 28, 1972.

68. James Cavanaugh, memo to Kenneth Cole, May 30, 1972, White House Central File/Staff Member and Office Files/James Cavanaugh, Box 18, Subject File: Health Care, National Archives, College Park, Maryland.

69. President Richard Nixon, audiotape, conversations in the Oval Office, Conversation No. 786-21, 12:49 P.M.–1:09 P.M., September 25, 1972.

70. October 18, 1972.

71. Richard Nixon, "Radio Address on Health Policy, November 3, 1972," Presidency Project, www.presidency.ucsb.edu/ws/index.php?pid=3683.

72. Reeves, *President Nixon,* 541.

73. Reeves, *President Nixon,* 558.

74. James Cavanaugh, interview with the authors, August 1, 2007.

75. Stuart Altman, PhD, interview with the authors, July 23, 2007. Altman served as deputy assistant secretary for Health Planning and Evaluation at Heath, Education, and Welfare.

76. Kenneth Cole, White House Central File, Staff Member and Office Files, Cavanaugh Subject File, Box 11: Domestic Council, Nixon Library.

77. Stuart Altman, PhD, interview with the authors, July 23, 2007.

78. Secretary Casper Weinberger, memo to the President, December 7, 1973, White House Central File/Subject File/Domestic Council, Box 5: October 1973–December 1973, National Archives, College Park, Maryland.

79. Secretary Casper Weinberger, memo to the President, December 7, 1973, White House Central File/Subject File/Domestic Council, Box 5: October 1973–December 1973, National Archives, College Park, Maryland.

80. White House Central File, Subject File Domestic Council, Box 5: October 1973–December 1973, Nixon Library.

81. Stuart Altman, PhD, interview with the authors, July 23, 2007.

82. White House Central File/Staff Member and Office Files, Cavanaugh Subject File, Box 23, Folder: Health Proposal, Nixon Library.

83. White House Central File/Staff Member and Office Files: James H. Cavanaugh, Box 6: Chronological Files, Folder: December 1973, Chronological File, Nixon Library.

84. White House Central File, Staff Member and Office Files, Cavanaugh Subject File, Box 23, Folder: Health Proposal, Nixon Library.

85. Richard Nixon, State of the Union address, January 30, 1974, President's Personal File, President's Speech File, Box 90, Folder: Wednesday, January 30, 1974: State of the Union Message [II, 1 of 3], Nixon Library.

86. Richard Nixon, February 5, 1974, President's Personal File, President's Speech File, Box 90, Folder: Tuesday, February 5, 1974: American Hospital Associate House of Delegates, Nixon Library.

87. Richard Nixon, "Address of President Richard Nixon to the American Hospital Association, February 5, 1974," Presidency Project, www.presidency .ucsb.edu/ws/index.php?pid=4336.

88. "Further Notes on Nixon's Downfall," *Time*, April 5, 1976; Bob Woodward and Carl Bernstein, *The Final Days* (New York: Simon & Schuster, 1976), 394–96, 403–4.

89. Bill Stanley Jones, interview with the authors, August 6, 2007.

90. Bill Stanley Jones, interview with the authors, August 6, 2007. Fullerton, was a Washington legend. As chief health aide to the Ways and Means Committee, he was influential in drafting health care legislation.

91. Stanley Jones, interview with the authors, August 6, 2007.

92. Stanley Jones, interview with the authors, August 6, 2007.

93. Richard Nixon, May 22, 1974, White House Central File/Staff Member and Office Files: James H. Cavanaugh, Box 7: Chronological Files, Folder: May 1974, Nixon Library.

94. Stuart Altman, PhD, interview with the authors, July 23, 2007; Stanley Jones, interview with the authors, August 6, 2007.

95. "The Fall of Chairman Wilbur Mills," *Time*, December 16, 1974, www .time.com/time/magazine/article/0,9171,911535,00.html.

## 7. JIMMY CARTER

1. Jimmy Carter, *Keeping Faith: Memoirs of a President* (New York: Bantam, 1982), 23.

2. Pat Caddell, memo to Governor Carter, "Additions to December 10 Working Paper," December 21, 1976, Staff Secretary [Presidential Handwriting] File, Box 1, Folder: Caddell, Patrick, 12/76–1/77, Carter Library.

3. Pat Caddell, memo to Governor Carter, "Additions to December 10 Working Paper," December 21, 1976, Staff Secretary [Presidential Handwriting] File, Box 1, Folder: Caddell, Patrick, 12/76–1/77, Carter Library.

4. Stephen Skowronek, "Presidential Leadership in Political Time," in *The Presidency and the Political System*, ed. Michael Nelson (Washington, D.C.: CQ Press, 2006), 125.

5. Jimmy Carter, *An Hour before Daylight* (New York: Simon and Schuster, 2001), 26.

6. Carter, *An Hour before Daylight*, 18 [Civil War], 65–66 [New Deal], 200 [Earl].

7. Carter, *An Hour before Daylight*, 79–80.

8. Carter, *An Hour before Daylight*, 194.

9. Carter, *An Hour before Daylight*, 193–94.

10. Carter, *An Hour before Daylight*, 83.

11. Joseph Califano, interview with the authors, October 6, 2006.

12. Carter, *Keeping Faith*, 85.

13. Peter G. Bourne, *Jimmy Carter: A Comprehensive Biography from Plains to Postpresidency* (New York: Scribner, 1997), 432–33.

14. Jimmy Carter, Carter Presidency Project interview with Charles O. Jones, H. Clifton McCleskey, Kenneth W. Thompson, James Sterling Young, Richard E. Neustadt, David B. Truman, Richard F. Fenno Jr., and Erwin C. Hargrove, Plains, Georgia, November 29, 1982 (©2003, The Miller Center).

15. Carter, *An Hour before Daylight*, 258; Bourne, *Jimmy Carter*, 77–82.

16. Denise Grady, "In a Former First Family, Cancer Has a Grim Legacy." *New York Times*, August 17, 2007, D6; Bourne, *Jimmy Carter*, 77–82.

17. Jimmy Carter, Carter Presidency Project interview.

18. Carter, *Keeping Faith*, 102.

19. Bert Karp, interview with the authors, August 10, 2006.

20. Jimmy Carter, Carter Presidency Project interview.

21. Carter, *Keeping Faith*, 198.

22. Jimmy Carter, "Inaugural Address, January 20, 1977," Presidency Project, www.presidency.ucsb.edu/ws/index.php?pid=6575.

23. Joseph Califano, *Inside: A Public and Private Life* (New York: Public Affairs, 2004), 333.

24. Joseph Califano, interview with the authors, October 6, 2006. Califano often used this story. For a printed version, see Joseph Califano, HCFA oral history, taken by Edward Berkowitz, August 31, 1995, www.cms.hhs.gov/about /history/califano2.asp; Burt Lance, quoted on PBS: *The American Experience: Jimmy Carter*, November 11, 2002 [quid pro quo].

25. Rostenkowski, quoted in Peggy Noonan, *When Character Was King* (New York: Penguin, 2001), 244 [smallness]; Joseph Califano, *Inside*, 334–35.

26. Jimmy Carter, Carter Presidency Project interview.

27. Benjamin Heineman, HCFA oral history, taken by Edward Berkowitz, October 24, 1995, www.cms.hhs.gov/about/history/heineman.asp.

28. Fred Greenstein, *The Presidential Difference: Leadership Style from FDR to Clinton* (Princeton, NJ: Princeton University, 2001), 135; Joseph Califano, *Governing America* (New York: Simon & Schuster, 2007), 126 [Rostenkowski quoted] 431 [Harris].

29. Joseph Califano, HCFA oral history, taken by Edward Berkowitz, August 31, 1995, www.cms.hhs.gov/about/history/califano2.asp [lunch]; Califano, *Governing America*, 148 [cost us votes].

30. Ben W. Heineman Jr. and Curtis A. Hessler, *Memorandum for the President: A Strategic Approach to Domestic Affairs in the 1980s* (New York: Random House, 1980), xix.

31. HEW Transition Team, memo to the President-elect, November, 1976, Staff Secretary Handwriting File, Box 3, Folder: Meeting with Ford Cabinet, 11/76, Carter Library [carries the Carter "C" denoting that the president had read the memo].

32. Joe Onek and Bob Havely, memo to Stuart Eizenstat, September 27, 1977, White House Central File, Box IS-2, Folder: 1/20/77–6/30/77, Carter Library.

33. Robert Berenson, interview with the authors, June 22, 2006; Karen Davis, personal correspondence with the authors, July 21, 2008.

34. Jimmy Carter, Carter Presidency Project interview.

35. Bourne, *Jimmy Carter*, 433.

36. Joseph N. Onek, HCFA oral history, taken by Edward Berkowitz, August 10, 1995, www.cms.hhs.gov/about/history/onek.asp.

37. Jimmy Carter, Carter Presidency Project interview; box score from Andrew Rudalevige, "The Executive Branch and the Legislative Process," in *The Executive Branch,* eds. Joel Aberbach and Mark Peterson (New York: Oxford, 2005), 419–451 (data cited from 431).

38. Greenstein, *The Presidential Difference,* 142.

39. Bourne, *Jimmy Carter,* 432.

40. *The Presidential Campaign 1976, Volume 1: Jimmy Carter* (Washington, D.C.: U.S. Government Printing Office, 1978).

41. Bourne, *Jimmy Carter,* 433.

42. Governor Carter, memo to Stuart Eizenstat, undated, Staff Secretary Handwriting File, Box 1, Folder: Confidential, File: 11/76–1/77, Carter Library.

43. Pat Caddell [surmised], memo to Jimmy Carter, undated, Staff Secretary Handwriting File, Box 3, Folder: Political Problems, Political File: 8/76–1/77, Carter Library.

44. Unsigned, memo to Jimmy Carter, undated, Staff Offices, Bourne, Box 4, Folder: Health Issues 12/20/76–1/31/77, Carter Library.

45. Richard D. Lyons, "Carter to Delay Health Insurance Plan," *Washington Post,* January 14, 1977, A1.

46. Heineman Jr. and Hessler, *Memorandum for the President,* 281.

47. Heineman Jr. and Hessler, *Memorandum for the President,* 290 [haphazard]; Bert Karp, interview with the authors, August 10, 2006 [out of time].

48. Richard D. Lyons, "Carter Proposes Law for Tough Controls on Hospital Charges," *New York Times,* April 26, 1977, A1.

49. Lawrence Meyer, "'Target Date' in '77 Sought on Health Bill," *Washington Post,* May 17, 1977, A4.

50. Peter Bourne, letter to Hamilton Jordan, August 1, 1977, DPS: Eizenstat, Box 240, Folder: National Health Insurance, Carter Library.

51. Joseph Califano, letter to Jimmy Carter, "re. meeting on November 9, 1977 on NHI," undated, DPS: Eizenstat, Box 240, Folder: National Health Insurance, Carter Library (underlining in original).

52. Robert G. Kaiser, "Carter Presidency to Date: Many Initiatives, Few Results," *Washington Post,* October 14, 1977, A10.

53. Tom Wicker, "The Health Insurance Minefield," *The New York Times,* December 20, 1977, 35.

54. Califano, *Governing America,* 106 [Ulman], 107 [Rostenkowski].

55. Peter Bourne, letter to Hamilton Jordan, and Landon Butler, April 17, 1978, White House Central File, IS-2, Folder: 4/1/78–6/30/78, Carter Library.

56. Stuart Eizenstat, briefing memo to President Carter, May 31, 1978, Staff Secretary File, Box 88, File: 6/1/78, Carter Library.

57. Stuart Eizenstat, briefing memo to President Carter, May 31, 1978, Staff Secretary File, Box 88, File: 6/1/78, Carter Library.

58. Joseph Califano, interview with the authors, October 20, 2006 [bombshell]; see also White House Central File, Insurance, Box IS-2, Folder: IS 1/20/77–1/20/81, Carter Library.

59. A summary of the meeting on June 15, 1978 in White House Central File, Insurance, Box IS-2, Folder: IS 1/20/77–1/20/81, Carter Library (underlining in original).

60. Jimmy Carter, note on a memo from Stuart Eizenstat to the president, June 19, 1978, DPS: Eizenstat, Box 242, Folder: National Health Insurance, 6/78, Carter Library.

61. Joe Califano and Stuart Eizenstat, memorandum to the President, July 22, 1978, Staff Secretary File, Box 94, Folder: 7/10/78, Carter Library.

62. Stuart Eizenstat, memo to President Carter, July 22, 1978, Staff Secretary File, Box 94, Folder: 7/10/78, Carter Library.

63. Senator Edward Kennedy, "Statement on National Health Insurance," July 28, 1978, DPS: Eizenstat, Box 242, Folder: National Health Insurance, Carter Library.

64. Carter, *Keeping Faith,* 87.

65. Edward Walsh, "Lackluster Convention Lights Up," *Washington Post,* December 10, 1978, A1.

66. Joe Califano, memo to the president, January 8, 1979, Staff Secretary File, Box 115, Folder: 1/19/79, Carter Library.

67. Jimmy Carter, "State of the Union Address, Delivered before a Joint Session of the Congress, January 23, 1979," Presidency Project, www.presidency.ucsb.edu/ws/index.php?pid=32657.

68. Stuart Eizenstat, letter to Jimmy Carter, February 22, 1979, White House Central File, Box IS-2, Folder: 1/1/79–4/30/79, Carter Library.

69. Jimmy Carter, Announcement of National Health Plan, June 12, 1979, Staff Secretary File, Box 136, Folder: 6/13/72 (2), Carter Library.

70. Victor Cohn, "Carter, Long Closer on Health Plan," *Washington Post,* June 14, 1979, A1.

71. "On Who Will Whip Whom," *Time,* June 25, 1979, www.time.com/time/magazine/article/0,9171,912449-1,00.html.

72. James Mongan, memo to Stuart Eizenstat, May 15, 1980, DPS: Eizenstat, Box 242, Folder: National Health Plan [CF O/A 729 (2)], Carter Library.

73. Jimmy Carter, "Address to the Nation on Energy and National Goals, July 15, 1979," Presidency Project, www.presidency.ucsb.edu/ws/index.php?pid=32596.

74. See Adam Clymer, *Edward M. Kennedy: A Biography* (New York: William Morrow and Co., 1990) [the malaise speech]; Greenstein, *The Presidential Difference,* 138 [emotional stability]; Lewis Gould, *The Modern American Presidency* (Lawrence: University of Kansas, 2003), 187 [on the firings].

75. Gradison, quoted by Jill Quadagno, *One Nation Uninsured* (New York: Oxford, 2005), 127.

76. Jimmy Carter, "Remarks on the Outcome of the 1980 Presidential Election, November 4, 1980," Presidency Project, www.presidency.ucsb.edu/ws/index.php?pid=45462.

77. Benjamin Heineman, HCFA oral history, taken by Edward Berkowitz, October 24, 1995, www.cms.hhs.gov/about/history/heineman.asp.

## 8. RONALD REAGAN

1. On the shooting, see Ronald Reagan, *An American Life* (New York: Pocket Books/Simon and Schuster, 1990), ch. 42; Ronald Reagan's diary, Monday, March 30, 1981. For a dramatic description based on interviews with the main characters, see Peggy Noonan, *When Character Was King* (New York: Penguin Books, 2001), 167–79.

2. Bob Woodward, *Veil: The Secret Wars of the CIA, 1981–1987* (New York: Simon and Schuster, 1987), 122–24.

3. Ronald Reagan, "Proposal For Economic Recovery: Address to a Joint Session of Congress, April 28, 1981," Presidency Project, www.presidency.ucsb.edu/ws/index.php?pid=43756.

4. Ronald Reagan's diary, Tuesday, April 28, 1981 [third ovation], March 29, 1981 [good about country].

5. Marilyn Berger, "Clark Clifford, A Major Advisor to Four Presidents is Dead," *New York Times,* October 11, 1988 [dunce]; Haynes Johnson, *Sleepwalking through History: American in the Reagan Years* (New York: Norton, 1991); David Stockman, *The Triumph of Politics: How the Reagan Revolution Failed* (New York: Harper and Row, 1986), 11; McFarland made his comment to George Schultz, who reported in George Schultz, *Turmoil and Triumph: My Years as Secretary of State* (New York: Charles Scribner's Sons, 1993), 1135; Donald Regan, *For the Record* (New York: Harcourt, Brace Jovanovich, 1988); John Patrick Diggins, *Ronald Reagan* (New York: Norton, 2007), xvii.

6. Ronald Reagan's diary, March 29, 1981.

7. Reagan, *An American Life,* 715.

8. Reagan, *An American Life,* 115 [hand-to-hand]; Peter Robinson, *How Ronald Reagan Changed My Life* (New York: Regan Books, 2003), 69–72 [we win].

9. Ronald Reagan, "Address to the National Association of Evangelicals, Orlando, Florida, March 8, 1983" Presidency Project, www.presidency.ucsb .edu/ws/index.php?pid=41023 [demons].

10. Ronald Reagan, "Inaugural address, January 20, 1981," Presidency Project, www.presidency.ucsb.edu/ws/index.php?pid=43130.

11. Reagan, *An American Life,* ch. 18; for an extended account of The Speech, see Thomas Evans, *The Education of Ronald Reagan* (New York: Columbia, 2006).

12. Ronald Reagan, letter to Lorraine Wagner, August 16, 1962, and letter to Professor Vsevold Nikolaev, November 13, 1979, both reprinted in *Reagan: A Life in Letters,* eds. K. Skinner Kiron and Annelise Anderson (New York: Free Press, 2003), 343, 344.

13. Stockman, *The Triumph of Politics,* 8–11.

14. Ronald Reagan, with Richard Hubler, *Where's the Rest of Me?* (New York: Karz-Segil, 1965), 3.

15. Reagan, *Where's the Rest of Me?* 7; Reagan, *An American Life,* 33–34, 94.

16. Reagan, *An American Life,* 12–13.

17. Reagan, *An American Life,* 40.

18. Reagan, *Where's the Rest of Me?* 66–67; Reagan, *An American Life,* 73.

19. Diggins, *Ronald Reagan,* 68–69; Dinesh D'Souza, *Ronald Reagan: How an Ordinary Man Became an Extraordinary Leader* (New York: Simon and Schuster, 1997), 42.

20. Reagan, *An American Life,* 43.

21. For examples, see Michael Rogan, *Ronald Reagan: The Movie* (Berkeley: University of California, 1987), 1–43.

22. Noonan, *When Character Was King,* 242, 243, 245, 249.

23. Reagan, *An American Life,* 145; Ronald Reagan, letter to Lorraine and Elwood Wagner, July 13, 1961, in Kiron and Anderson, eds., *Reagan.*

24. Ronald Reagan, "Address at the Commencement Exercise at Notre Dame, South Bend, Indiana, May 17, 1981," Presidency Project, www.presidency.ucsb .edu/ws/index.php?pid=43825. Reagan recycled the story from Reagan, *Where's the Rest of Me?* 94–95.

25. For a string of Gipper examples and a superb analysis, see Rogan, *Ronald Reagan,* 15–6; Congressman from Reagan, "Address as the Commencement Exercise at Notre Dame."

26. Reagan, *Where's the Rest of Me?* 3–7.

27. Lawrence Altman, MD, "The Doctor's World, a Recollection of Early Questions About Reagan's Health," *New York Times,* June 15, 2004.

28. William Chafe, *Private Lives/Public Consequences* (Cambridge, MA: Harvard University Press, 2005), 303.

29. Lou Cannon, *The Role a of Lifetime* (New York: Public Affairs, 2000), 478.

30. Cannon, *The Role of a Lifetime*, 480.

31. Altman, "The Doctor's World," *New York Times*, June 15, 2004.

32. Regan, *For the Record*, 15; Ronald Reagan's diary, March 30, 1981; Altman, "The Doctor's World," *New York Times*.

33. Robinson, *How Ronald Reagan Changed My Life*, 8.

34. Ronald Reagan's diary, January 4, 1987; Regan, *For the Record*, 71.

35. Quoted in Richard Reeves, *President Reagan: Triumph of the Imagination* (New York: Simon and Schuster: 2005), 56–57.

36. Jeffrey Tulis, *The Rhetorical Presidency* (Princeton: Princeton University Press, 1987), 197.

37. Stockman, *The Triumph of Politics*, 182.

38. Stockman, *The Triumph of Politics*, 13 [bazooka], 161, 189.

39. Stockman, *The Triumph of Politics*, 191.

40. Stockman, *The Triumph of Politics*, 193; Cannon, *The Role of a Lifetime*, 209.

41. See Alan Greenspan, *The Age of Turbulence* (New York: Penguin, 2007), 94–96.

42. See Rick Mayes and Robert Berenson, *Medicare Prospective Payment and the Shaping of US Health Care* (Baltimore: Johns Hopkins, 2006), esp. 43–46; James Morone and Andrew Dunham, *The Politics of Innovation: The Introduction of DRGs* (Princeton, NJ: HRET Press, 1983).

43. For analysis and measurement of how hospitals shifted costs from Medicare to private payers, see Jon Oberlander, The Political Life of Medicare (Chicago: The University of Chicago, 2003), 125.

44. Ronald Reagan, letter to Professor Vsevolod Nikolaev, November 3, 1979, in Kiron and Anderson, eds., *Reagan*, 344.

45. Ronald Reagan, "Address before a Joint Session of the Congress on the State of the Union, January 25, 1983," Presidency Project, www.presidency. ucsb.edu/ws/index.php?pid=41698; Otis Bowen, oral history, "Interview with Otis Bowen MD," Charlottesville, VA, taken as part of the Ronald Reagan Oral History Project, page 57, November 8–9, 2001, Miller Center for Public Affairs, Charlottesville, Virginia.

46. Otis Bowen and Thomas Burke, "A Cost Neutral Catastrophic Care Proposal for Medicare Recipients," *Federation of American Hospitals Review* (November/December 1985): 12–25.

47. Richard Himmelfarb, *Catastrophic Politics: The Rise and Fall of the Medicare Catastrophic Coverage Act of 1988* (University Park: Pennsylvania State University Press, 1995), 11.

48. Ronald Reagan, "Address Before a Joint Session of Congress on the State of the Union, February 4, 1986," Presidency Project, www.presidency .ucsb.edu/ws/index.php?pid=36646.

49. Otis Bowen, oral history, "Interview with Otis Bowen MD," Charlottesville, Virginia, taken as part of the Ronald Reagan Oral History Project, page 57, November 8–9, 2001, Miller Center for Public Affairs, Charlottesville, Virginia; Carolyn Rinkus Thompson, "Presidential Transition and Public Policy: The Repeal of Medicare Catastrophic Coverage," in *Principle over Politics: The Domestic Policy of the George H. W. Bush*

*Presidency,* eds. Richard Himmelfarb and Rosanna Perotti (Westport, CT: Praeger Publishers, 2004), 264, Himmelfarb, *Catastrophic Politics,* 19–21.

50. Robert Pear, "Political Medicine," *The New York Times,* February 15, 1987.

51. Himmelfarb, *Catastrophic Politics,* 22.

52. November 6, 1986, Office of the President, the President Briefing Papers: Records, Case File 509306, Box 14, Loc: 153/08/01, Reagan Library.

53. Ronald Reagan's diary, November 12, 1986.

54. Regan, *For the Record,* 36.

55. Ronald Reagan's diary, November 24, 1986.

56. Ronald Reagan, *An American Life,* 532; Noonan, *When Character Was King,* 277; Cannon, *The Role of a Lifetime,* 639–41.

57. Ronald Reagan's diary, January 6, 1987; Regan, *For the Record,* 71.

58. Otis Bowen, oral history, 57.

59. Ronald Reagan's diary, December 15, 1986, December 23, 1986.

60. Otis Bowen, oral history, 57.

61. Cannon, *The Role of a Lifetime,* 630–34.

62. Ronald Reagan, radio talk: "Catastrophic Illness," WHOOF: Research Office, February 14, 1987, ID# oA 18093, Loc: 147/15/3, Reagan Library.

63. Himmelfarb, *Catastrophic Politics,* 25.

64. Ronald Reagan, "Radio Address on Catastrophic Illness Medical Insurance, July 25, 1987," Presidency Project, www.presidency.ucsb.edu/ws/index .php?pid=34603.

65. Bruce Bartlett, White House memo to Gary Bauer and Ken Cribb, September 10, 1987, Catastrophic File, 614530PD, IS 001, HE.LE.FG006–07, Reagan Library.

66. Deborah Steelman and Tim Muris, draft memo to Jim Miller, WHORM Subset File ISoo1: 603995, Reagan Library.

67. Jim McCrery and Clyde Holloway, letter to Ronald Reagan, June 21, 1988; Herbert Bateman, letter to Ronald Reagan, June 9, 1988; Larry Craig, letter to Ronald Reagan; Peter DeFazio, letter to Ronald Reagan, June 9, 1988; Ohio State University, letter to Ronald Reagan; The Committee to Save Social Security, Letter to Ronald Reagan: all in WHORM Subset Files FE 010 PR 013 IS LE008: 57295, 572640, 584572, 583027, 599376 (in order of quotation), Reagan Library.

68. Beryl Sprinkle, letter to James M. Frey, assistant director for legislative reference, OMB, June 15, 1988, 609277, ISoo1, LE.FG00603, FG 00611, Reagan Library; T. Kenneth Cribb Jr., "White House Staffing Memorandum," June 29, 1988, ISoo1, 576435, Reagan Library.

69. Ronald Reagan, "Remarks by the President at Signing Ceremony of the Medicare Catastrophic Coverage Act of 1988, July 1, 1988," Presidency Project, www.presidency.ucsb.edu/ws/index.php?pid=36074.

70. Himmelfarb, *Catastrophic Politics,* 36.

71. Greg Monfils, "What Clinton Could Learn from the Catastrophic Health Care Catastrophe," *Washington Monthly,* March 1993.

## 9. GEORGE HERBERT WALKER BUSH

1. George H. W. Bush, February 7, 1992, Appointments and Scheduling, White House Office of Presidential Diary/Backup Box 92 Folder—Presidential daily backup 2/7/92 CF OA 1788, Bush Library.

2. Herbert S. Parmet, *George Bush: The Life of a Lone Star Yankee* (Piscataway, NJ: Transaction Books, 2000), 26–27.

3. Parmet, *George Bush*, 21, 28.

4. Parmet, *George Bush*, 23, 30.

5. Parmet, *George Bush*, 68.

6. Donnie Radcliffe, *Simply Barbara Bush: A Portrait of America's Candid First Lady* (New York: Warner Books, 1989), 105.

7. Parmet, *George Bush*, 73.

8. Parmet, *George Bush*, 119.

9. www.youtube.com/watch?v=E5DZBFbMdjI.

10. Michael Dukakis, conversation with the authors, May 1, 2003, Providence, Rhode Island.

11. Richard Himmelfarb and Rosanna Perotti, *Principle over Politics? The Domestic Policy of the George H. W. Bush Presidency* (Westport, CT: Praeger, 2004), 285.

12. Ryan J. Barilleaux and Mark J. Rozell, *Power and Prudence: The Presidency of George H. W. Bush* (College Station: Texas A&M Press, 2004), 51 [press conferences], 6-7 [sports]; William Lammers and Michael Genovese, *The Presidency and Domestic Policy: Comparing Leadership Styles, FDR to Clinton* (Washington, D.C.: CQ Press, 2000), 282 [call to service].

13. Charles Kolb, *White House Daze: The Unmaking of Domestic Policy in the Bush Years* (New York: The Free Press, 1995), 9.

14. Charles Krauthammer, "Where's the Rest of Bush?" *Washington Post* December 27, 1991, A21.

15. George H. W. Bush, "Inaugural Address, January 20, 1989," Presidency Project, www.presidency.ucsb.edu/ws/index.php?pid=16610.

16. Barilleaux and Rozell, *Power and Prudence*, 66.

17. Lammers and Genovese, 285 [bored]; Gail Wilensky, interview with the authors, September 25, 2006.

18. Barilleaux and Rozell, *Power and Prudence*, 30.

19. Radcliffe, *Simply Barbara Bush*, 153; Parmet, *George Bush*, 79–80.

20. Radcliffe, *Simply Barbara Bush*, 117.

21. Parmet, *George Bush*, 79–80.

22. George Bush, *All the Best, George Bush: My Life in Letters and Other Writings* (New York: Scribner, 1999), 81.

23. Jim McGrath, ed., *Heartbeat: George Bush in His Own Words* (New York: Scribner, 2001), 271.

24. Johannes Kuttner, interview with the authors, October 4, 2006; Kolb, *White House Daze*, 83.

25. Kolb, *White House Daze*, 331.

26. Kolb, *White House Daze*, 330–31.

27. Unsigned memo to President-Elect George H. W. Bush, January, 1989, Robert Grady Files, Box 14, Folder: Memoranda Concerning Various White House Initiatives Including Health Care 0A/ID 08841, Bush Library.

28. George H. W. Bush, "Remarks at the Swearing-in Ceremony for Louis W. Sullivan as Secretary of Health and Human Services, March 10, 1989," Presidency Project, www.presidency.ucsb.edu/ws/index.php?pid=16759&st= health+care&st1=.

29. Associated Press, "House Panel Leader Jeered by Elderly in Chicago," August 19, 1989; Waxman , quoted in Jill Quadagno, *One Nation Uninsured: Why the US Has No National Health Insurance* (New York: Oxford University Press, 2005), 158.

30. Otis Bowen, with William Du Bois Jr., *Doc: Memories from a Life in Public Service* (Bloomington: Indiana University Press, 2000), 60.

31. George H. W. Bush, "State of the Union, January 31, 1990," Presidency Project, www.presidency.ucsb.edu/ws/index.php?pid=18095.

32. George H. W. Bush, "Remarks at the Centennial Celebration of the Johns Hopkins University Medical Institutions in Baltimore, Maryland, February, 22, 1990," Presidency Project, www.presidency.ucsb.edu/ws/index .php?pid=18178.

33. Hans Kuttner, memo to Roger B. Porter, May 28, 1990, J. Kuttner Files, Computer Diskettes 1992, Kuttner Files Backup (Disk), TTRVOL002/ Director: TT-Jul006.002 [2] [Health Strategy], OA/ID 08768, Box 62, Bush Library; Johannes [Hans] Kuttner, memo to Roger B. Porter and James Pinkerton, Kuttner Files, Box 28, Folder: DPC study, Bush Library.

34. Roger B. Porter, memo to the president, November 8, 1990, J. Kuttner Files Computer Diskette—1992 Kuttner Files Backup {Disk: TTRVOL0005/Director: TT-Jul006.004} Health Care Issues, OA/ID 08768, Box 63, Bush Library.

35. Bill Gradison and Nancy Johnson, letter to President George H. W. Bush, December 17, 1990, Korfanta Files, DPC, Subject file: Health Care Reform OA/ID 01861, Bush Library.

36. George H. W. Bush, "State of the Union Address, January 29, 1991," Presidency Project, www.presidency.ucsb.edu/ws/index.php?pid=19253.

37. Hans Kuttner, memorandum to Roger B. Porter, Kuttner Memos 1990-1991 [Out of Order] [OA/ID 08768], Box 61.

38. Johannes Kuttner, memo to Roger B. Porter, April 16, 1991, J. Kuttner Files, Box 82: Health Care Reform—4/16/91, Kuttner, Porter Meeting on Status, Progress, OA/ID 09799, Bush Library.

39. George D. Lundberg, "National Health Care Reform," *Journal of the American Medical Association* 265, no. 19 (1991): 2567.

40. Roger B. Porter, memo to President Bush, May 30, 1991, J. Kuttner Files Computer Disks—1992 Kuttner Files and Backup {Disk: TT_RVOLOOO3/ Directory: TT_Jul06.001}[Health proposals] OA/ID 08768, Box 62, Bush Library.

41. George H. W. Bush, "Address to the National Federation of Independent Businesses, June 3, 1991," in *Public Papers of the President: George Bush, 1989–1993* (Washington, D.C.: Government Printing Office, 1991).

42. Ann Devoy, *Washington Post,* September 26, 1991, 1.

43. Michael Decourcy Hinds, "Race for Senate Shows Big Split on Health Care," *New York Times,* October 31, 1991; Jacob Hacker, *Road to Nowhere* (Princeton, NJ: Princeton University Press, 1999), 10 [40-point lead].

44. George H. W. Bush, "Statements at Press Conference," November 8, 1991, FOIA Box 39: OPD JKF Folder Health Reform—Inside the Complex OA/ID 08189, Bush Library.

45. Janice Castro, Mary Cronin, Barbara Dolan, and Hayes Gory, "Condition: Critical," cover story, *Time,* November 25, 1991, www.time.com/time/magazine/article/0,9171,974331,00.html.

46. Gail Wilensky, interview with the authors, September 25, 2006.

47. Gail Wilensky, interview with the authors, September 25, 2006.

48. Johannes Kuttner, interview with the authors, October 4, 2006.

49. Stephen H. Wildstrom and Susan B. Garland, "Health Care: Finally a Pulse at the White House," *Businessweek,* January 20, 1992, 43.

50. George H. W. Bush, "State of the Union Address, January 28, 1992," Presidency Project, www.presidency.ucsb.edu/ws/index.php?pid=20544.

51. George H. W. Bush, "Remarks to the Greater Cleveland Growth Association in Cleveland, Ohio, February 6, 1992," Presidency Project, www.presidency.ucsb.edu/ws/index.php?pid=20570.

52. Kathy Jeavons through Bobbie Kilberg, memo to Sherrie Rollins, "Health Care," February 14, 1992, Kilberg Files, Box 91, Health Care 1991–2/14/92 OA/ID 05303, Bush Library.

53. Michael Wines, "Bush Unveils Plan for Health Care," *New York Times,* February 7, 1992, 1; Karen Hosler, "Bush Vague on Financing for Health Care Proposal," *Baltimore Sun,* February 7, 1992, 14A.

54. Alixe R. Glen, memorandum to the Secretary, February 19, 1992, Kuttner Files Health Care Reform, '92 Proposal-Marketing Efforts OA/ID 08977, Kuttner Files, Computer Diskettes 1992, Kuttner Files (Disk) TTRVOL0003/Directory: TT_Jul06.004[2][Health Care Finance] OA/ID 08768, Box 62, Bush Library.

55. Alixe Glenn, memo to Dave Carney, Bush–Quayle Campaign, "Health Care Town Meeting," March 2, 1992, Kuttner Files, Health Care Reform—92 Proposal—Marketing Efforts OA/ID 08799, Bush Library.

56. Unsigned minutes of meeting, undated, presumed Johannes Kuttner, Kuttner Files, Health Care Reform—Intra-Administration Policy Development—Post Announcement 1992 OA/ID 08799, Bush Library.

57. George H. W. Bush, "The President's News Conference, April 10, 1992," in *Public Papers of the President: George Bush, 1989–1993* (Washington, D.C.: Government Printing Office, 1992).

58. Communications staff, undated, memo from communications staff to Gail Wilensky. Kuttner Files, 1992, OA/ID 08799, Bush Library.

59. Authors interview with Gail R. Wilensky, September 25, 2006.

60. George H. W. Bush, "Remarks to the Health Care and Business Community in Baltimore, MD, May 13, 1992," Presidency Project, www.presidency.ucsb.edu/ws/index.php?pid=20963.

61. George H. W. Bush, "Remarks to the Health Care and Business Community in Baltimore, MD, May 13, 1992," Presidency Project, www.presidency.ucsb.edu/ws/index.php?pid=20963.

62. Robert Grady Files, Memoranda concerning Various White House Initiatives Including Health Care [no order—retrieved from Burn Bag], Box 15 08841, Bush Library.

63. George H. W. Bush, "Radio Address to the Nation on Health Care Reform, July 3, 1992," in *Public Papers of the President: George Bush, 1989–1993* (Washington, D.C.: Government Printing Office, 1992).

64. Kevin Moley, Press Briefing by Deputy Assistant to the President for Policy Development Gail Wilensky and Deputy Secretary of the Department of Health and Human Services Kevin Moley, August 4, 1992, Press Office, White House, Fitzwater, Marlin Files Folder Health Care [2] 6791, Bush Library.

65. George H. W. Bush, "Presidential Debate in St. Louis, October 11, 1992," Presidency Project, www.presidency.ucsb.edu/ws/index.php?pid=21605.

66. Health Care Briefing Document, April 10, 1992, J. Kuttner Files Health Care Reform—Intra-Administration: Policy Development—Post Announcement 1992 OA/ID 08799, Bush Library.

67. "The Guts to Reform Health Care," editorial, *New York Times,* August 2, 1992.

10. BILL CLINTON

1. Haynes Johnson and David S. Broder, *The System: The American Way of Politics at the Breaking Point* (Boston: Back Bay/Little Brown, 1997), 33.

2. Bill Clinton, *My Life* (New York, Vintage, 2005), 5.

3. G. Weingarten, "The First Father: W.J. Blythe Died in a Ditch before His Son Was Born. He Left behind a Mystery. And a President," *Washington Post,* June 20, 1993, F1.

4. Clinton, *My Life,* 7.

5. David Maraniss, *First in His Class: The Biography of Bill Clinton* (New York, Simon and Schuster, 1995), 349.

6. Clinton, *My Life,* 10.

7. Clinton, *My Life,* 17.

8. John F. Harris, *The Survivor: Bill Clinton in the White House* (New York, Random House, 2005), xx.

9. Clinton, *My Life,* 26 [bordello], 30 [churches].

10. Harris, *The Survivor,* xx.

11. Clinton, *My Life,* 20.

12. Clinton, *My Life,* 45.

13. Clinton, *My Life,* 48.

14. Maraniss, *First in His Class,* 41.

15. Maraniss, *First in His Class,* 419.

16. Maraniss, *First in His Class,* 421.

17. Maraniss, *First in His Class,* 234.

18. William W. Lammers and Michael A. Geneovese, *The President and Domestic Policy: Comparing Leadership Styles, FDR to Clinton* (Washington, D.C.: CQ Press, 2000), 305.

19. Clinton, *My Life,* 15.

20. Maraniss, *First in His Class,* 144.

21. Maraniss, *First in His Class,* 280–81, cited in Nigel Hamilton, *Bill Clinton: An American Journey* (New York, Random House, 2005), 268–69.

22. Hamilton, *An American Journey,* 339.

23. Harris, *The Survivor,* 53.

24. Harris, *The Survivor*, xxviii.

25. Harris, *The Survivor*, 117.

26. Harris, *The Survivor*, xxi.

27. Harris, *The Survivor*, xiv.

28. Harris, *The Survivor*, xv.

29. Jacobs and Shapiro, *Politicians Don't Pander: Political Manipulation and the Loss of Democratic Responsiveness* (Chicago: University of Chicago Press, 2000), 79.

30. Clinton, *My Life*, 49.

31. Clinton, *My Life*, 33.

32. Clinton, *My Life*, 91.

33. Clinton, *My Life*, 105.

34. Clinton, *My Life*, 112.

35. Clinton, *My Life*, 223.

36. Clinton, *My Life*, 267.

37. Clinton, *My Life*, 260.

38. Johnson and Broder, *The System*, 33.

39. Johnson and Broder, *The System*, 92–93.

40. Theda Skocpol, *Boomerang: Clinton's Health Security Effort and the Turn against Government in U.S. Politics* (New York, Norton, 1997), 37.

41. Jacob Hacker, *The Road to Nowhere: The Genesis of President Clinton's Plan for Health Security* (Princeton, NJ: Princeton University Press, 1997), 69.

42. Johnson and Broder, *The System*, 75.

43. Johnson and Broder, *The System*, 82.

44. Hacker, *The Road to Nowhere*, 48.

45. Hacker, *The Road to Nowhere*, 108–11.

46. Jacobs and Shapiro, *Politicians Don't Pander*, 83–84.

47. Hacker, *The Road to Nowhere*, 110.

48. Clinton, *My Life*, 521.

49. Hacker, *The Road to Nowhere*, 119.

50. Hacker, *Road to Nowhere*, 119.

51. The meeting is nicely described by Hacker, *Road to Nowhere*, 119–21, and Johnson and Broder, *The System*, 109.

52. Johnson and Broder, *The System*, 109.

53. Johnson and Broder, *The System*, 109.

54. Johnson and Broder, *The System*, 105.

55. Clinton, *My Life*, 482.

56. Skocpol, *Boomerang*, 54; Jacobs and Shapiro, *Politicians Don't Pander*, 88.

57. Hacker, *Road to Nowhere*, 112.

58. Jacobs and Shapiro, *Politicians Don't Pander*, 89.

59. Clinton, *My Life*, 467.

60. Harris, *The Survivor*, 57.

61. Robert Woodward, *The Agenda: Inside the Clintons' White House* (New York: Simon and Schuster, 1994), 73 [bond traders]; Lammers and Geneovese, *The President and Domestic Policy*, 311.

62. For a marvelous account from the losing side, see Robert Reich, *Locked in the Cabinet* (New York: Knopf, 1997); Johnson and Broder, *The System*, 122.

63. Gwen Ifill, "The 1992 Campaign: Political Memo; Clinton's 4-Point Plan to Win the First Debate," *The New York Times*, October 9, 1992, http://query.nytimes .com/gst/fullpage.html?res=9E0CE4DD143EF93AA35753C1A964958260& sec=&spon=&pagewanted=1.

64. Harris, *The Survivor*, 80; Hacker, *Road to Nowhere*, 127.

65. Johnson and Broder, *The System*, 119.

66. Harris, *The Survivor*, 80.

67. www.youtube.com/watch?v=NRCWbFFRpnY

68. Johnson and Broder, *The System*, 122.

69. Clinton, *My Life*, 492.

70. Skocpol, *Boomerang*, 81.

71. Jacobs and Shapiro, *Politicians Don't Pander*, 93.

72. Johnson and Broder, *The System*, 127.

73. Johnson and Broder, *The System*, 147.

74. Johnson and Broder, *The System*, 134.

75. Johnson and Broder, *The System*, 135.

76. Johnson and Broder, *The System*, 136.

77. Johnson and Broder, *The System*, 113.

78. For a vivid description of the debate, see Jacobs and Shapiro, *Politicians Don't Pander*, 76.

79. Johnson and Broder, *The System*, 145.

80. Johnson and Broder, *The System*, 157–58.

81. Johnson and Broder, *The System*, 157.

82. Skocpol, *Boomerang*, 63.

83. William J. Clinton, "Address to a Joint Session of the Congress on Health Care Reform, September 22, 1993," Presidency Project, www.presidency.ucsb .edu/ws/index.php?pid=47101&st=&st1.

84. Johnson and Broder, *The System*, 196.

85. Johnson and Broder, *The System*, 205.

86. Personal communication, Senator John Chafee, March 1993.

87. Harris, *The Survivor*, 56.

88. Johnson and Broder, *The System*, 264.

89. Monthly public opinion polls, reported at the Presidency Project, www .presidency.ucsb.edu/data/popularity.php.

90. See Lawrence Brown, "Dogmatic Slumbers: American Business and Health Policy," in *The Politics of Health Care Reform*, eds. James Morone and Gary Belkin (Durham, NC: Duke University Press, 1994), 206–23.

91. Johnson and Broder, *The System*, 231.

92. Skocpol, *Boomerang*, 90.

93. Johnson and Broder, *The System*, 232.

94. Johnson and Broder, *The System*, 196.

95. On BTUs, see Mark Peterson, "The Congressional Graveyard for Health Reform," in *Healthy, Wealthy and Fair*, eds. James Morone and Lawrence Jacobs (New York: Oxford University Press, 2005), 221.

96. William J. Clinton, "Address Before a Joint Session of the Congress on the State of the Union, January 25, 1994," Presidency Project, www.presidency .ucsb.edu/ws/index.php?pid=50409.

97. Harris, *The Survivor*, 113.

98. Harris, *The Survivor*, 111.

99. Johnson and Broder, *The System*, 451.

100. Johnson and Broder, *The System*, 456; Harris, *The Survivor*, 118; William J. Clinton, "Address to the National Governor's Association, July 19, 1994," in *Public Papers of the Presidents of the United States: William J. Clinton* (Washington, D.C.: Government Printing Office, 1994), 1285.

101. Harris, *The Survivor*, 118.

102. Johnson and Broder, *The System*, 461.

103. Alliance for Health Reform: Lessons Learned—the Health Reform Debate of 1993–1994, April 2008, www.allhealth.org/publications/uninsured/health_reform_debate_of_1993-94_81.pdf.

104. Johnson and Broder, *The System*, 521.

105. Clinton, *My Life*, 621.

106. Clinton, *My Life*, 631.

107. Paul Starr, "What Happened to Health Care Reform?" *The American Prospect*, no. 20 (Winter 1995): 20–31.

108. Hacker, *Road to Nowhere*, 179.

## 11. GEORGE W. BUSH

There are not yet any archives for the Bush presidency. The research in this chapter was based, in part, on interviews with sources—both Democratic and Republican—who were promised anonymity. We cite records and documents in the public record, but our understanding of President Bush himself came from some of the men and women who worked for—and against—his health care policies.

1. Hubert Humphrey, March 6, 2005, 11:25 A.M., C.7024–7025, LBJ Library.

2. Fred Barnes, *Rebel-in-Chief: Inside the Bold and Controversial Presidency of George W. Bush* (New York: Three Rivers Press, 2006), 31.

3. Jacob Weissberg, *The Bush Tragedy* (New York: Random House, 2008), xvii; Bill Minutaglio, *First Son* (New York: Times Books, 1999), 85.

4. Minutaglio, *First Son*, 51.

5. Minutaglio, *First Son*, 29, 43.

6. Elizabeth Mitchell, *W.: Revenge of the Bush Dynasty* (New York: Hyperion, 2000), 31.

7. Minutaglio, *First Son*, 45–46.

8. Mitchell, *W.: Revenge of the Bush Dynasty*, 34 [standing on her head]; Minutaglio, *First Son*, 46–47.

9. Minutaglio, *First Son*, 46.

10. Minutaglio, *First Son*, 46.

11. Mitchell, *W.: Revenge of the Bush Dynasty*, 45.

12. Weissberg, *The Bush Tragedy*, 48.

13. Mitchell, *W.: Revenge of the Bush Dynasty*, 45.

14. Weissberg, *The Bush Tragedy*, 37.

15. Weissberg, *The Bush Tragedy*, 56.

16. Weissberg, *The Bush Tragedy*, 39.

17. Mitchell, *W.: Revenge of the Bush Dynasty*, 50.

18. Minutaglio, *First Son,* 73, 92, 99, 113.

19. Weissberg, *The Bush Tragedy,* 39.

20. Minutaglio, *First Son,* 69, 101.

21. Weissberg, *The Bush Tragedy,* 83 [drinking], 76–77 [Jesus].

22. Minutaglio, *First Son,* 225, 232 [enforcer], 221 [evangelicals], 260 [Maitlan], 278 [Ellis].

23. Weissberg, *The Bush Tragedy,* 122.

24. Barnes, *Rebel-in-Chief,* 127.

25. Weissberg, *The Bush Tragedy,* 127.

26. Weissberg, *The Bush Tragedy,* 92.

27. Weissberg, *The Bush Tragedy,* 92.

28. T. R. Oliver, P. R. Lee, and H. I. Upton, "A Political History of Medicare and Prescription Drug Coverage," *Milbank Quarterly* 82, no. 2 (2004): 283–354.

29. Oliver, Lee, and Upton, "A Political History of Medicare," 297.

30. Robert Pear, "Clinton's Plan to Have Medicare Cover Drugs Means a Big Debate Ahead in Congress," *New York Times,* January 24, 1999, A24.

31. Robert Pear, "Democrats Seek Medicare Coverage for Prescription Drugs," *New York Times,* April 21, 1999, A20.

32. "Excerpts from Prepared Remarks by George W. Bush," *New York Times,* May 16, 2000, A18.

33. Kevin Sack, "The 2000 Campaign: The Vice President; Gore, in Attack on Drug Industry, Focuses on 2 Medicines," *New York Times,* August 29, 2000, A19.

34. "The 2000 Campaign; Transcript of Debate between Vice President Gore and Governor Bush," *New York Times,* October 4, 2000, A30.

35. www.youtube.com/watch?v=RO2xiOuLnj8

36. Scott McClellan, *What Happened: Inside the Bush White House and Washington's Culture of Deception* (New York: Public Affairs, 2008), 63.

37. Robert Pear, "Bush Proposes Aid on Medicare Drugs," *New York Times,* January 30, 2001, A18.

38. Pear, "Bush Proposes Aid on Medicare Drugs," *New York Times,* January 30, 2001, A18.

39. Robert Pear, "Bush Drug Plan Calls for Using Discount Cards," *New York Times,* July 11, 2001, A1.

40. Nancy Johnson, interview with the authors, September 10, 2008.

41. President George H. W. Bush, "Remarks at Truman High School, Independence, Mo., August 21, 2001," Presidency Project, www.presidency.ucsb.edu/ws/index.php?pid=62637.

42. David Broder, "Bush's Domestic Agenda Takes Back Seat; Education Reform, Faith-based Initiatives Vie for Attention with Terrorist Fight," *Washington Post,* October 15, 2001, A4.

43. Robert Pear, "GOP Drug Plan for Elderly Nears Passage in House," *New York Times,* June 21, 2002, A1.

44. Robert Pear, "2 Parties' Plans on Drug Costs Falter in Senate," *New York Times,* July 24, 2002, A1.

45. President George W. Bush, "Remarks at a Dinner Honoring Senatorial Candidate Elizabeth Dole, Greensboro, N.Ca., July 25, 2002," Presidency Project, www.presidency.ucsb.edu/ws/index.php?pid=63139.

46. See, for example, Ron Suskind, *The Price of Loyalty* (New York: Simon and Schuster, 2004); Bob Woodward, *The War Within* (New York: Simon and Schuster, 2008).

47. Robert Pear and Elisabeth Bumiller, "Doubts Are Emerging as Bush Pushes His Medicare Plan," *New York Times,* January 30, 2003, A18.

48. Amy Goldstein, "On Medicare Bush Left Details to the Congress," *Washington Post,* April 20, 2003, A4.

49. M. T. Heaney, "Brokering Health Policy: Coalitions, Parties, and Interest Group Influence," *Journal of Health Politics, Policy & Law* 31, no. 5 (2006): 887–944.

50. Robert Pear, "Bush Will Accept Identical Benefits On Medicare Drugs," *New York Times,* June 10, 2003, A1.

51. Robin Toner and Robert Pear, "Senate Move to Increase Federal Role in Drug Benefits Fails," *New York Times,* June 19, 2003, A18.

52. Robert Pear, "Tentative Medicare Pact Offers Drug Benefits to Elderly," *New York Times,* November 13, 2008, A28.

53. John Rother, interview with the authors, September 15, 2008; David Broder and Amy Goldstein, "AARP Decision Followed a Long GOP Courtship," *Washington Post,* November 20, 2003, A1.

54. Elisabeth Bumiller, "Sharply Split, House Passes Broad Medicare Overhaul; Forceful Lobbying by Bush," *New York Times,* November 23, 2003, N1.

55. Jeffrey Smith, "GOP's Pressing Question on Medicare Vote: Did Some Go Too Far to Change a No to Yes?" *Washington Post,* December 23, 2003, A1.

56. President George W. Bush, "Radio Address to the Nation, November 22, 2003," Presidency Project, www.presidency.ucsb.edu/ws/index.php?pid=25092.

CONCLUSION: EIGHT RULES FOR THE HEART OF POWER

1. For an analysis of alcoholism and Ronald Reagan, see Robert Gilbert, *The Mortal Presidency* (New York: Fordham, 1998), 259–65 (see also ch. 9).

2. Franklin Delano Roosevelt, first inaugural address, March 4, 1933; Ronald Reagan, First inaugural address, Tuesday, January 20, 1981.

3. Lee Hamilton, personal conversation with the authors, the Woodrow Wilson International Center for Scholars, Washington, D.C., October 3, 2007.

4. For an overview of the crucial congressional dimensions, see Mark Peterson, "The Congressional Graveyard for Health Reform," in *Healthy, Wealthy and Fair,* eds. James Morone and Lawrence Jacobs (New York: Oxford, 205–33).

5. Ronald Reagan's diary, February 16, 1981.

6. President Richard Nixon, audiotape, Conversation No. 66-2, tape 3 of 7, July 23, 1971.

7. A summary of the meeting on June 15, 1978 in White House Central File, Insurance, Box IS-2, Folder: IS 1/20/77–1/20/81, Carter Library (underlining in original).

# Index

AARP. *See* American Association of Retired
  Persons (AARP)
access to health care
  local efforts to improve, 109
  as a right, 52
  value Americans place on, 54
Ackley, Gardner, 193
Adams, Brock, 258, 277
Adams, Sherman, 112
Addison's disease, 134, 135
adequate medical care, as inherent right, 52
affirmative action, 223
Agnew, Spiro, 222, 229
Agriculture, U.S. Department of, 74, 80
AIDS patients, subsidies for, 313, 314
Aid to Families with Children, 195
Aiken, George, 89, 154
Albert, Carl, 163, 170, 172, 186, 189, 244
Al Caldy economics, 191–192
alcoholics, children of, 290
Allen, Richard, 287
Altman, Dr. Lawrence, 295, 296
Altman, Stuart, 237, 239, 243, 244, 360, 361
Altmeyer, Arthur J., 32, 35, 51, 94
Ambrose, Stephen, 100
American Association of Retired Persons
  (AARP), 312, 374, 401, 403
American Bar Association, 77
American College of Surgeons, 36
American Hospital Association, 240
American Medical Association (AMA), 12
  "aura of inevitability" editorial, 334
  Medical Advisory Committee (MAC) to the
  Committee on Economic Security, 33
  and Medicare, opposition to, 198–201
  opposition to government-sponsored health
  insurance, 33, 45, 160
  promises made to, 194

public relations campaign, 73, 90–93, 152,
  188
role of in defeating Medicare, according to
  John Kennedy, 112
Roosevelt's relations with, 54
tax credits vs. employer mandates plan, 239
voluntary health insurance coverage, accep-
  tance of, 36
Americans with Disabilities Act of 1990, 326,
  342
"The American Way," 16–18
Anderson, Clinton, 126, 154, 155, 156, 169,
  171
Anderson, Martin, 300
Anderson–Javits health care bill, 157, 161
antiwar protests, 220
Appel, James, 199
Ash, Roy, 215
Association of American Physicians and
  Surgeons, 200
autonomous physicians, 304

Badger, Douglas, 398
balanced budget
  achievement of, 393
  Clinton's commitment to, 366, 381
  Eisenhower's commitment to, 102
  importance of, 366, 381
  role of health care in, 264
  tax cuts as means to, 301–302
Ball, Robert, 145, 157, 161, 196
Barnett, Rose, 142
Bartlett, Bruce, 313
Bateman, Herbert H., 314
Bator, Francis, 192
Baucus, Max, 401
Bauer, Gary, 313
Bay of Pigs invasion, 141, 142, 147

Begin, Menachem, 272
Bell, David, 145
Bell, Griffin, 258
Bentsen, Lloyd, 313, 323
Berlin airlift, 97
Berlin Wall, fall of, 331
Beveridge report, 50
Biemiller, Andrew, 243
Blue Cross and Blue Shield health plans, 36
Blumenthal, Michael, 258, 266
Blythe, William Jefferson, Jr., 347
Boggs, Hale, 186
Book of Promises, 260–261, 265, 282
Bourne, Peter, 252, 254, 265, 266, 267
Bowen, Dr. Otis, 5, 6, 19, 305, 306, 309, 315, 316, 317, 331, 418
Bowles, Erskine, 354
Bradley, Gen. Omar, 75
Breaux, John, 401
Bretton Woods agreement, 223
Brezhnev, Leonid, 220
Brock, Bill, 310
Bryant, Farris, 197
Buchanan, Patrick, 218, 219, 246
budget deficits, reducing, 299, 326, 328, 329
budget reconciliation, 366
budget surplus, 393
bully pulpit, 4, 153, 332, 383
Bureau of the Budget, 76
Burke, Tim, 305
Burkley, Adm. George, 136
Burns, Arthur, 215
Burroughs, Robert, 121
Bush, Barbara, 322, 326, 386, 388
Bush, George Herbert Walker (Bush 1), 418
    catastrophic insurance amendments, repeal of, 330, 331
    congressional relations, 330, 341–342
    diplomatic career, 323–324
    domestic initiatives, 320, 326, 328–329
    evangelical right, connection to, 390, 391
    failure to fully develop, package, and "sell" health reforms, 12, 319, 329, 334–335, 339, 340, 341–342, 344
    financing for health reforms, lack of, 339, 341
    first 100 days, 329
    flawed policy process, 328
    foreign policy, affinity for, 323, 325–326, 329, 333
    and Franklin Roosevelt compared, 328
    Gradison–Johnson warning re: health care initiatives, 332–333, 334, 343
    Gulf War, management of, 326, 333
    health care cost containment, emphasis on, 330, 331, 334, 336
    health history, 321
    health insurance plan, essential elements of, 338–339
    illness/death of daughter Robin, 326–328
    and Jimmy Carter compared, 329, 332
    legislative success (congressional votes won), 217
    and Lyndon Johnson compared, 326
    management style, 324, 325–326, 334, 391
    military service, 321–322
    move to Texas, 322–323
    multiple health care bills, introduction of, 340, 341
    partisan tensions, 329
    passion for health care reform, lack of, 6, 319–320, 326, 330, 340, 345
    personal history, 320–323
    political rise of, 323–324
    presidential campaign tactics, 324
    presidential debates, failure to articulate health reforms, 342
    Presidential Library, 328
    press conferences, 325
    "read my lips" pledge, 326
    rebellious streak, 321–322
    Skull and Bones Society, membership in, 322
    State of the Union address (1990), 331
    State of the Union address (1992), 338
    sudden interest in health care reform, reasons for, 335–337
    and tax credits for purchase of health insurance, 337
    "two George Bushes," 326
    vision for health care, lack of, 325, 329, 342, 345
Bush, George W. (Bush 2), 2, 7, 9, 20
    academic performance, 389
    advocacy of funding to combat AIDS in developing countries, 408
    affinity for health care issues, 386, 405
    approval ratings, 405
    "axis of evil," 397
    big picture, ability to see, 391, 395
    childhood in Texas, 385, 386–389
    coming to Christ, 390
    compassionate conservatism, 392
    congressional relations, 406, 416–417
    desire to serve, 392
    domestic issues, focus on, 391, 397
    economic competition as basis for health care plan, 19
    education, passion for, 391
    environmental issues and, 223
    events of 9/11, and domestic initiatives, 397
    going public with plans for health care reform, 396–397
    illness/death of sister Robin, 326, 387–388
    insecurity, feelings of, 390
    leadership style, 4, 389–390
    lessons learned about health care reform, 406
    management skills, lack of, 394
    Medicare expansion, 413
    Medicare Modernization Act of 2003, 194, 227, 385–386, 392–404, 405
    Medicare reform, plans for, 395, 399, 405
    political rise of, 390
    presidential campaign (2000), 393–394
    prescription drug benefit, call for, 194, 395, 400
    rebellious streak, 389, 391
    reelection of, 405
    role as family caretaker, 387, 388
    State Children's Health Insurance Program (SCHIP), veto to extend/expand, 408
    State of the Union address (2002), 397

State of the Union address (2003), 400
and tax credits for purchase of health insurance, 337
tax cuts, 395
Bush, John Ellis (Jeb), 326, 387
Bush, Marvin, 388
Bush, Neil, 388
Bush, Prescott, 320–321
Bush, Robin, 326–327, 387
Byrd, Harry, 14, 146, 158, 190, 193, 196
Byrd, Robert, 193, 366, 382
Byrnes, John, 188, 231, 232

Cabinet
   call for an agency devoted to health, 94
   failure to work with, 9, 140, 174
Caddell, Pat, 248, 249, 262
Cain, Dr. James, 169, 170, 187
Califano, Joseph, 273
   California Proposition 13, thoughts on, 269
   health care reform proposals, 279, 357
   influence of in Jimmy Carter's Cabinet, 265
   and Lyndon Johnson, relationship with, 166, 174, 202, 252, 363
   Medicare drug benefits, support for, 392
   Model Cities program, design of, 9
   sacking of by Jimmy Carter, 10, 257, 258, 277
California Proposition, 13, 269
Camp David Peace Accords, 272–273, 275
Cannon, Lou, 308, 311
Card, Andy, 398
Carter, Jimmy
   admiration for Harry Truman, 279
   approval ratings, 248, 269
   attention to detail, 5, 253–254, 279, 317, 417–418
   backing from organized labor, 261
   balanced budget, as paramount domestic goal, 264
   big picture, failure to see, 281
   Book of Promises, 260–261, 265, 282
   boundless self-confidence, 253, 254
   campaign promises, 254, 260, 279, 415
   Camp David Peace Accords, 272–273, 275
   chief of staff, absence of, 11
   communication, failures of, 261
   congressional relations, 256–257, 269, 271
   contempt for medical establishment, 252
   and Dwight Eisenhower compared, 279
   early years, 249–253
   energy initiatives, 266, 276–277
   failure to deliver on health care, 346, 355
   foreign policy achievements, 261, 272–273, 275
   and George H. W. Bush compared, 329, 332
   health care policy, emphasis on hospital cost containment, 263–264, 271, 277
   leadership style, 4, 249, 258–260, 276–277, 281
   legislative success (congressional votes won), 260
   lessons to be drawn from, 280–282
   and Lyndon Johnson compared, 303
   Medicare, failure to embrace, 289
   national health insurance plan, failure to embrace, 261–270

pancreatic cancer, family history of, 254–255
passion for health care reform, lack of, 252, 267, 276–278, 345
personal health issues, 251–252
political decline, 276–277
and Richard Nixon compared, 270, 275–276
rigid commitment to principle, 273–278
rise to presidency, 254–255
sacking of Joseph Califano, 10, 257, 258, 277
split with Ted Kennedy over health care issues, 270, 271, 273–274, 276, 278
stagflation under, 275
State of the Union address (1979), 274
tenacity, 254
as a Washington outsider, 255–258, 266, 352
Carter, Lillian, 251
Catastrophic Coverage Act, collapse of, 392
catastrophic illness insurance
   amendments to Medicare, repeal of, 330, 331, 332, 392
   Clinton proposal for, 370
   efforts to draft legislation re, 145, 233, 274, 275, 311
   Reagan's plan for, 304–307, 314, 392
Cater, Douglas, 196, 200, 201
Catholic Hospital Association, 77
Cavanaugh, James, 229, 236
Celebreeze, Anthony, 158, 187
Celler, Emmanuel, 95, 96
Center for Medicare and Medicaid Services, 398, 402
Central High School (Little Rock, Arkansas), desegregation of, 116
Central Intelligence Agency, 324
centralization of power, 108
Chafee, John, 372, 378
Cheney, Richard (Dick), 398
chief of staff
   absence of, 11, 174
   delegation by, 418
   importance of, 11, 259
   president acting as, dangers of, 281–282
Children's Bureau, 74, 78
CHIP. See Comprehensive Health Insurance Plan (CHIP)
chronic illness, cost of managing, 403
civil rights
   Democratic party and, 139
   desegregation, schools, 116, 226
   Eisenhower and, 116
   under Kennedy administration, 132, 139
   legislation, introduction of, 143
   1960s protests, 132, 142
   segregation, effects of on passage of Medicare, 195–198
   Truman's defense of, 81, 98
Civil Rights Act of, 1964
   passage of, 163, 196
   Title VI, 196
Civil War and Reconstruction, 250
Clean Air Act, 223, 326
Clean Water Act, 223
Clements, Earle, 181
Cleveland, Grover, 25

Clifford, Clark, 79, 84, 140, 285
Clinton, Bill, 227
  ability to listen, 350
  affinity for medicine and health, 352–353
  attention to detail, 270, 418
  balanced budget, importance of, 365, 366,
    381, 393
  budget reconciliation, attachment of health
    care reform to, 366
  campaign promises, 415
  congressional relations, 373, 376–381, 416
  diabetes, personal experience with, 354
  domestic violence, personal history of, 347,
    348
  early childhood, 347–349
  erosion of support from key constituencies,
    373, 374
  extemporaneous speaking, 371
  failure to deliver on health care, 346, 411,
    418
  financial effects of illness, personal experi-
    ence with, 354
  first 100 days, 359
  going public to promote health care reform,
    372–373
  health care, commitment to reforming, 355,
    381–384
  health care plan, George H. W. Bush's
    response to, 342
  health care reform, mismanagement of, 5,
    380, 382
  health care task force, appointment and
    work of, 32, 363, 367–368
  image, ability to remake, 351
  insecurity, feelings of, 351, 352
  intellectual debates about health care ("Ox-
    ford on the Potomac"), 10, 369
  intelligence of, 350–351
  legislative success (congressional votes won),
    217
  management style, 364, 382
  Medicare prescription drug benefit, plan for,
    393
  military mission to Mogadishu, 373
  mother, relationship with, 349
  North American Free Trade Agreement
    (NAFTA), 373, 374, 381, 411
  passion for health care issues, 346, 410
  personal health history, 353
  political rise of, 351, 353
  presidential campaign (1992), 356–359
  procrastination, as a pattern of behavior,
    352, 357, 370
  public relations blunders, 373–374
  rebellious streak, 351–352
  self-destruction, tendencies toward, 355
  State of the Union address (1999), 393
  "tollgate" meetings, 368
  transition to office, 381–382
  universal health coverage, commitment to,
    370, 376–377, 379
  as a Washington outsider, 351
  welfare reform, 344
  White House direction of health care policy,
    362
  Whitewater investigation, 374, 375

Clinton, Hillary
  Health Security Express, 379
  image, remaking of, 351
  passion for health care issues, 354, 356, 362,
    368
  role of in health care reform planning,
    360–362, 375
Clinton, Roger, 348
Clinton, Virginia, 354
closet socialism, 300
coal strike, United Mine Workers, 78–79
Coggleshell, Lowell T., 110
Cohen, Wilbur, 242, 256
  advisor to Harry Truman, 94, 117
  in Johnson administration, 13, 162, 164,
    171, 172, 173, 189, 199, 200
  in Kennedy administration, 144, 154, 157,
    159, 187
  as Medicare champion, 156, 162, 201
  tying Social Security to health care, 50
coinsurance, 243
Cold War, 97
Cole, Kenneth, 216, 233, 237
Colmer, William, 138
Committee for the Nation's Health, 92
Committee on Economic Security (CES), 30,
    31–33
  AMA Medical Advisory Committee to, 33
Committee to Save Social Security and Medi-
    care, 314
communism
  decline of, 331
  Hungarian revolt against, 116
  Reagan's rhetoric about, 286–287
  "red scare," 80, 286
communist witch hunts, 97
community health centers, 331
Comprehensive Health Insurance Plan (CHIP),
    235–246, 356
Congressional Budget Office, 191, 384, 414
congressional relations
  Bush, George H. W., 330, 341–342
  Bush, George W., 406, 416–417
  Carter, Jimmy, 256–257, 269, 271
  Clinton, Bill, 373, 376–381, 416
  Eisenhower, Dwight, 9, 148
  importance of in securing health care reform,
    130, 203–204, 383, 406, 416–417
  Johnson, Lyndon, 6, 165, 172–174,
    181–183, 202, 317, 367, 416
  Kennedy, John, 7, 139, 146, 155, 159
  legislative liaison teams, 417
  Nixon, Richard, 216–217, 235, 383, 417
  Reagan, Ronald, 257, 383, 416
  Roosevelt, Franklin, 30, 147
  Truman, Harry, 70, 98
Constitutional Convention, 3
Cooper, James, 357, 358, 377
Cooper, Ted, 244
Copeland, Aaron, 72
Council of Economic Advisers, 8, 76, 193, 204,
    216, 239, 268, 306
Cox, Edward, 241
Cox, James, 24
cradle-to-grave national health insurance
  proposals, 50, 225

Craig, Larry, 314
creative chaos, as a presidential management style, 28–29, 104, 139
Cribb, T. Kenneth, 314, 317
cross-subsidies, 316
Cruikshank, Nelson, 145
Cuban missile crisis, 141, 158
Cushing, Dr. Harvey, 33, 34, 54, 55

Danforth, John, 378
Darman, Richard, 328, 334, 336, 337, 382
Davis, Dr. Daniel, 135
Davis, Michael, 71, 72
deductibles, 157, 243
DeFazio, Peter, 314
deficit spending, 301
Democratic Leadership Council (DLC), 352
Democratic Party
  break in over national health insurance, 267
  national health insurance, failure to secure, 248
  ownership of health care issue, 117–119, 332, 405
desegregation, schools, 116, 226
Dewey, John, 72, 83
Dewire, Jeff, 354
Diagnosis Related Groups (DRGs), 302, 303, 317
Diggins, John, 286
Dingell, John, 50, 69, 88, 93, 95, 96, 111
Dingell, John, Jr., 96, 377, 383
Dirksen, Everett, 94
disability benefits, Social Security, 50, 118, 223
disability insurance, 70
disability programs, 44
disease prevention, 331
disengaged executive, 6
Disraeli, Benjamin, 218
The Doctor, 91
Dole, Elizabeth, 398
Dole, Robert, 313, 372, 377, 380
Domestic Council, 215, 222–223, 398
  Subcommittee on Health, 228
Doughton, Robert Lee, 70
Douglas, Justice William, 83
Downey, Sheridan, 94
DRGs. See Diagnostic Related Groups (DRGs)
D'Souza, Dinesh, 292
Dubinsky, Dave, 151
Duffy, Joseph, 350
Dukakis, Michael, 324, 329
Dungan, Ralph, 139, 141
Durenberger, David, 378

Early, Steven, 37
Earth Day, 223
economic bill of rights, 22, 52
economists
  "fiscal drag" of health care plans, concerns about, 414
  managing, 204, 384, 405, 413–415
  rise of, 7–9
  separating economics from health care policy, 165, 191
Eisenhower, Dwight, 83
  balanced budget, commitment to, 102, 110, 126

civil rights movement and, 116–117
  as a compassionate conservative, 105, 119
  congressional relations, 9, 148
  crises faced by, 116–117
  and Democratic Party position on health insurance, 117–119
  Department of Health, Education, and Welfare, creation of, 109–110
  employer-based health insurance, tax benefits for, 17, 113–114, 128, 407, 413
  exit strategy, need for, 115
  health care exception to budget constraints, 102–103
  health history, influence of on health care policy, 3, 105–108
  illness while in office, 3, 127
  and Kennedy compared on health care, 162
  Kerr–Mills bill, signing of, 126
  lost health year, 114–116
  management style, 103–105, 127, 139
  personal interest in health care, 108, 128–129, 328
  place in history, 100
  political values, 101–103
  Bush, Prescott, backing of, 321
  presidential term limits and, 116
  push for private insurance, 110–112
  reinsurance plan, 111, 116, 128
  and Republican Party position on health care, 99, 122–126, 407
  role of in shaping of American attitudes about health care, 109
  State of the Union address (1954), 110–111
  vision for health care reform, 343
  warnings about growth of military-industrial complex, 102
Eizenstat, Stuart, 258, 260, 262, 266, 270, 273
elections. See midterm elections; presidential elections
Ellis, John, 390
Emergency Banking Bill, 22
employer-based health insurance, 377
  federal incentives to offer, 101
  OMB plan to eliminate tax breaks for, 337
  requirement to provide, 238
  small business mandates, 245
  tax benefits for, 17, 113–114, 128, 407, 413
energy crisis, 276–277
Enthoven, Alain, 357
environmental movement, emergence of, 223
Environmental Protection Agency, creation of, 223
Equal Employment Opportunity Enforcement Act of 1972, 223
Erlichman, John, 214, 216, 221, 226, 244, 259, 417
Ewing, Oscar, 65, 81, 86, 88, 92, 94–95
Ewing report. See The Nation's Health–A Ten-Year Program
Executive Office of the President, 29, 215, 414

Fair Deal, 68, 85, 97
Falk, Isidore, 34, 42, 50, 94, 117
Fallows, James, 290
Family Health Insurance Plan, 230
farm subsidies, 330

Faubus, Orval, 116
Feder, Judy, 358, 359, 360
Federal Council on Aging, 118
Federal Emergency Agency, 197
Federal Emergency Management Agency
    (FEMA), 197
Federal Employees Health Benefits Program,
    119, 128, 396
Federal Security Administration (FSA), 74,
    86, 94
Ferguson, Homer, 80
Ferrara, Peter J., 307
Finch, Robert, 217, 225, 226
first 100 days (presidential term), 22, 145, 226,
    329, 359, 412
Fleischer, Ari, 395
Flemming, Arthur, 103, 108, 119
Flemming Plan ("Medicare Program for the
    Aged"), 120, 124–125, 128
Foley, Tom, 258, 378
Folsom, Marion B., 118
Forand, Aime, 118
Forand Bill, 118, 120, 123, 124, 126, 144
Ford, Gerald, 245, 323
foreign oil, U.S. dependence on, 277
Foreign Relations Committee, 353
"Forty Little Hospitals Bill," 49
Foxe, Fanne, 245
Fraser, Douglas, 265
Frist, Bill, 401, 403
Fullbright, William, 352
Fullerton, Bill, 242, 244

Gaither, James, 171
Gardner, John, 197, 200
Gawande, Atul, 357, 359, 360
General Electric Theater, 288
George, Walter, 46, 51, 55, 70
Gephardt, Richard, 365, 367, 383
Gibbons, Sam, 377
Gingrich, Newt, 372
global climate change, 223
going public on health care reform, 11, 52,
    143, 148–151, 154, 156, 160, 372–373,
    396–397, 415–416
Goldman, Lee, 242
Goldwater, Barry, 121, 125, 129, 182, 186,
    221, 288
Goodpaster, Gen. Andrew, 121
Goodwin, Richard, 172
goo-goos, 5, 281
Gorbachev, Mikhail, 286
Gore, Al, 365, 393
Gore, Albert Sr., 182
Gore, Thomas, 37
Gore Amendment, 182
government-sponsored health insurance
    AMA opposition to, 33, 45, 160
    Beveridge report, 50
    European models for, 33
    and quality of medical care, 36, 403
    state-run programs for low-income Ameri-
        cans, 37
Gradison, Bill, 277, 332–333, 337, 343
Graham, Col. Wallace, 65, 75
Grassley, Charles, 395, 402

Great Depression, 21, 250, 409
Great Society, 4, 163, 177–178, 187, 255, 412
"The Greenhouse Compact," 363
Green, William, 78, 87
Greenspan, Alan, 302
Greenspan Commission. See National Commis-
    sion on Social Security
Greenstein, Fred, 175
Griffin, Robert, 241
Gulf War, 326, 333

Hacker, Jacob, 382
Hague, Frank, 83
Haig, Alexander, 221–222, 237, 241
Haldeman, Robert, 216, 221, 244, 259
Hamilton, Alexander, 2
Hamilton, Lee, 411
Handler, Milton, 52
Hannigan, Robert, 62
Harding, Warren G., 24
Harlow, Bryce, 122, 123, 171, 216, 221
Harness, Forest, 81
Harris, John, 348
Harris, Louis, 148, 156, 160
Harris, Patricia, 257
Harris, Richard, 151, 186, 199
"Harry and Louise" ads, 372, 412
Hastert, Denny, 403
Hayden, Carl, 182
Health and Human Services, U.S. Department
    of, 305, 330, 331, 333–334, 335, 402
health care in general
    access to, 54, 109
    adequate, as inherent right, 52
    affordable, public concern about, 332
    costs and coverage, Americans' fears about, 231
    health security, American paths to, 15–20
    purging waste from, 262–263
    quality improvement, 332
health care reform, 420
    as a campaign issue, 415
    compromises, need for, 204
    congressional relations, importance of in se-
        curing, 130, 203–204, 383, 406, 416–417
    congressional inaction on, 234
    consistent message, need for, 416
    creating political momentum for, 203, 381
    economists, managing, 204, 384, 405, 413–415
    eight keys to enacting, 410–420
    financing, pay-or-play approach to, 356, 358
    garnering public support for, 371, 383,
        415–416
    having a plan ready, 406, 412–413
    intrusion of other events into, 411
    learning how to lose on, 384, 418–420
    limits of history, 383–384
    Massachusetts program for, 344
    need for speed in enacting, 203, 280, 381,
        405, 406, 411–412
    organization vs. creativity, 382
    partisan politics and, 384, 405
    policy hubris, danger of, 382
    politics of, 375
    presidential passion about, need for, 203,
        410–411
    PSROs, 417–418

sharing the credit for, 204
substance vs. technique, 281
taking advantage of opportunities, 412
vision, need for, 417
Health, Education, and Security, U.S. Department of, 94
Health, Education, and Welfare, U.S. Department of
Carter administration, tension with, 258–259
Civil Rights Division, 226
efforts to cut waste in, 238
formation of, 74, 109–110
Health Insurance Association of America (HIAA), 333, 371–372
Health Maintenance Organizations (HMOs), 17, 227, 234, 246
Health Security Express, 379
Hearst, William Randolph, Jr., 94
Heineman, Ben, 2180
Heinz, John, death of, 335
Helm, William, 63
Heritage Foundation, 309
Hill, Lister, 89
Hill–Aiken hospital construction bill, 89
Hill–Burton. See Hospital Survey and Reconstruction Act (Hill Burton)
Hinkley, John Jr., 284
HMOs. See Health Maintenance Organizations (HMOs)
Hobby, Oveta Culp, 103, 107, 110
Hodel, Don, 310
Hodges, Luther, 9, 175
Hoffman, Dr. Charles, 211
Holloway, Clyde, 314
Holmes, Oliver Wendell, 28
Hoover, J. Edgar, 80
Hopkins, Harry, 30, 34, 35, 53
Horton, Willie, 324
hospital construction, 44, 70, 79, 111
Hospital Cost Containment bill, 263–264, 271, 277, 303
Hospital Survey and Reconstruction Act (Hill Burton), 79, 111
Hospital Trust Fund, 187
House Committee on Expenditures in the Executive Department, 80
House Un-American Activities Committee, 80
Housing and Urban Development, U.S. Department of, 257
Howe, Harold, 197
Humphrey, Hubert, 8, 88, 95, 96, 163, 166, 171, 173, 197, 204, 219
Hussein, Saddam, 333
Hutschnecker, Dr. Arnold A., 212, 229

Ickes, Harold, 374, 375
indigent health care, 44. See also Medicaid
individual and small group insurance markets, reforming, 338, 344
infant mortality rate, 331
inflation, 220, 223
information technology
to empower consumers, 343–344
to improve insurance claims processing efficiency, 338
to transform medical care, 344

Initial White House Study Group on Health, 226
Interdepartmental Committee for the Coordination of Health and Welfare Activities, 40–41, 45
Internal Revenue Service, 28
investment tax credits, 223
Iran–Contra scandal, 297, 298–299, 308, 311

Jacobs, Lawrence, 358
Jacobson, Dr. Max, 136
Jacobson, Eddie, 60
Javits, Jacob, 126, 154, 155, 204, 225
Jeffords, James, 395
Jennings, Chris, 379
Jim Crow rules, 250
job loss, 332
Johnson, Clay, 394
Johnson, Haynes, 285
Johnson, Lyndon, 140
aid to education, 143
Achilles' heel, 176–177
administrative skills, 202
admiration for Franklin Roosevelt, 23
Cabinet, failure to work with, 9, 174
chief of staff, absence of, 174
Civil Rights Act of 1964, passage of, 163
congressional relations, 6, 165, 172–174, 181–183, 202, 317, 367, 416
crudeness, 176
domestic issues, preference for, 166
economic forecasts, suppressing, 165, 191
financing Medicare, cavalier attitude toward, 8, 414
Forand bill, support for, 124
foreign policy failures, 175–176, 205
and George H. W. Bush compared, 326
governing style, 172–177
Great Society, 4, 163, 167, 177–178, 255, 412
health history, 168–170
insecurity of, 176
intuition, 171
and Jimmy Carter compared, 303
Kennedy's assassination, 171, 177
landslide election of (1964), 164, 202
legislative success (congressional votes won), 173, 260
media, failure to use, 177
Medicare, successful passage of, 164, 178–185, 203–205
Model Cities program, 9, 174, 175
organizational capacity, 173, 174–176
passion for health care issues, 97, 164, 165–170, 203, 291, 410, 415
personal history, 166–168
personality, 170–172
political ambition, 167, 171–172
signing of Medicare into law, 95, 380
State of the Union Address (1964), 187
tax cuts won by, 163
tenacity, 170
Vietnam and, 175
War on Poverty, 143, 163
working with Wilbur Mills, 177, 179–181, 189, 204, 368, 414, 417
Johnson, Nancy, 332–333, 343, 396, 399

Johnson, Sam, 166
Jones, Stan, 224, 242, 243
Jordan, Hamilton, 257, 265, 267

Kaiser, Edgar, 227
Kaiser, Robert, 266
Kaiser Permanente Health Plan, 226, 357
Karp, Bret, 255
Katzenbach, Nicholas, 197
Kearns, Doris, 167, 171, 177
Kee, John, 66
Keen Dr. W. W., 25
Kennedy, Edward (Ted), 8, 17, 204, 273
    and Bush's Medicare modernization plan,
        396, 401, 407
    early support for Medicare, 383
    and Jimmy Carter, relationship with, 269,
        271
    joint health care proposal with Wilbur Mills,
        238, 242–243, 244
    Nixon–Mills–Kennedy partnership, 245,
        247, 270
    passion for health care issues, 224–225, 248,
        268, 307, 310, 331, 355, 401
    run for the presidency, 267
Kennedy, John
    access to health care services, views on,
        137–138
    Addison's disease, 134, 135
    approval ratings, 132
    assassination, 171, 177
    Bay of Pigs invasion, 141, 142, 147
    Cabinet, failure to work with, 140
    capacity to move and inspire, 142
    charisma, 132, 140, 159
    civil rights and, 132, 139
    congressional relations, 7, 139, 146, 155,
        159
    Cuban missile crisis, 141, 158
    and education, 143, 148
    and Eisenhower compared on health care,
        162
    extemporaneous speaking, 152
    father's illness, influence of on health care
        views, 138
    first 100 days, 145
    foreign policy, affinity for, 141, 160
    going public on health care reform, 143,
        148–151, 154, 160
    grassroots health care campaign, 143, 148,
        150, 154
    health care initiatives, 143–148, 157–159
    health history, 3, 133–138, 328
    intellectuals, employment of, 140
    legacy, 132–133
    legislative success (congressional votes won),
        148, 260
    Madison Square Garden Rally for health
        care, 149, 151, 161
    management style, 137, 159
    margin of victory, 1960 election, 138
    Medicare, defeat of, 112, 156
    meeting with Khrushchev, 141
    national security staff, reorganization of,
        141
    New Frontier, 140, 143, 178
    omnibus bill on problems of the elderly, 144

    passion for health care issues, 97, 133, 161
    personal appeal of, 28
    political ambitions, 120
    popularity of, 148, 159
    presidential campaign, 126
    presidential priorities, 147, 148, 160
    press conference, first televised, 12
    press leaks, 148
    Profiles in Courage, 131
    reelection, plans for, 142, 158
    setting the stage for future success of Medi-
        care, 143–148, 160
    sophistication of, 139
    State of the Union address (1961), 145
    State of the Union address (1962), 150
    stature as an international leader, 141
    tax cuts, 158
    transition task force on health and Social
        Security issues, 144
Kennedy, Joseph P., Sr., 4, 137
Kennedy, Robert, 136, 142, 219
Kennedy–Anderson bill, 126, 144
Kennedy–Mills health care proposal, 238, 243,
    244
Kent State University, antiwar protests at,
    220
Kernell, Samuel, 140
Kerr, Robert, 126, 146, 155
Kerrey, Robert, 356
Kerr–Mills bill, 126, 129, 144, 195
Khrushchev, Nikita, 136, 141
King, Martin Luther Jr., 142, 219
King–Anderson bill, 179, 182, 188
Kings Row, 295
Kissinger, Henry, 207, 213, 215, 220, 221
Knowles, Dr. John, 225
Knute Rockne–All American, 294
Kolb, Charles, 325, 328–329
Korean War, 93, 97
Kraft, Joseph, 166
Kraus, Dr. Hans, 136
Krauthammer, Charles, 325

Labor, U.S. Department of, 74
labor unions
    backing of Jimmy Carter by, 261
    nationwide strikes, 97
    opposition to health insurance copayments,
        243
    support for comprehensive health care cover-
        age, 50
    United Mine Workers, coal strike, 78–79
La Guardia, Mayor Fiorello, 72
Laird, Melvin, 207
Lea, Clarence F., 78
League of Women's Voters, 78
Lee, Dr. Burton, 325
Lee, Dr. Philip, 168, 169, 170
    legislative liaison teams, 417. See also congres-
        sional relations
Lehrer, Jim, 342
Lewis, James Hamilton, 43
life expectancy, 331
Lincoln, Abraham, 22
Long, Huey, 37, 55
Long, Russell, 113, 182–183, 185–187, 233,
    245, 262

long-term care, coverage for, 305, 312
Lovett, Dr. Robert, 25
Lowi, Theodore, 140
Lucas, Scott, 93

Magaziner, Ira, 357, 358, 382
Maguire, Dick, 149
malpractice reform, 331, 338, 342
managed care, 227, 333, 370
managed competition, 356, 357, 369, 370
Mansfield, Mike, 146, 182, 244
market-based health care plans, 413
market competition, 227, 396
Marmor, Theodore, 12
Martin, Joseph, 69, 80
Matalin, Mary, 390
Maternal and Child Health Bureau, 49
maternal and child health services, 44, 70, 331
McCain, John, 19, 337
McCarthy, Agent Tim, 283
McCarthy, Eugene, 219
McCarthy, Joseph, 93, 94, 105
McClellan, John, 94
McClellan, Mark, 398
McClellan, Scott, 394
McCormack, John, 189
McCoy, Donald, 76
McCrery, Jim, 314
McCullough, David, 64
McDermott, Rose, 135
McFarland, Robert (Bud), 285, 286, 297, 311
McGovern, George, 234
McIntire, Ross, 33, 37, 54
McInturff, Robert, 334
McIntyre, James, 266
McIntyre, Marvin, 43
McNamara, Patrick, 157, 172
Meany, George, 261
media
    blitz, 97
    effects of on commitment to health reform,
        415
    Kennedy's health care proposals in, 152
    press conferences, presidential, 12, 29–30,
        325
Medicaid
    adjustments to original plan, 44
    economics of, 190–191
    origins of, 164, 188
    plan for greater flexibility in, 339
    as a vehicle for supporting maternal and
        child health, 331
Medicare
    adjustments to original plan, 44
    AMA opposition to, 198–201
    "bombshell," Wilbur Mills, 179
    beneficiaries, initial signup, 201
    boycotts against, 198, 200, 204
    catastrophic illness amendments, repeal of,
        330, 332, 392
    conference committee debates on, 183–185
    cost of drug coverage under, 399
    coupling with Social Security, 16
    drug benefit, administration by private plans,
        401
    economics of, 190–192, 193, 197, 204
    eligibility for, 193

expansion of to include catastrophic illness
        insurance, 5, 193–194, 392
    as federal intrusion into the practice of
        medicine, 199
    Flemming Plan ("Medicare Program for the
        Aged"), 120, 124–125, 128
    future of, 407
    gap in coverages, 305
    implementing, 195–202
    incorporating private-sector innovations
        into, 403
    as instrument of social change, 196
    Kennedy's influence on, 133, 143–148, 160
    Lyndon Johnson's involvement in passage of,
        6, 178–185
    Part A, 188, 201
    Part B, 164, 188, 201
    Part D (prescription drug benefit), 194,
        393, 419 (see also Medicare Moderniza-
        tion Act of)
    passage of, 185–195
    paving the way for, Oscar Ewing's prelimi-
        nary work, 94–95
    private sector role, move to increase, 393
    segregation challenge, 195–198
    self-funded benefits, 312, 315
    and shortages of hospital facilities, 201–202
    as third rail of American politics, 289
    Wilbur Mills in passage of, 12, 146, 154,
        155, 164, 179–181, 189, 202
    wrapping in mantle of Social Security, 151
Medicare Modernization Act of 2003, 227,
        385–386, 392–404
Meese, Ed, 306, 308, 309, 310
Mercer, Lucy, 26
Meredith, James, 142
Messal, Vick, 63
midterm elections
    1946, 79
    1950, 93
    1986, 307
    1994, 379
    2002, 397, 399
Milbank Fund, 34, 36
Miller, James, 306, 310
Miller, Warren, 75
Miller, Watson, 74, 75
Mills, Wilbur
    "bombshell," 184
    CHIP program, introduction of, 242
    Fanne Foxe scandal, 245
    Forand bill, opposition to, 118, 124, 125
    hearings on health care, 120, 188, 231
    influence of on George H. W. Bush's congres-
        sional career, 323
    joint health care proposal with Ted Kennedy,
        238, 242–243, 244
    and John Kennedy, relationship with, 158, 162
    and Lyndon Johnson, relationship with, 177,
        189, 204, 368, 414, 417
    Nixon–Mills–Kennedy partnership, 245,
        247, 270
    and Richard Nixon, relationship with, 18,
        232, 383
    role of in passage of Medicare, 12, 146, 154,
        155, 164, 179–181, 189, 202
    three-pronged approach to healthcare, 180, 188

Mills–Anderson–Ribicoff healthcare proposal, 183
minimum wage, 7
minority businesses, federal set-asides, 224
"missile gap," 117
Mitchell, George, 365, 379, 383, 384
Model Cities program, 9, 174, 175
Moley, Kevin, 342
Mondale, Walter, 269, 289, 296
Mongan, James, 276
Monroe, Marilyn, 152
Moore, Edward H., 84
Moore, Frank, 258
Morgan, Gerald, 38
Morgenthau, Henry, 29, 51, 69
Morse, Wayne, 79
Moyers, Bill, 183, 196
Moynihan, Daniel Patrick, 215, 223, 301, 377, 383
Murray, James E., 50, 60, 71, 76, 87, 88, 95, 96, 111
Murray–Wagner–Dingell bill, 71, 77, 377

NAACP, 80
NAFTA. See North American Free Trade Agreement (NAFTA)
National Association of Manufacturers, 320
National Commission on Social Security, 301, 302
National Conference on Economic Security, 35
National Council of Senior Citizens, 148
national debt, efforts to reduce, 301, 302
National Economic Council, 398
National Federation of Independent Business (NIFB), 334, 371–372
National Grange, 77
National Health Conference, 45
national health insurance
inevitability of, 98
misrepresentation of, 93
as prepayment of medical costs, 70
Roosevelt's proposal for, 23
Truman's plan for, 67–79, 94–95
National Health Program, 42, 48, 49
National Medicare Enrollment Month, 201
National Oceanic and Atmospheric Administration, creation of, 223
national security advisor, origins of, 104
National Security Council, 215
National Youth Administration, 167
The Nation's Health–A Ten-Year Program, 82, 96
Nestingen, Ivan, 149, 157
Neustadt, Richard, 7, 23, 29, 140
New Deal, 2, 16, 23, 101, 268
New Frontier, 140, 143, 178
Nixon, Richard, 142
anti-ballistic missile treaty, 220
attention to details, 409
campaign promises, 219, 222
character, formation of, 213–219, 291
charisma, lack of, 214
childhood, 207–208
childhood traumas, effects of on health care innovation, 224, 241
Comprehensive Health Insurance Plan (CHIP), 235–246, 356

congressional relations, 216–217, 235, 383, 417
cultural differences, exploitation of, 139
desire for solitude, 214, 418
détente with USSR, 220
domestic initiatives, 218, 222–224
driving ambition, 210, 211
and Dwight Eisenhower, relationship with, 103
emotional health, colleagues' concerns about, 221
environmental issues, stance on, 223
failure to secure health care reforms, 18, 235, 242–243, 247
Family Health Insurance Plan, components of, 230
first 100 days, 226
foreign policy, affinity for, 217
going public with a policy, fear of, 12, 247
health care legacy, 246–247, 412
health care reform, early efforts, 223–235
health history, 209–213
influence of on George H. W. Bush's political career, 323
inner thoughts and impulses, revelations of, 207
intelligence of, 213
invasion of Cambodia, 220
isolation, feelings of, 167, 208, 213
legislative success (congressional votes won), 217
management style, 214–215
motivation for pursuing health care reform, 230, 234
national health insurance, redefinitions of, 233, 413
Nixon–Mills–Kennedy partnership, 245, 247, 270
obstruction of justice, 221
opening of China, 213, 220
paranoia, 219, 220–221
personal health issues, 206, 241, 328
Philadelphia Plan, 223–224
political ascent, 214
popularity of, 219
presidency of, overview, 219–224
presidential campaign (1960), refusal to play up Kennedy's health issues, 135
presidential campaign (1968), 219
presidential campaign (1972), 227–228, 235, 236, 246
presidential leadership, lack of, 235
press leaks, 239
public advocacy for health care plan, 240
public image, management of, 214
public-private universal insurance plan, call for, 236
race relations, record on, 223
resignation of, 221, 245
school desegregation, stand on, 222
State of the Union address (1970), 226
State of the Union address (1973), 240
support for health care reform as a Senator, 89
tuberculosis, family history of, 1, 17, 209, 241

uncoupling health care from Social Security, 96
as vice president under Eisenhower, 106, 107
Vietnam War, efforts to end, 220, 222
vindictiveness, 9, 28
vision for health care reform, 343, 344
wage and price controls, 223
Watergate scandal, 18, 221, 244–245
Noonan, Peggy, 257, 308
North American Free Trade Agreement (NAFTA), 373, 374, 381, 411
nursing home care, insurance coverage for, 305

Obama, Barak, 119, 226, 344
O'Brien, Larry, 258
    health care policy, development and promotion of, 154, 157
    and John Kennedy, relationship with, 138, 139, 146, 149, 159
    in the Johnson administration, 162, 173, 182, 187, 193, 196
O'Donnell, Kenneth, 149, 150
Office of Education, 80
Office of Management and Budget (OMB)
    creation of, 8, 191, 214
    and money for health care reform, 268, 337, 384
    role of in formulating health care policy, 306, 317, 328
Office of War Mobilization and Reconversion, 75
oil prices, rise in, 275
old-age pensions, 32
O'Neill, Tip, 256, 257, 258, 299, 382, 416
Onek, Joe, 259, 260, 266

Pace, Frank, 76
Packwood, Robert, 241, 379
Panetta, Leon, 226
Parkel, James, 403
Parr, Agent Jerry, 283
Parran, Dr. Thomas, 48
Parson, Gen. Jerry, 122
passion for health care reform
    Bush, George H. W., 6, 319–320, 326, 330, 340, 345
    Carter, Jimmy, 252, 267, 276–278, 345
    Clinton, Bill, 346, 410
    Clinton, Hillary, 354, 356, 362, 368
    Johnson, Lyndon, 97, 164, 165–170, 203, 291, 410, 415
    Kennedy, John, 97, 133, 161
    Kennedy, Ted, 224–225, 248, 268, 307, 310, 331, 355, 401
    need for, 203, 410–411
    Roosevelt, Franklin, 32, 54, 56, 419
    Truman, Harry, 11, 58, 65–67, 166, 380, 410
pay-as-you-go budgeting, 341
pay-or-play approach to financing health reform, 356, 358
Pear, Robert, 395
Pendergast, Jim, 60
Pendergast, Tom J., 60
Pepper, Claude, 74, 79, 88, 313
Pepper–Rockefeller Commission, 356

Perkins, Frances, 23, 26, 33, 34, 37, 50
"permanent campaign," 9, 97, 215
Persons, Gerry, 124
Pharmaceutical Manufacturers Association, 314
Philadelphia Plan, 223–224
Phillips, Cabell, 64
Phillips, Howard, 208
physiatry, 25
physicians
    access to medical information, 55
    autonomous, 305
    opposition to government-sponsored health insurance, 33, 45, 160
Pierce, Samuel, 296
Pierpoint, Robert, 107
pink Communism, 83
"Pink-Whiskers," 43
poliomyelitis (polio), 24–26, 107
political capital, erosion of, 411
populism, 66, 168
Porter, Roger, 328, 332, 333, 334, 343
prepaid group practice, 226–227, 246. See also Kaiser Permanente Health Plan
prescription drug benefits, 312, 397, 406, 411. See also Medicare Modernization Act of, 2003
presidency
    as bully pulpit, 4, 153, 332, 383
    Cabinet, 9, 140, 174
    caretaker, 285, 330
    chief of staff and, 11, 174, 259, 281–282
    first 100 days, 22, 145, 226, 329, 359, 412
    individual presidents, health of, 3, 20
    leadership, need for, 11–14
    limitations of, 418–419
    modern, invention of, 90, 97
    need to confront health reform, 419–420
    "permanent campaign" for, 9, 97, 215
    role of in shaping history, 194
    transition period between election and inauguration, 144, 381–382, 412
    winning large-scale domestic policy reforms, 129–130
presidential elections
    1960, 120
    1964, 164, 202
    1968, 219
    1972, 235
    2000, 393–394
press conferences, presidential, 12, 29–30, 325
private health insurance
    combined with federal and state insurance plans, 270
    complexity of, 157
    Eisenhower's support for, 110–112, 119
    incentives for marketing to near-poor and elderly, 101
    Nixon's support for, 230
    as outcome of tension between compassion and conservatism, 101
    provisions for the poor, 89, 96
    shortcomings of, 82
    tax deductions for purchase of, 338
Professional Standard Review Organization (PRSO), 270, 417–418

*Profiles in Courage*, 131
Progressive Citizens of America, 83
Progressive era, 5
Protestant Hospital Association, 77
Prouty, Winston, 154
PSRO. *See* Professional Standard Review
    Organization (PRSO), 270, 417–418
psychosomatic illness, 212, 229
Public Health Service, 48, 49, 74, 80, 202
Public Welfare, U.S. Department of, 74

Quayle, Dan, 365

racial quotas, 197
Randolph, Jennings, 155
Rasco, Carol, 364
Rather, Dan, 239
Rayburn, Sam, 14, 57, 124, 139, 140, 146,
    190
Reagan, Jack, 290
Reagan, Nancy, 296, 297, 308, 409
Reagan, Ronald
    age of, as a health issue, 295–297
    Alzheimer's, diagnosis of, 296
    Anti-Ballistic Missile Treaty, 311
    assassination attempt on, 283–285
    aura of heroism, 299
    big government, aversion to, 4
    budget cuts, 299–302
    budget deficits incurred by, 329
    building public support for policies, 12
    catastrophic insurance amendments to Medi-
        care, 194, 330, 406
    congressional relations, 257, 383, 416
    core beliefs, influence of on decision-making,
        286–288
    cultural differences, exploitation of, 139
    decline of support from key constituencies,
        307
    dementia, signs of, 295
    "Dutch" persona, 290–293
    health care legacy, 315–318
    "hidden health care revolution," response to,
        302–304
    image, protecting, 292, 295, 298
    inattention to details, 317
    Iran–Contra scandal, 293, 297, 308, 311
    legislative success (congressional votes won),
        217, 260
    management style, 325
    and Medicare, expansion of, 304, 309, 392,
        413
    movie images, use of, 294–295, 316
    personal appeal of, 28
    personal health issues, 293–299, 309
    political rise of, 18, 261
    and press, interactions with, 325
    private diary, 316, 409
    reelection campaign (1984), 296
    small government, commitment to, 287,
        289, 303
    "the speech" on behalf of Barry Goldwater,
        288
    State of the Union address (1986), 305
    as a storyteller, 284, 292
    vision, 286–290

Reaganomics, 301, 324, 329
"red scare," 80, 286
redistribution of wealth, 37, 312
Redway, Dr. L. D., 39
Reedy, George, 176
Regan, Donald, 286, 297, 308, 310
Reich, Robert, 360
reinsurance, 111, 116, 128
Republican National Committee, 323
Republican Party
    Southern strategy, 222
    stealing health care issue from the Demo-
        crats, 336–337, 344–345
    tax rebellion, 269
    vision for health care reform, 343
Reuther, Walter, 125, 174
Revenue Act of 1954, 113
revenue sharing, 223
Ribicoff, Abraham, 154, 181
Ribicoff Amendment, 182
Richardson, Elliot, 213, 227, 233, 236
Robinson, Peter, 298
Roche, Josephine, 38, 44
Rockefeller, Jay, 347, 355, 361, 375
Rockefeller, Nelson, 114
Roosevelt, Eleanor, 24, 36, 45, 57, 72
Roosevelt, Franklin, 2, 7, 10, 218
    ability to restore confidence, 409
    alphabet agencies and programs, 30
    congressional relations, 30, 147
    denial of illness, 27
    economic bill of rights, 22, 52
    economic collapse, commitment to prevent-
        ing, 29
    executive power, notions about, 30
    Fireside Chats, 22
    first 100 days, 22
    four freedoms, 22
    and health care, general attitudes toward,
        27, 32, 53–56
    legacy of, 20
    legislative success (congressional votes won),
        147
    lost opportunity for health care reform, 344
    management style, 23, 28–29, 139
    national health care, proposals for, 15
    National Heath Conference, 45
    New Deal, 2, 16, 23, 101, 268
    passion for health care issues, lack of, 32,
        54, 56, 419
    personal appeal of, 28
    personal disability, handling of, 328
    and physicians, personal relations with, 54–55
    polio, personal experience with, 24–26
    political intuition, 28
    presidential nomination and election of
        (1932), 21
    press conferences, 29–30
    as a product of the times, 29–31
    reelection of (1936), 42
    reelection of (1944), 31, 52
    relationship between health policy and own
        illness, 28
    rise to political prominence, 24
    Social Security program, 30, 31–40
    State of the Union address (1945), 52

Supreme Court, expanding the size of, 30
unemployment insurance, 27, 32, 34
universal health care, public views on, 39
as a war president, 31, 48
Roosevelt, Theodore, 4, 24, 218, 328
Rosenman, Samuel, 21, 23, 52, 68, 73, 79
Rosenman Commission, 66
Roshe, Josephine, 41–42
Rostenkowski, Dan
    attacks on by elderly voters, 330
    Carter administration, relationship with,
        256, 263, 382
    Clinton administration, relationship with,
        367, 383
    financing for health care reform, 267
    resignation of, 377
    Ronald Reagan, relationship with, 293, 302
Rove, Karl, 391, 392, 398, 401
Rovere, Richard, 140
Rowling, J. K., 206
Rubin, Robert, 360, 365
Russell, Dick, 8, 155, 191–192

Sadat, Anwar el-, 272
Salk, Dr. Jonas, 107
Saltonstall, Leverett, 154
savings and loan bailout, 330
SCHIP. See State Children's Health Insurance
    Program (SCHIP)
Schlesinger, Arthur, 1, 137, 139, 173
Schlesinger, James, 258
Schulz, Charles, 266
Schweiker, Richard, 300
Scully, Tom, 398, 402
segregation, effects of on passage of Medicare,
    195–198
"shadow welfare state," 17, 101
Shalala, Donna, 351, 360, 361, 363
Shapiro, Robert, 358
Shultz, George, 228
Sidey, Hugh, 327
"silent majority," 220
Simon, William, 241
"single-payer model," 16
Skinner, Sam, 337
Skocpol, Theda, 370
Skowronek, Stephen, 6
Smathers, George, 6, 181, 188
Smith, David Barton, 195, 198
Smith, Al, 21
Smith, Howard, 138
Snyder, Dr. Howard, 105, 121
social justice, 22
Social Security
    Committee on Economic Security (CES)
        recommendation for, 30
    disability benefits, 50, 118, 223
    hospital cost containment and, 303
    indexing of payments to inflation, 223
    linking national health insurance with, 96,
        168, 412–413, 415
    National Commission on, 302
    overview, 15–16
    passage of under Roosevelt, 31–40
    as a precursor to universal health care,
        371

proposals for expansion of to cover health
    care, 11, 51, 118, 121, 180, 182, 188
proposed cuts in, under Ronald Reagan,
    300–301
separating health bill from, 23, 35
signed into law, 38
task force on, Kennedy administration, 144
Social Security Act, 150, 168
Social Security Administration, 201
social welfare
    American pattern of, 101
    policy, 115
    spending for, lack of interest in, 332
    state, 67
socialized medicine
    defense of, 153, 210
    denouncement of, 109, 125
    Eisenhower's opposition to, 111
    Eleanor Roosevelt's call for, 45
    Franklin Roosevelt's attitudes toward, 39
    military health care as, 123
    as a misnomer for universal health care, 71,
        80, 150
Solidarity movement, Poland, 283
*Son of Gobbledegook*, 303
Sorensen, Theodore, 136, 138, 145, 152, 154
Sprinkel, Beryl, 5, 306, 309, 310, 312, 314,
    316
Sputnik, 117
Staats, Elmer, 182
stagflation, 275
Stans, Maurice, 123, 125
Starr, Paul, 358
"Star Wars" antimissile shield, 311
State Children's Health Insurance Program
    (SCHIP), 339, 380, 408
Stevenson, Adlai, 106, 140
Stockman, David, 19, 285, 286, 289, 299,
    301, 317
Student National Medical Association, 261,
    275
Suez Canal crisis, 116
Sullivan, Dr. Louis, 330, 333, 335
Summers, Lawrence, 360
Sununu, John, 332, 333, 334, 337, 343, 390
supply-side economics, 329
survey of American health care, first national,
    42
Swope, Gerard, 72
Sydenstricker, Edgar, 34

Taft, Howard, 24
Taft, Robert, 76, 79, 83, 100
Taft–Smith Act, 78, 84
taxes
    credits for purchase of private health insur-
        ance, 337, 338
    cuts (George W. Bush), 395
    cuts (Lyndon Johnson), 163
    and employer-based health insurance, 337,
        407
    progressive, as remedy for economic crisis
        (Franklin Roosevelt), 27
    "read my lips" pledge (George H. W. Bush),
        326
Taylor, Zachary, 219

Technical Committee on Medical Care, 42
Teeter, Robert, 236
10th Ward Democratic Club, 60
Thomas, Bill, 402, 403
Thomas, Elbert, 88
Thomas, Helen, 340
Thompson, Tommy, 402
Thornburgh, Dick, 335
Thorpe, Ken, 360
Thurmond, Strom, 83, 129
Timmons, William, 216
"tollgate" meetings, 368
Tower, John, 298, 311
Tower Commission, Iran–Contra investigation,
    298–299, 311
Townsend, Francis, 37, 55
Trading with the Enemy Act, 21
Travell, Dr. Janet, 136
Truman, Harry, 8, 291
    civil rights, defense of, 81, 98
    congressional relations, 70, 98
    crises faced by, 97
    early years, 59–62
    failure to secure health care reform, 89–90,
        117
    Fair Deal, 68–69, 85, 97
    first Medicare card recipient, 201
    fitness routine, 64
    "give 'em hell" campaign style, 84, 151
    health care policy, specific elements of, 70,
        95–96
    health history, 63–65
    invention of the modern presidency by, 90, 97
    and machine politics, 60–61
    management style, 59, 62, 87
    military service, 60
    mother's health, influence of on ideas for
        health care reform, 64–65
    national health insurance, call for, 81, 88
    passion for health care issues, 11, 58, 65–67,
        166, 380, 410
    picking up where Roosevelt left off, 15, 23,
        31, 51, 53, 57, 70, 419
    popularity of, 58
    presence at signing of Medicare bill, 95, 194,
        380
    presidential campaign (1948), 82–83
    public speaking ability, 85–86, 97
    Reconversion Program, 68
    "red scare," 80
    from senator to president, 62
    State of Union address (1948), 81
    State of the Union address (1949), 85
    United Mine Workers' coal strike, response
        to, 78–79
Tsongas, Paul, 356
tuberculosis, 1, 17, 209, 241
Turoff, Ben, 66
Twenty-Second Amendment (presidential term
    limits), 116

U-2 spy planes, 117, 124
Udall, Morris, 153
Ullman, Al, 257, 258
unemployment, 143
unemployment insurance, 27, 32, 34

United Auto Workers, 261, 265
United Mine Workers, 78
United Nations, 116
United Negro College Fund, 321
universal health insurance
    Clinton's commitment to, 370, 376–377, 379
    disappearance of from public agenda, 49
    dreams of, 8
    Kennedy's plan for, 4, 144
    organized medicine's opposition to, 33
    paid for by market competition, 357
    public support for, 40
    Roosevelt's public views on, 31, 39

Valenti, Jack, 193
Veterans Affairs, U.S. Department of, 74, 78,
    202
Vietnam War, 175, 192, 202, 219, 220
voluntary health insurance coverage
    AMA acceptance of, 36
    limitations of, 120
The Voluntary Way Is the American Way, 92
Voting Rights Act of 1965, 166
Voting Rights Act of 1970, 223
vouchers for health care, 5, 6, 38, 309, 317, 377

wage and price controls, 223
Wagner, Robert, 48, 50, 69, 96
Walker, Dr. John, 326
Walker, George Herbert, 320
Wallace, George, 197, 219
Wallace, Henry, 83
War on Poverty, 143, 163
Warm Springs, Georgia, 25
Washington, George, 3, 22
Watergate scandal, 18, 221, 244–245
Waxman, Henry, 312, 315, 330
Weinberger, Casper (Cap), 236, 237, 244
welfare reform, 154, 223, 263, 344, 377, 380,
    318
Whitaker and Baxter (public relations firm), 91
White, Dr. Paul Dudley, 105
White, Lee, 196
The White House, as an institution, 7–14
White House Domestic Policy Council, 306
Whitewater investigation, 374, 375
Whitman, Ann, 123, 124
Wicker, Tom, 266
Wilensky, Gail, 326, 336, 342
Wilson, Dr. H. P., 209
Wilson, Henry Hall, 159
Wilson, Woodrow, 24, 105
Witte, Edwin, 32
Wofford, Harris, 335, 336, 355
Woodcock, Leonard, 243
workplace insurance. See employer-based
    health insurance
World Health Organization, 81
Wright, Betsey, 351
Wright, Jim, 299, 313

Yankee Brahmin code, 328
Yarborough, Ralph, 323
Yom Kippur War, 221

Zapata Petroleum Corporation, 387